EFFECTS OF ANTIDEPRESSANTS

Edited by **Ru-Band Lu**

Effects of Antidepressants
Edited by Ru-Band Lu

Published by InTech
Janeza Trdine 9, 51000 Rijeka, Croatia

Publishing Process Manager Romina Skomersic

Technical Editor Teodora Smiljanic

Cover Designer InTech Design Team

Additional hard copies can be obtained from orders@intechopen.com

Effects of Antidepressants, Edited by Ru-Band Lu
p. cm.
ISBN 978-953-51-0663-0

For EU product safety concerns:
IN TECH d.o.o., Prolaz Marije Krucifikse Kozulić 3, 51000 Rijeka, Croatia, info@intechopen.com or visit our website at intechopen.com.

Meet the editor

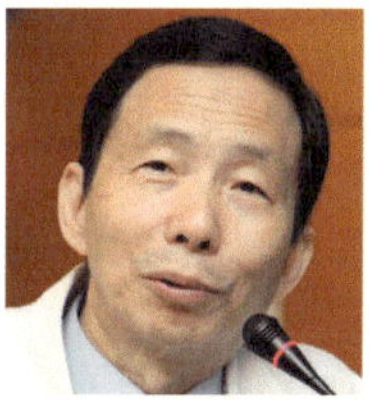

Professor Ru-Band Lu graduated from National Defense Medical Center (NDMC) in 1972, following that he completed his resident training, as well as being a lecturer of NDMC in 1980. He gained a clinical fellowship of psyphamachology in Baylor Medical College, Huston, Texas, USA between 1981 and 1982, and he became a clinical psychopharmacologist in the USA. He became a professor of Psychiatry at NDMC in 1989. From 1992 to 1993, he was a visiting research scientist in Human Genetics at Yale University, New Haven, CT, USA. From 2003 to 2009, he was the director of the Institute of Behavioral Medicine and chairman of the Department of Psychiatry, National Cheng Kung University, Tainan, Taiwan. Now he is a distinguished professor in university. Dr. Lu was the President of the Taiwanese Psychiatry Association from 2003 to 2005. He received an Academic Achievement Award, Taiwanese Society of Psychiatry in 2007 and K.T. Lee Science and Humane Award - Gold Medal in 2011.

Contents

Preface XI

Chapter 1 **Evaluation of the Humoral Immune Response of Wistar Rats Submitted to Forced Swimming and Treated with Fluoxetine 1**
Eduardo Vignoto Fernandes, Emerson José Venancio and Célio Estanislau

Chapter 2 **Effects of Antidepressants on Inhibitory Avoidance in Mice: A Review 23**
Concepción Vinader-Caerols, Andrés Parra and Santiago Monleón

Chapter 3 **Participation of the Monoaminergic System in the Antidepressant-Like Actions of Estrogens: A Review in Preclinical Studies 47**
Carolina López-Rubalcava, Nelly Maritza Vega-Rivera, Nayeli Páez-Martínez and Erika Estrada-Camarena

Chapter 4 **Antidepressants and Morphological Plasticity of Monoamine Neurons 73**
Shoji Nakamura

Chapter 5 **Serotonin Noradrenaline Reuptake Inhibitors (SNRIs) 91**
Ipek Komsuoglu Celikyurt, Oguz Mutlu and Guner Ulak

Chapter 6 **Antidepressants Self-Poisoning in Suicide and Suicide Attempt: Acute Toxicity and Treatment 109**
Sara Santos Bernardes, Danielle Ruiz Miyazawa, Rodrigo Felipe Gongora e Silva, Danielle Camelo Cardoso, Estefânia Gastaldello Moreira and Conceição Aparecida Turini

Chapter 7 **Rational Polypharmacy in the Acute Therapy of Major Depression 131**
Per Bech and Claudio Csillag

Chapter 8 **Antidepressant Drugs and Pain 143**
Blanca Lorena Cobo-Realpe, Cristina Alba-Delgado, Lidia Bravo, Juan Antonio Mico and Esther Berrocoso

Chapter 9 **Antidepressant Drug Use in Patients with Diabetes Mellitus Type 1 – The Effect of Medication on Mental Problems and Glycemic Control 163**
Jana Komorousová and Zdeněk Jankovec

Chapter 10 **Effects of Fluoxetine and Venlafaxine on the Salivary Gland – Experimental Study 181**
Silvana da Silva, Luciana Reis de Azevedo, Antônio Adilson Soares de Lima, Beatriz Helena Sottile França, Maria Ângela Naval Machado, Aline Cristina Batista Rodrigues Johann and Ana Maria Trindade Grégio

Preface

Depression could be called the black death of the twenty-first century due to its high prevalence (life time prevalence could be 10-15% or higher). It often occurs in people during their middle age, 30-50 years old, and costs much because of the medical resources used to treat it and the higher suicide and rate of recurrence. In addition, people with depression are often comorbid with anxiety disorders and lack of efficient treatment. Even for the patients with anxiety disorders, the most useful medications are antidepressants.

From 1970 to 1990, antidepressants drug delivery has developed rapidly, including monoamine oxidase inhibitors (MAOIs), tricyclic antidepressants (TCAs), tetracyclic antidepressants (TCAs), selective serotonin reuptake inhibitors (SSRIs) and serotonin-norepinephrine reuptake inhibitors (SNRIs), being the most commonly used. These medications are among the most commonly prescribed by psychiatrists and other physicians, and their effectiveness and adverse effects are the subject of many studies and competing claims. As more studies are carried out more evidence of the other effects of antidepressants have been reported; antidepressants are no longer anti-depressant/mood only, but provide other effects.

The editor tried to integrate various aspects of treatment for depression and the effects of antidepressants. In recent years, more and more researchers are exploring the mechanisms in psychiatry and psychopharmacology of treating psychiatric illnesses. Some hypotheses have been challenged through various points of view, but, the hypothesis on monoamine still plays an important role in treating depression. From the viewpoint of traditional psychopharmacology, animal models to clinical trials in humans, a comprehensive review was carried out to understand the possible pathology of depression. In addition, the other therapeutic effects of antidepressants, as well as side effects, are also reported in this book. Moreover, psychotherapy has also been reported to have similar effects, especially cognitive-behavioural therapy; these treatments are also reported to work for depression. On the fundamental understanding of pharmacological effects and the relationship with depression, the therapeutic effect of psychotherapy could be more applicable.

The editor tried to help the readers who are beginners in this field to have a comprehensive and basic knowledge of antidepressants and further, have inspiration for their future studies.

Ru-Band Lu
Department of Psychiatry, National Cheng Kung University & Hospital, Tainan, Taiwan

1

Evaluation of the Humoral Immune Response of Wistar Rats Submitted to Forced Swimming and Treated with Fluoxetine

Eduardo Vignoto Fernandes,
Emerson José Venancio and Célio Estanislau
State University of Londrina,
Brazil

1. Introduction

The term stress was introduced into the biomedical field by Hans Selye (1936) in reference to a General Adaptation Syndrome which would consist of all non-specific systemic reactions that occur during an intense and chronic exposure to a stressor (e.g., pressure at work and poor diet). This syndrome would be different from the specific adaptive reactions (such as muscle hypertrophy caused by exercise performed on a regular basis) and immune responses (Selye, 1936).

A study evaluating occupational stress in nurses presented the most common symptoms involved: a feeling of fatigue, headache or muscle pain due to tension (neck and shoulders), decreased sexual interest, a feeling of discouragement in the morning, sleep difficulties, upset stomach or stomach pain, muscle tremors, feeling short of breath or shortness of breath, decreased appetite, tachycardia when under pressure, sweating and flushing (Stacciarini & Tróccoli, 2004). The main psychological symptoms present in people with stress are anxiety, tension, insomnia, alienation, interpersonal difficulties, self-doubt, excessive worry, inability to concentrate, difficulty relaxing, anger and emotional hypersensitivity (Lipp, 1994).

Stress has been considered one of the biggest causes of depression. After a situation of great stress, approximately 60% of individuals develop depression. Psychosocial problems (work pressure, job loss and debt) can also be preconditions for its emergence (Kendler et al. 1995; Post, 1992).

Major depression is a mood disorder whose prevalence throughout life, depending on the population, is estimated at between 0.9 to 18% and involves a significant risk of death (Waraich et al., 2004). It is estimated that men and women with depression are 20.9 and 27 times, respectively, more likely to commit suicide than those without depression (Briley & Lépine, 2011).

Multiple environmental factors have been associated with the etiology of depression. Adverse events during childhood and everyday stress are described as important factors for the development of depression (Kessler, 1997). Children with a history of sexual abuse, living in troubled homes or who receive little attention from parents have a high risk of becoming depressed adults (Kessler, 1997). Stressful events such as the loss of a loved one, job loss, or partner separation are factors associated with the onset of depression (Kessler, 1997). Individual personality is also a predisposing factor to depression, as evidenced by the higher frequency of depression in people with a tendency to be sad when they experience a stressful event (Fava & Kendler, 2000). Gender is strongly associated with depression. Studies have shown that depression is on average twice as common in women as in men (Bromet et al., 2011). Interestingly, a decrease in the female/male proportion of depression has been observed in young adults (18 to 24 years), possibly due to greater gender equality in today's society (Seedat et al., 2009). Besides environmental factors, individual genetic characteristics also contribute to susceptibility to depression (Jabber et al., 2008).

In addition to the psychological changes associated with depression, immune system changes are often found in depressed individuals (Altenburg et al., 2002). Several studies have indicated that stress and depression involve the individual in a chronic process that results in host defense failure against microorganisms and a higher likelihood of developing certain cancers. These alterations are probably associated with profound changes in the functioning of the immune system of individuals suffering from depression (Reiche et al., 2004; Irwin et al., 2011). Epidemiological and experimental evidence shows that changes in the defense capability of the individual are related to decreased proliferative capacity of peripheral blood lymphocytes stimulated with mitogens in vitro (Schleifer et al., 1985; Schleifer et al., 1996), a decrease in the cytotoxic activity of natural killer cells (NK) (Schleifer et al., 1996; Calabrese et al., 1987; Nunes et al., 2002), the suppression of T-cell activity due to increased apoptosis and decreased cell proliferation in response to antigens (Szuster-Ciesielski et al., 2008; Schleifer et al., 1984). Moreover, imbalance in cytokine levels is often observed, such as increased levels of interleukin 2 (IL-2), interleukin 6 (IL-6) and interferon-alpha (IFN-α) (Seidel et al. 1995; Vismari et al., 2008). The results have been conflicting regarding humoral immune response and immunoglobulin levels in the blood. A significant increase in IgM levels in patients with depression was observed by Kronfol (1989) and Song et al. (1994), although other studies have been unable to detect significant changes in immunoglobulin levels in the peripheral blood of patients with depression (Bauer et al., 1995; Nunes et al., 2002). These changes in the immune system probably directly and/or indirectly compromise host immunity against microorganisms (Miller, 2010). On the other hand, the immune system changes observed in individuals with depression may not be caused by changes in the central nervous system of these individuals but instead may be directly related to the origin of such changes, including the development of a pro-inflammation state directly related to the onset of a depressive state, which is suggested by the hypothesis that macrophages act as a cause of depression (Miller, 2010). This hypothesis is related to an increased secretion of proinflammatory cytokines such as interleukin 1 (IL-1), IFN-α, and the resulting change in production of corticotrophin-releasing factor (CRF) and adenocorticotrophic hormone (ACTH) (Smith, 1991).

Importantly, animal models of stress and depression have shown immune system changes, including increased production of IL-1, the number of circulating neutrophils and lowered resistance to infection by bacteria. Mice that had been transgenically modified to exhibit a depressive type of behavior (catalepsy) and were inoculated with sheep red blood cells

(SRBC) had lower amounts of platelet-forming cells and antigen-specific T lymphocytes than their parents without this disorder. In rats with high levels of anxiety, lower concentrations of specific T lymphocytes were also found five days after inoculation with SRBC (Kubera et al., 1996; Pedersen & Hoffman-Goetz, 2000; Altenburg et al., 2002; Robles et al., 2005; Alperin et al., 2007; Loskutov et al., 2007; Miller, 2010).

Because this disorder severely compromises the functioning of individuals, several alternative treatments for depression have been proposed, including psychotherapy and pharmacotherapy, as well as a combination of both types. The use of antidepressant drugs for treating patients with depression began in the late 1950s. Since then, many drugs with potential antidepressants have been made available and significant advances have been made in understanding their possible mechanisms of action (Stahl, 1997). Only two classes of antidepressants were known until the 80's: tricyclic antidepressants and monoamine oxidase inhibitors. Both, although effective, were nonspecific and caused numerous side effects (Lichtman et al., 2009). Over the past 20 years, new classes of antidepressants have been discovered: selective serotonin reuptake inhibitors, selective serotonin/norepinephrine reuptake inhibitors, serotonin reuptake inhibitors and alpha-2 antagonists, serotonin reuptake stimulants, selective norepinephrine reuptake inhibitors, selective dopamine reuptake inhibitors and alpha-2 adrenoceptor antagonists (Bezchlibnyk-Butler & Jeffries, 1999). Serotonin reuptake inhibitors belong to this new generation of antidepressant drugs; fluoxetine is the most commonly prescribed drug for treating depression and anxiety because of its efficacy, safety and tolerability (Egeland et al., 2010).

Despite the current extensive use of antidepressant drugs, few studies have investigated the effects of antidepressant drugs on the immune system (Janssen et al., 2010). Experimental and clinical evidence suggests that changes in the immune system in patients with depression can be reversed by the use of antidepressant drugs (Leonard, 2001).

In animal models the use of fluoxetine has been associated with significant changes in immunity. Laudenslager & Clarke (2000) inoculated rhesus monkeys (*Macaca mulatta*) with tetanus toxoid and found increased levels of IgG anti-tetanus. When analyzing the effect of the antidepressant desipramine and fluoxetine, it was observed that animals treated with these antibodies showed higher plasma levels than those treated with saline.

Some studies with mice have showed the effects of fluoxetine on humoral immune response. Kubera et al. (2000) observed that continuous administration of fluoxetine in C57BL/6 mice for four weeks results in decreased IL-4 production and in increased IL-6 and IL-10 production. Genaro et al. (2000) found that fluoxetine has an inhibitory action on the proliferation of B lymphocytes induced by lipopolysaccharide (LPS) or anti-IgM. On the other hand, fluoxetine increases the proliferative action of B lymphocytes, being stimulated by suboptimal concentrations of anti-IgM. In an experimental model of depression in BALB/c, Edgar et al. (2002) observed a decrease in lymphoproliferative response induced by mitogens (phytohemagglutinin and concavalina A), an increase in the proliferative response of B lymphocytes to lipopolysaccharide (LPS) and that the chronic administration of fluoxetine reverses these immune changes.

The experimental investigation of depression in humans is largely ethically unfeasible. Thus, animal models of depression have been developed for this purpose, such as the olfactory bulbectomy, learned helplessness, restraint stress and forced swimming (Willner, 1990). Forced swimming is a widely used model for preclinical evaluation of the possible effects of antidepressant drugs (Porsolt et al., 1977). Its widespread use is mainly due to its ease of implementation, the reliability of its results confirmed in various laboratories and its ability to detect the action of almost all classes of currently available antidepressants (Borsini & Meli, 1988).

In this study we evaluated the humoral immune response of rats chronically submitted to a model of stress/depression, i.e., forced swimming for twenty-five days and daily treatment with fluoxetine. Antibody production was assessed five days after the rats were inoculated with sheep red blood cells and, after the last day of forced swimming, the animals were euthanized and the adrenal glands, thymus and spleen were removed and weighed.

A growing number of people are diagnosed with stress and depression, for which antidepressant drugs are increasingly prescribed. Although many of their effects on individuals are known, there have been few studies reporting the effects of antidepressants on human and/or animal immune systems, especially regarding humoral immunity. Although experimental, this study has great social significance principally due to the large number of people vaccinated annually who are also undergoing regular treatment with antidepressants. The objective of this study was to evaluate the humoral immune response of Wistar rats submitted to forced swimming and treated with fluoxetine.

2. Methodology

2.1 Animals and experimental groups

A sample of 72 male Wistar rats with a body mass of about 300 grams was obtained from the Central Vivarium of the State University of Londrina's Center of Biological Sciences for use in the experiment.

The experiment was conducted at the vivarium of the Department of General Psychology and the Behavior Analysis Center of Biological Sciences of the State University of Londrina. The rats were housed in polypropylene cages (40 cm x 34 cm x 17 cm) with up to six animals per cage. Water and feed were provided ad libitum throughout the experiment, the vivarium temperature was maintained at approximately 25°C and a 12 hour light/dark cycle was established (light from 7:00 am). The animals' body weight was measured daily before the forced swimming session.

In order to study the effects of chronic forced swimming, chronic fluoxetine treatment and an immunization protocol, roughly half of the animals were submitted to chronic forced swimming sessions and the rest were kept in the vivarium. Each of these groups was subdivided and treated chronically with fluoxetine or saline. Again, each of the four groups was subdivided with part of the animals submitted to the immunization protocol and the other part not. Thus, the following eight groups were involved in the procedure: control saline not immunized (Ctl-Sal-n-Im, n=10); control saline immunized (Ctl-Sal-Im, n=10); control fluoxetine not immunized (Ctl-Fxt-n-Im, n=9); control fluoxetine immunized (Ctl-Fxt-Im, n=9); swimming saline not immunized (Swm-Sal-n-Im, n=10); swimming saline immunized (Swm-Sal-Im, n=10); swimming fluoxetine not immunized (Swm-Fxt-n-Im, n=7); swimming fluoxetine immunized (Swm-Fxt-Im, n=7).

The experimental procedures were approved by the Ethics Committee on Animal Experimentation of the State University of Londrina, Project No. 6977, Case No. 16828/2010.

2.2 Protocol of forced swimming

The forced swimming model was performed in accordance with Lucki (1997) to evaluate the acute effect. In the current study, forced swimming sessions were performed daily for twenty-five days and the behavior of the animals was rated on the first and last day. Forced swimming was performed in a black plastic cylinder (50 cm high and 22 cm in diameter) in which the water was 30 cm deep and kept at 25 ± 2°C. The sessionss were performed individually for 15 minutes between 12 and 2 pm. At the end of the session, each animal was removed from the cylinder and dried. The cylinder was cleaned and the water replaced between use by different groups.

2.3 Fluoxetine: Dilution and application

We used the drug Daforin® (fluoxetine hydrochloride 20mg/ml) diluted 1:2 in saline solution for the experiment. Thirty minutes after the end of each forced swimming session, the animals received 10 mg/kg/day of fluoxetine or saline intraperitoneally (i.p.). The injections began at the first session (pretest) and finished on the penultimate day of the experiment (the 24th day).

2.4 Behavioral evaluation

For behavioral analysis, the animals were filmed during the first five minutes of the 1st and the 25th session of forced swimming. After the tests, the videos were stored on a computer for further analysis.

The amount of time the animals spent in the following behaviors was recorded: floating (complete immobility or faint movements, i.e., the minimum necessary to keep the nose/head above the surface), climbing (vigorous movements with forepaws above the surface or against the cylinder wall) and swimming (horizontal movement without the front legs breaking the surface of the water). The behavioral data were recorded by a trained observer (minimal intra-observer agreement: 0.85).

2.5 Blood collection and immunization

On days 5, 10 and 25 of the study at the end of the forced swimming session, all animals were sedated by non-lethal inhalation of ethyl ether and approximately 1 mL of blood was collected by cardiac puncture. The collected blood was stored in 1.5 ml plastic tubes containing 50 µL of 5% EDTA. On days 5 and 20 the animals belonging to subgroups Ctl-Sal-Im, Ctl-Fxt-Im, Swm-Sal-Im and Swm-Fxt-Im, were inoculated i.p. with a 250 µl solution of 2.5% SRBC.

2.6 Preparation of antigen

The following protocol was used to extract proteins from sheep erythrocytes: the sheep red blood cells were centrifuged in test tubes at a speed of 1000g for 15 minutes. The cell pellet was then suspended in saline, centrifuged at 1000g for 15 minutes and the leukocyte layer was removed (this process was repeated twice more). After the third wash, the supernatant was removed and 30 ml of Tris-EDTA [5 mM buffer 2-Amino-2-hydroxymethyl-propane-1,3-diol/hydrochloric acid (Tris-HCl), pH 7.6, containing 1 mM Ethylenediamine tetraacetic acid (EDTA)] was added. The tubes were subjected to centrifugation at 25000g for 30 minutes (this process was repeated until the supernatant had turned pink). The contents of the tubes were then filtered through cheesecloth and underwent a final wash with Tris-EDTA. The pellet obtained was suspended in 0.1% Sodium Dodecyl Sulfate (SDS) in Phosphate Buffered Saline (PBS) at a volume three times that of the pellet. The suspension was dialyzed for 24 hours at room temperature and the PBS/SDS solution was changed at least twice. Aliquots of the suspension were stored at -20°C. The protein suspension dosage followed Bradford (1976).

2.7 Sacrifice

On the 25th day of study, after finishing the forced swimming test, the animals were again non-lethally sedated by inhalation of ethyl ether for blood collection, after which the animals were sacrificed by lethal ethyl ether inhalation. The spleen, thymus and adrenal glands of each rat were subsequently removed to assess the relative weight.

2.8 ELISA

To assess the production of antibodies (IgM, IgG1 and IgG2a), an enzyme-linked immunosorbent assay (ELISA) containing 100 µl of a solution of 2.5 mg/ml sheep erythrocyte proteins obtained in the above-described manner was added to each well. The plasma was diluted 1:100. The dilutions of peroxidase conjugated anti-IgM, anti-IgG1 (Zymed) and anti-IgG2a (BETHYL) were 1:10000, 1:20000 and 1:5000, respectively.

ELISA was conducted according to the following protocol: first, the 96-well plates were coated with 100 µl of the antigen diluted in carbonate-bicarbonate pH 9.6 and incubated overnight at 4°C. The plates were then washed 3 times with PBS-Tween 0.05% and blocked with 150 µl of PBS with skim milk (PBS-milk) 5% in each well for 1 h at 25°C. After 3 washes with PBS-Tween 0.05%, plasma samples diluted in PBS-milk 1% (100 µl of 1:100 diluted sample per well) were incubated for 1 h at 25°C. The plates were then washed 3 times with PBS-Tween 0.05% and the conjugate (100 µl of conjugate diluted in PBS-milk 1% per well) anti-IgM, anti-IgG1, or anti-IgG2a was incubated for 1 h at 25°C, washed 3 times with PBS-Tween 0.05%, and then the substrate (sodium acetate buffer 0.1 M pH 5, containing TMBZ – tetramethylbenzidine of 1% and H_2O_2 - hydrogen peroxide 0.005%) was added (100 µl of substrate/well). After incubation in the dark for 15 minutes at 25°C, 50 µl of 1N H_2SO_4 was added per well. Reading was performed in a microplate reader at 450 nm.

2.9 Statistical analysis

Statistical analysis was performed with Statistica 5.0®. To evaluate homogeneity and normality, the Levene and Kolmogorov-Smirnov tests were used. To evaluate antibody production (IgM, IgG1 IgG2a), four-way repeated-measures ANOVA was performed including the effects of the swimming sessions (Ctl X Swm), fluoxetine treatment (sal X fxt), immunization (n-Im X Im) and repeated measurement factor of blood sampling time (preImmunization X after the 1st immunization X after the 2nd immunization). Behavioral comparisons were also performed by means of four-way ANOVAs, but with a different repeated-measures factor (Session 1 x Session 25). Repeated-measures comparisons of the following masses were conducted: body (fluctuation), spleen, adrenal gland and thymus. Therefore, the above described remaining factors were analyzed in three-way ANOVAs run for this purpose. When interactions of main effects were found to be significant, Tukey post hoc tests were applied. The significance level was set at $P < 0.05$.

3. Results

Figure 1a shows the production values of IgM antibody groups. The results show no effects for stress (F [1.64] = 0.348, P> 0.05), but effects for immunization (F [1.64] = 20.050, P <0.001), drug (F [1.64] = 6.673, P <0.05), time (F [2.128] = 32.208, P <0.001), interaction between immunization and time (F [2.128] = 21.710, P <0.001), drug and time (F [2.128] = 7.383, P <0.001) and immunization, drug and time (F [2.128] = 9.268, P <0.001). Comparing the pre, post1 and post2 immunization periods, the Tukey test showed that there was an increase in IgM production only for the Ctl-Sal-Im and Swm-Sal-Im groups. We observed that only animals treated with saline responded to inoculation with SRBC, while fluoxetine inhibited the production of antibodies.

The production of IgG2a antibody (Figure 1b) appeared to be similar to the values observed for IgM. Four-way ANOVA showed no stress effect (F [1.64] = 1.188, P> 0.05), but effects for immunization (F [1.64] = 26.326, P <0.001), drug (F [1.64] = 7.139, P <0.05), time (F [2.128] = 25.483, P <0.001) , immunization and drug interaction (F [1.64] = 7.814, P <0.01), immunization and time (F [2.128] = 25.734, P <0.001), drug and time (F [2.128] = 6.578, P < 0001) and immunization, drug and time (F [2.128] = 6.630, P <0.01). In the pre, post1 and post2 immunization periods, the Tukey test showed increased production of IgG2a only in Ctl-Sal-Im and Swm-Sal-Im. Only non-stressed animals treated with saline responded to inoculation with sheep red blood cells, while fluoxetine inhibited the production of antibodies.

Figure 1c shows the production values for IgG1 antibody. There were no effects for stress (F [1.64] = 0.404, P> 0.05) drug (F [1.64] = 0.001, P> 0.05), but effects for immunization (F [1.64] = 48.908, P <0.001), time (F [2.128] = 81.116, P <0.001), interaction between stress and drug (F [1.64] = 9.370, P <0.01), immunization and time (F [2.128] = 67.428, P <0.001), stress, immunization and drug (F [1.64] = 11.223, P <0.01), stress, drug and time (F [2.128] = 18.953, P <0.001) and stress, immunization, drug and time (F [2.128] = 20.187, P <0.001). Comparing the pre, post1 and post2 immunization periods, an increase in IgG1 production was observed only for the Ctl-Sal-Im and Swm-Fxt-Im groups. It was observed that stress and fluoxetine in isolation inhibit the production of IgG1, but that stress and drugs together interacted to cause antibody production similar to that of the control group (Ctl-Sal-Im).

The variation in rat body mass was not altered by immunization (F [1.64] = 0.34, P> 0.05), although stress (F [1.64] = 19.948, P <0.001) and drug effects (F [1.64] = 111.595, P <0.001) were observed. There was no significant interaction between variables. Intergroup comparison revealed that fluoxetine was responsible for reducing body mass (Figure 2).

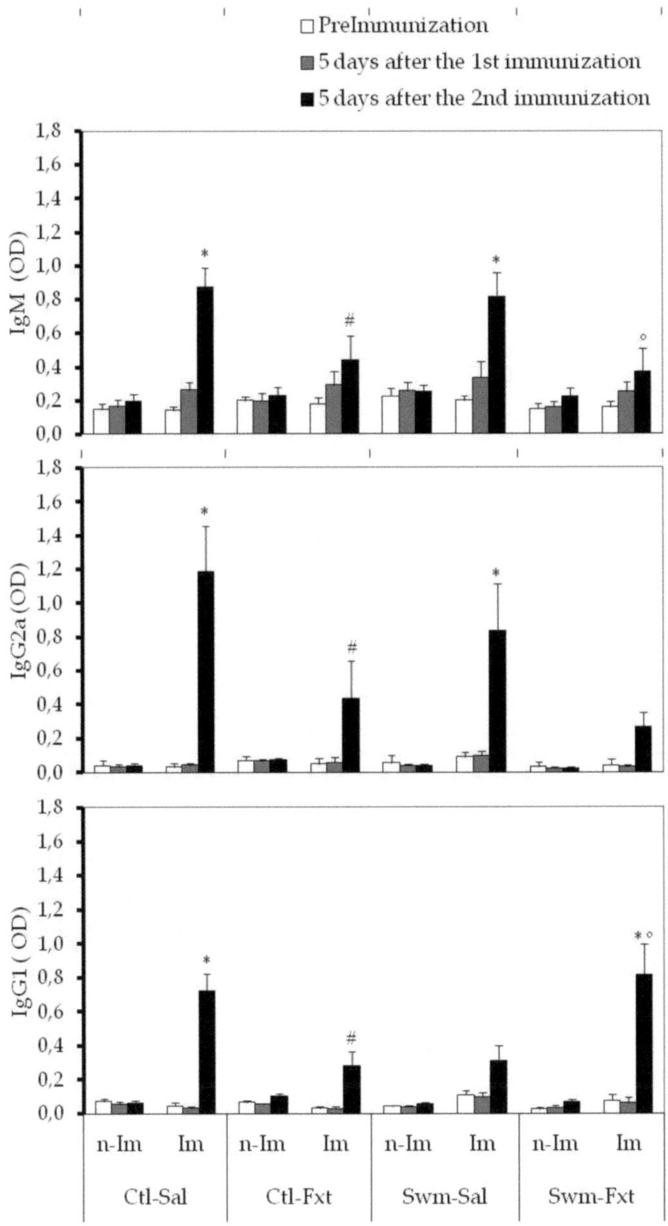

Fig. 1. Variation (mean ± SEM) in the production of antibody. We analyzed the variation in the production of antibodies (IgM, IgG2a and IgG1) at three different points in time (pre-immunization, five days after the first immunization and 5 days after the second immunization). Fluoxetine was responsible for suppressing the production of IgM (a) and IgG2a (b). In relation to IgG1 (c), the administration of only stress and fluoxetine impaired antibody production. However, the interaction between these variables did not impair production. * Different the pre-immunization and 5 days after the first immunization (P <0.001); #Different from Ctl-Sal-Im 5 days after the second immunization (P <0.001); ° Different Swm-Sal-Im 5 days after the second immunization (P <0.002).

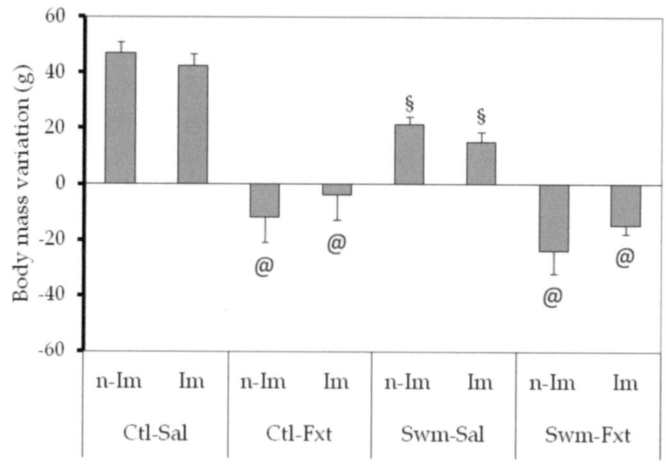

Fig. 2. Variation (mean ± SEM) in body mass. It was observed that both fluoxetine and swimming resulted in reduced body mass. @ Different the saline group that underwent the same treatment (P < 0.05); § Different from the control group that underwent the same treatment (P < 0.05).

There was no stress (F [1.64] = 2.660, P> 0.05) or immunization effect (F [1.64] = 0.373, P> 0.05) on the relative mass of the adrenal glands. There was a significant effect for drug (F [1.64] = 38.558, P <0.001) and interaction between drugs and immunization (F [1.64] = 2.479, P <0.05). The Tukey test showed an increase in relative mass of the adrenal group Swm Fxt-n-Im compared to its control Swm-Salt-n-Im (Table 1).

There was no stress effect on the relative mass of the spleen (F [1.64] = 0.728, P> 0.05), but there was a drug effect (F [1.64] = 19.534, P <0.001, Table 1). Nevertheless, there was no significant difference between groups in post hoc comparisons.

There was no stress (F [1.64] = 0.276, P> 0.05) or immunization effect (F [1.64] = 0.704, P> 0.05) on relative thymus mass, but a drug effect (F [1.64] = 32.504, P <0.001) and an interaction between stress and drug (F [1.64] = 7.535, P <0.05) was detected. It was observed that the drug reduced the relative mass of the thymus in unstressed animals treated with fluoxetine (Table 1).

Organ	Control				Swim			
	Saline		Fluoxetine		Saline		Fluoxetine	
	n-Im	Im	n-Im	Im	n-Im	Im	n-Im	Im
Adrenals	6.6 ± 0.6	7.6 ± 0.3	9.7 ± 0.7	10.0 ± 0.8	6.9 ± 0.8	7.7 ± 0.8	13.1 ± 1.6	9.8 ± 0.5
Spleen	158.4 ± 3.4	150.4 ± 5.6	222.2 ± 27.7	206.8 ± 26.8	143.4 ± 5.2	164.0 ± 7.6	202.0 ± 20.5	189.5 ± 18.0
Thymus	66.2 ± 4.3	71.5 ± 3.8	36.0 ± 7.3	36.1 ± 5.0	54.9 ± 5.1	57.4 ± 5.7	42.1 ± 7.9	47.2 ± 3.4

Table 1. Relative mass of the adrenal glands, spleen and thymus of rats at the end of the experiment. It was observed that fluoxetine was responsible for changing the relative mass of the three organs analyzed, with the adrenal glands and thymus increased and the spleen reduced (P <0.05). Measure (1 = 0.001% of the body mass).

Figure 3a shows the duration of floating behavior. Statistical analysis showed no effects for immunization (F [1.30] = 0.078, P> 0.05) or drug (F [1.30] = 1.099, P> 0.05) but effects for time

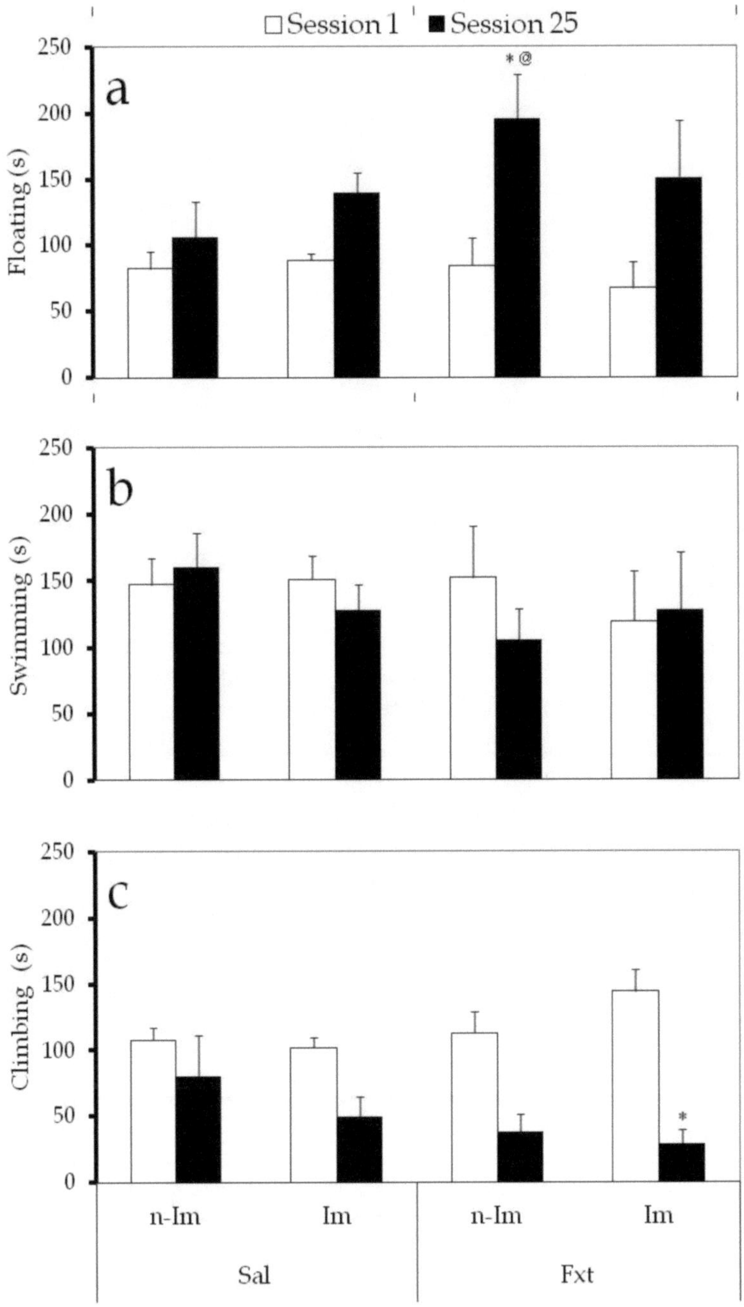

Fig. 3. Variation in the time of analyzed behaviors. Fluoxetine treatment increased floating (a) and reduced climbing (c) behavior between Session 1 and 25; no alteration was found in swimming behavior (b). The animals treated with saline did not show significant alterations in behavior between sessions. *, significant difference compared to Session 1 ($P < 0.01$). @, significant difference in the same session compared to the saline group that had been otherwise submitted to the same treatment ($P < 0.05$).

($F [1. 30] = 30.010$, $P < 0.001$). An interaction between factors occurred only with drug and time ($F [1.30] = 5.989$, $P < 0.05$). Comparing the 1st and the 25th session, a reduction was observed only in the nonimmunized, drug treated group. There was also a distinction observed between the Fxt-n-Im and Sal-n-Im groups at the 25th session.

For swimming, statistical analysis revealed no effects for immunization ($F [1.30] = 0.208$, $P > 0.05$), drug ($F [1.30] = 0.861$, $P > 0.05$), time ($F [1.30] = 0.563$, $P > 0.05$) or interaction of factors (Figure 3b).

Figure 3c shows the time of analyzed behaviors. There were no effects for immunization ($F [1.30] = 0.081$, $P > 0.05$) or drug ($F [1.30] = 0.091$, $P > 0.05$) and effects for time ($F [1. 30] = 32.243$, $P < 0.001$). There was an interaction between drug and time ($F [1.30] = 5.338$, $P < 0.05$). Comparing the 1st and 25th sessions, an increase in climbing time was detected in the Fxt-Im group.

4. Discussion

The current study investigated the effects of chronic stress and the administration of the drug fluoxetine on humoral immune response. It assessed primary and secondary immune response against sheep red blood cells, variation in body mass and the relative mass of the adrenal glands, thymus and spleen, as well as the behavior of rats subjected to a daily forced swimming protocol, which is an model used to assess depression-like behavior in rodents.

In general, stress is considered to be an immunosuppressant. Elenkov & Chrousos (1999) conducted an extensive review on the influence of stress on the immune system and found that acute stress produced subacute or chronic immunosuppressive activity on cellular immune response. On the other hand, stress also was found to have an immunostimulating effect on humoral immune response. Another literature review Segerstrom & Miller (2004) that included research from the last 30 years on the effects of stress on immune function in men and women found no relationship between acute and subacute stress regarding modulation of humoral immune response. Nevertheless, it was observed that stress is associated with chronic immunosuppression in that it lowered antibody capacity against an influenza virus.

The ability of stress to inhibit cellular immune response (Th1) is probably related glucocorticoid and catecholamine suppression of pro-inflammatory cytokines, IL-12, IFN-γ and TNF-α (Elenkov & Chrousos, 1999). Regarding the suppression of cellular immune response, several studies have shown that stress can cause a predisposition to autoimmune diseases (rheumatoid arthritis and type 1 diabetes), allergies (asthma, food allergies and emphysema), and some types of cancer, including Kaposi's sarcoma and Epstein-Barr virus associated B-cell lymphomas (Reiche et al., 2004).

On the other hand, the modulation of humoral immune response by stress is a controversial topic in the literature because studies differ regarding the possible modulation. Baldwin et al. (1995) submitted rats to a stress regime that can be considered subchronic (forced swimming for 3-5 days, 60 minutes each session) and found no differences in the production of anti-sheep red blood cells between stressed and unstressed rats. Besides studies that have found no increase, others have observed a decrease. Kennedy et al. (2005) submitted rats to acute restraint stress and found that it did not alter the production of IgG1 (Th2) but suppressed the production of IgM and IgG2a (Th1) antibodies. Stanojevic et al. (2003)

verified the effects of shock stress for five days in rats and, after immunization with bovine serum albumin (BSA), found that there was suppressed production of IgG anti-BSA compared to controls upon second exposure to the antigen. Hawley et al. (2006) showed that stress caused by high social competition in birds involves a lower production of anti-sheep erythrocytes. Rammal et al. (2010) found that anxious mice produced fewer IgA and IgE antibodies than their nonanxious counterparts, and when both groups were subjected to restraint stress, it appears that all studied antibodies (IgA, IgE and IgG) were suppressed in both groups. On the other hand, Guéguinou et al. (2011) analyzed the natural antibodies of mice subjected to a rotational velocity model (2 and 3 G-force) for 21 days and found an increase in IgG levels of animals subjected to 2Gs. Thus, it can be inferred that the type and length of exposure to the stressor has a direct relationship with the modulated production or elimination of certain antibodies.

In our study, the chronic stress of forced swimming did not interfere in the production of antibody classes IgM and IgG2a, although the production of IgG1 was suppressed. These results are similar to those of Kennedy et al. (2005). The modulation of IgG1 antibody production in mice suggests a suppression of the Th2-type response, which in rats is associated with the production of antibodies to this class of immunoglobulins. On the other hand, the results suggest that the Th1 immune response is not affected by forced swimming since we did not observe a change in the levels of IgG2a antibodies. It is important to note that the production of antibodies in response to an antigen derived from a complex network of cellular interactions that involve the production of molecules with opposite effects, such as cytokine IFN-γ in mice, which has a stimulating effect on cellular immune response and IgG2a antibody production as well as an inhibiting effect on humoral immune response and the production of IgG1 antibody, whereas IL-4 has the opposite effect. The fact that the forced swimming model results in the removal of IgG1 antibodies from production suggests that, by mechanisms not yet understood, stress results in the modulation of signals involved in Th2 response without changing the Th1 response. Whereas there is an antagonistic relationship between IFN-γ and IL-4, these results suggest that the stress-modulated molecular mechanism does not directly involve the main molecules responsible for modulation of antibody production. Recent studies have shown that the role of neurotransmitters in immune system function may be more important than previously considered (Rosas-Ballina et al., 2011).

Besides the relationship between stress and humoral immune response, we investigated the action of fluoxetine on this relationship. Although the 25 days of forced swimming in the present study did not affect the normal production of IgM or IgG2a but inhibited IgG1, we can speculate that the chronic use of this model may stimulate cellular immune response. The administration of fluoxetine inhibited the production of all immunoglobulin classes studied, which shows its general immunosuppressive effect, both for Th1 and Th2. However, the interaction of forced swimming x fluoxetine normalized the production of IgG1. This suggests that stress alone diverts the immune response to Th1-type, while fluoxetine alone has an immunosuppressive effect on humoral immune response. On the other hand, administration of fluoxetine in animals subjected to forced swimming can modulate the immune response to a Th2 pattern. A study about the effects of fluoxetine on humoral immune response showed that mice with rheumatoid arthritis that were treated with fluoxetine (10 or 25 mg/kg/day) for seven days had no changes in the levels of anti-collagen antibodies (IgG1 and IgG2a) (Sacre et al., 2010). This result is at odds with the findings of this study since the time/effect analysis of fluoxetine showed immunosuppression of all studied classes of antibodies after twenty-four days of treatment. These results suggest that the effect of fluoxetine depends on the physiological state of the animal. It is important to note that fluoxetine administered concomitantly with stress can have an immunostimulatory effect. Frick et al. (2009) observed that chronic restraint stress in rats causes decreases in CD4 + T lymphocytes and no change in CD8 + T lymphocyte but when treated with fluoxetine, initial values of CD4 + T cells were restored. According to Freire-Garabal et al. (1997), stressed rats treated with fluoxetine had a higher number of circulating lymphocytes than their control counterparts (stressed and not treated with fluoxetine).

The reduction in specific antibody levels observed in our study is probably related to the action of fluoxetine on the production of cytokines and B lymphocytes, the cells responsible for producing antibodies, as has been observed in other studies. Kubera et al. (2000) demonstrated that the administration of fluoxetine for more than four weeks suppresses the production of IL-4, the main stimulus for differentiating T helper cells into Th2 cells. The decrease in Th2 production may influence isotype synthesis or immunoglobulin levels. Regarding the plasma level of antibodies, Laudenslager & Clarke (2000) observed an increase in immunoglobulin class IgM and IgG and a decrease in the levels of specific IgG antibodies against the tetanus toxoid immunogen in monkeys (*Macaca mulatta*). Therefore, fluoxetine can induce an increased level of total Ig and a decreased level of specific antibodies. However, Sluzewska et al. (1995), studying depressed patients treated with fluoxetine, showed a decrease in IL-6, the cytokine responsible for the growth of B lymphocytes, which differentiate into antibody producers. Moreover, Genaro et al. (2000) observed that fluoxetine had an inhibitory effect on the proliferation of B lymphocytes that had been stimulated by LPS.

The immunosuppressive action of fluoxetine cannot be restricted to the production of antibodies. Pellegrino & Bayer (2002) observed that the in vitro proliferation of lymphocytes from rats that had received fluoxetine via i.p. (5 mg/kg) was lower than their respective controls, suggesting that the antidepressant has an immunosuppressive role for lymphocytes. Fazzini et al. (2009) found that three weeks of continued fluoxetine use in rats triggered an increase in CD8 + T lymphocytes and reduced CD4 + T cells.

The immunomodulatory action of fluoxetine probably involves the participation of cytokines. Patients with major depression have high levels of IL-6, and treatment with fluoxetine for 8 weeks leads to normalization of the cytokine levels (Nishida et al., 2002). Frick et al. (2008), studying cancerous rats, observed that fluoxetine treatment has a direct relationship with increased production of anti-tumor cytokines (IFN-γ and TNF-α), which resulted in lower rates of tumor growth and, therefore, longer survival time. On the other hand, Roumestan et al. (2007) found that fluoxetine had an anti-inflammatory effect (5, 10, 15 and 20 mg/kg) when rats were treated thirty minutes prior to inoculation with LPS and reported reductions of 60% in TNF-α levels and 50% in mortality compared to controls. Sacre et al. (2010) also observed that fluoxetine had an anti-inflammatory effect in rats with rheumatoid arthritis that were treated with 25 mg/kg for seven days, as reflected in reduced levels of IL-12 and joint damage. On the other hand, some studies have failed to show a relationship between fluoxetine and the modulation of cytokine production (Kubera et al., 2004; Maes et al. 1995; Jazayeri et al., 2010). Grundmann et al. (2010) treated rats orally with 10 mg/kg/day of fluoxetine for 21 days and observed no changes in the production of proinflammatory cytokines (IL-6 and TNF-α).

The production of pro- and anti-inflammatory cytokines due to stress plus fluoxetine is dependent on the type of stress and route of drug administration. Sprague-Dawley strain rats, after 21 days of restraint stress and chronic oral treatment with fluoxetine (10 mg/kg), showed lower production of IL-6 than stressed-only animals, although TNF-α levels increased, reaching values similar to those of untreated stressed animals (Grundmann et al., 2010). On the other hand, Kubera et al. (2006) pre-treated rats with imipramine (5 mg/kg) 1, 5 and 24 hours before forced swimming and found that the splenocytes of treated animals produced more IL-10 than controls (stressed and treated with vehicle), with no IFN-γ differences observed in any group. Rogoz et al. (2009) treated rats 1, 5 and 24 hours before forced swimming with 10 mg/kg of fluoxetine i.p. and observed that the interaction between stress and fluoxetine did not alter the splenocyte production of IL-10 or IFN-γ.

There are reports that the chronic administration of fluoxetine either causes weight loss (Wellman et al., 2003) or prevents weight gain (Gutierrez et al., 2002). In the present study, the chronic administration of fluoxetine led to a reduction in body mass when compared with saline treatment; this reduction was more pronounced when the animals were treated with the drug and subjected to forced swimming. First et al. (2011) treated rats for five weeks with fluoxetine (5 mg/kg) and observed reduced body mass. However, when they were treated with the drug and submitted to chronic stress with multiple stressors, fluoxetine prevented weight loss due to this protocol. Zafir & Banu, (2007) also observed weight maintenance by chronic administration of fluoxetine in animals subjected to restraint stress. It is important to point out that the above-mentioned studies differed in the degree of stress generated. In this study 15 min/day of forced swimming did not prevent the animals from gaining weight, but First et al. (2011), using various types of stressors for five weeks and Banu & Zafir (2007), using four hours of restraint stress, observed reduced body mass. Thus, combined multiple stressors or prolonged restraint seem to be more stressful than forced swimming. Considered jointly, these studies indicate two seemingly opposite effects of fluoxetine: in the presence of severe stressors known to induce mass reduction, the drug prevents such losses, while in the presence of mild stressors, the drug leads to weight loss, which suggests an anorexic effect. Human studies have confirmed the anorectic effect of fluoxetine in that reductions in body mass from the chronic administration of fluoxetine were observed in obese individuals (Wise, 1992).

Stress affects the mass of the adrenal glands and lymphoid organs such as the thymus and spleen. Baldwin et al. (1995) investigated the effects of forced swimming (3 to 5 days, sixty minutes per session) and found that the number of rats housed together (one or five) influenced the relative masses of the adrenal glands, spleen and thymus, the production of corticosterone and body mass. They observed that forced swimming, regardless of the type of accommodation, reduced the spleen, thymus and body mass of animals, but did not alter the production of corticosterone or the relative mass of the adrenal glands. When the animals were subjected to social isolation and forced swimming, however, there was increased corticosterone production and adrenal mass in addition to the above-mentioned effects, showing that these two models administered separately do not lead to stress, but together are stressful. Regarding the chronic effect of forced swimming, Zivkovic et al. (2005a) found that after submitting rats to 21 days of this protocol, the thymus weight of stressed animals was lower than that of non-stressed animals. In another study by the same authors (2005b), blood was collected from rats after their final swimming session for analysis of circulating corticosterone levels and it was observed that, even after 21 days of chronic forced swimming, corticosterone values remained high.

In our study, the adrenal gland mass of Wistar rats submitted to swimming (15 min daily for 25 days) did not change, which was a further similarity with the findings of Baldwin et al. (1995), i.e., body mass reduction in animals submitted to swimming. Our study differed from the above-mentioned studies in that our stress model did not lead to changes in spleen or thymus mass. Moreover, Connor et al. (1998) observed no changes in Sprague-Dawley spleen weight after acute forced swimming, which shows that, depending on the strain and stress time, body mass values may or may not vary.

Fluoxetine is also responsible for changing the mass of the adrenal glands, spleen and thymus of rodents. Garabal-Freire et al. (1997) submitted mice to a sound stressor (100 dB, 1 to 3 hours per day, four to twelve days) and observed a decrease in the number of thymic and spleen cells; this stressor also contributed to a reduction in relative thymus weight, a condition reversed by treatment with fluoxetine (5 mg/kg). Kubera et al. (2006) treated rats with three doses of imipramine 1, 5 and 24 hours before forced swimming and found that acute treatment with this drug did not alter the relative thymus weight, but did reduce spleen weight. In the present study, 24 days of fluoxetine treatment (10 mg/kg) reduced the relative thymus weight and body mass of rats and increased spleen and adrenal gland mass. Thus, either chronic treatment with fluoxetine stressed the animals or the change in relative adrenal mass is merely a reflection of the change in body mass since the adrenal glands did not necessarily increase. However, the sudden loss of body mass would have led to this apparent increase.

The currently-used antidepressants have specific compounds that act on different regions of the central nervous system, so it is expected that their use in rats or mice would lead to improvement in depression symptoms, i.e., reduced time floating (passive behavior) and increased time climbing and/or swimming (active behavior) during a forced swimming stressor (Piras et al., 2010). However, increases in climbing and/or swimming are dependent on the type of drug administered (Cryan & Lucki, 2000). Page et al. (1999) observed a reduction in floating time and an increase in swimming time in rats treated with fluoxetine. Carr et al. (2010) used fluoxetine in rats (20 mg/kg) three times before forced swimming yielded similar results. Cryan & Lucki (2000) compared fluoxetine and reboxetine in a rat forced swimming model and found that both drugs led to reduced flotation time, although the former increased swimming time and the latter increased climbing time.

To investigate the effects of chronic treatment with fluoxetine (10 mg/kg), Hansen et al. (2011) treated Wistar rats for 48 days with subcutaneous injections, after which the animals were subjected to forced swimming. The results showed that the floating, swimming and climbing times of treated rats were similar to those observed when fluoxetine was administered 24 hours before the test (acute effect). Pedreañez et al. (2011), studying the effects of forced swimming as a chronic stressor, carried out fifteen 30-min forced swimming sessions and found that the animals' active behavior dropped by 84 percent between the first and last session.

In our experiment, forced swimming was performed over a chronic period (twenty-five days). The results were expected to be similar to those in the literature (with test-retest separated by 24 h) or to those of Pedreañez et al. (2011) for rats subjected to chronic swimming. We found that, after the chronic treatment period, the time values were different from those observed when the test and retest were separated by 24 h. Stressed animals treated with saline had no alterations in floating, swimming or climbing times, indicating that forced swimming, when performed on a chronic basis, is not an appropriate model for investigating behavioral changes in rats. It should be pointed out that different strains of rats exhibited different behavior in the two studies: the active behavior of Sprague-Dawley rats was reduced in Pedreañez et al. (2011) whereas, in the present study, Wistar behavior was constant throughout the protocol.

On the other hand, it was observed that animals treated with fluoxetine significantly increased floating time after treatment. Since climbing time was also reduced, we can infer that adaptation to the drug also leads to behavioral changes, contradicting expected behavior for this model of stress/depression. Two possibilities could explain this: first, chronic treatment with fluoxetine engenders passive behavior; second, their reduced body weight made them denser, which may have facilitated buoyancy and thus reduced effort expenditure.

5. Conclusion

We observed in this study that animals treated with fluoxetine and submitted to a 25 day forced swimming protocol had a reduced production of IgM and IgG2a and an increased production of IgG1. Considering the unique effect of the drug, the adrenal gland and relative spleen weight increased, while thymus weight was reduced. Drug-treated rats lost body mass compared to saline-treated rats. Regarding the analyzed behaviors, treatment with fluoxetine resulted in distinct changes in acute effect, indicating that swimming is not be trusted as a model chronic stressor in rats. However, the alterations observed in this study may have important implications for the treatment of depression in humans since fluoxetine appears to impair the production of antibodies. Thus the indiscriminate use of this drug for non-stressed individuals must be questioned.

6. Acknowledgments

To Dr. Solange de Paula Ramos, Department of Histology, State University of Londrina, PR, Brazil, for providing materials used in much of the study and also for the supervision and guidance in animal handling and the procedures for collecting blood, sacrifice and removing organs.

To Dr. Tiemi Matsuo, Department of Statistics, State University of Londrina, PR, Brazil for help with the experimental design and statistical analysis.

To the Coordenação de Aperfeiçoamento de Pessoal de Nível Superior (CAPES) for the scholarship granted to EVF.

7. References

Alperina, E. L.; Kulikov, A. V.; Popova, N. K. & Idova, G. V. (2007). Immune Response in Mice of a New Strain ASC (Antidepressants Sensitive Catalepsy). *Bulletin of Experimental Biology and Medicine*, Vol.144, pp. 221-223, ISSN 1573-8221

Altenburg, A. S. P.; Ventura, D. G.; Da-Silva, V. A.; Malheirosa, L. R.; Castro-Faria-Neto, H. C.; Bozza, P. T. & Teixeira, N. A. (2002) The role of forced swim test on neutrophil leukocytosis observed during inflammation induced by LPS in rodents. *Progress in Neuro-Psychopharmacology and Biological Psychiatry*, Vol.26, pp. 891–895, ISSN 0278-5846

Baldwin, D. R.; Wilcox, Z. C. & BAYLOSIS, R. C. (1995) Impact of Differential Housing on Humoral Immunity Following Exposure to an Acute Stressor in Rats. *Physiology and Behavior*, Vol.57, No.4, pp. 649-653, ISSN 0031-9384

Bauer, M. E.; Gauer, G. J.; Luz, C.; Silveira, R. O.; Nardi, N. B. & Von Mühlen, C. A. (1995). Evaluation of immune parameters in depressed patients. *Life Sciences*, Vol.57, pp. 665-674, ISSN 0199-9966

Bezchlibnyk-Butler, K. Z. & Jeffries, J. J. (1999) *Clinical handbook of psychotropic drugs*. Hogrefe & Huber, ISBN 0-88937-271-3 Ashland, OH, US

Borsini, F. & Meli, A. (1998) Is the forced swimming test a suitable model for revealing antidepressant activity? *Psychopharmacology*, Vol.94, pp.147–160, ISSN 1432-2072

Bromet, E.; Andrade, L. H.; Hwang, I.; Sampson, N. A.; Alonso, J.; De Girolamo, G.; De Graaf, R.; Demyttenaere, K.; Hu, C.; Iwata, N.; Karam, A. N.; Kaur, J.; Kostyuchenko, S.; Lépine, J. P.; Levinson, D.; Matschinger, H.; Mora, M. E.; Browne, M. O.; Posada-Villa, J.; Viana, M. C.; Williams, D. R. & Kessler, R. C. (2011) Cross-national epidemiology of DSM-IV major depressive episode. *BMC Medicine*, Vol.9, No.90, pp. 1-16 ISSN 1741-7015

Bradford, M. M. (1976) A rapid and sensitive method for the quantitation of microgram quantities of protein utilizing the principle of protein-dye binding. *Analytical Biochemistry*, Vol.7, No.72, pp. 248-254, ISSN 1096-0309

Calabrese, J. R.; Kling, M. A. & Gold, P. W. (1987) Alterations in immunocompetence during stress, bereavement, and depression: Focus on neuroendocrine regulation. *American Journal of Psychology*, Vol. 144, pp. 1123-1134, ISSN 1939-8298

Carr, G. V.,;Schechter, L. E. & Lucki, I. (2010). Antidepressant and anxiolytic effects of selective 5-HT6 receptor agonists in rats. *Psychopharmacology*, DOI 10.1007/s00213-010-1798-7, ISSN 1432-2072

Connor, T. J.; Kelly, J. P. & Leonard, B. E. (1998) Forced Swim Test-Induced Endocrine and Immune Changes in the Rat: Effect of Subacute Desipramine Treatment. *Pharmacology Biochemistry and Behavior*, Vol.59, No.1, pp. 171-177, ISSN 0091-3057

Cryan, J. F. & Lucki, I. (2000). Antidepressant-Like Behavioral Effects Mediated by 5-Hydroxytryptamine 2C Receptors1. *The Journal of Pharmacology and Experimental Therapeutics*, 295, 1120-1126, ISSN 1521-0103

Edgar, V. A.; Cremaschi, G.; Sterin-Borda, L. & Genaro, A. M. (2002) Altered expression of autonomic neurotransmitter receptors and proliferative responses in lymphocytes from a chronic mild stress model of depression: effects of fluoxetine. *Brain, Behavior and Immunity*, Vol.16, pp. 333-350, ISSN 0889-1591

Elenkov, I. J. & Chrousos, G. P. (1999) Stress Hormones, Th1/Th2 patterns, Pro/Anti-inflammatory Cytokines and Susceptibility to Disease. *Trends in Endocrinology and Metabolism*, Vol.10, No.9, pp. 359-368, ISSN 1043-2760

Egeland, M.; Warner-Schmidt, J.; Greengard, P. & Svenningsson, P. (2010). Neurogenic effects of fluoxetine are attenuated in p11 (S100A10) knockout mice. *Biological Psychiatry*, Vol.67, pp. 1048-1056, ISSN 0006-3223

Fava, M. & Kendler, K. S. (2000) Major Depressive Disorder. *Neuron*, Vol.28, pp. 335–341, ISSN 0896-6273

Fazzino, F.; Urbina, M.; Cedeño, N. & Lima, L. (2009). Fluoxetine treatment to rats modifies serotonin transporter and cAMP in lymphocytes, CD4+ and CD8+ subpopulations and interleukins 2 and 4. *International Immunopharmacology*, Vol.9, pp. 463–467, ISSN 1567-5769

First, M.; Gil-Ad, I.; Taler, M.; Tarasenko, I.; Novak, N. & Weizman, A. (2011) The Effects of Fluoxetine Treatment in a Chronic Mild Stress Rat Model on Depression-Related Behavior, Brain Neurotrophins and ERK Expression. *Journal of Molecular Neuroscience*, in press, ISSN 1559-1166

Freire-Garabal, M.; Nlifiez, M. J.; Losada, C.; Pereiro, D.; Riveiro, M. P.; Gonzalez-Patiao, E.; Mayan, J. M. & Rey-Mendez, M. (1997). Effects of fluoxetine on the immunosuppressive response to stress in mice. *Life Sciences*, Vol.60, pp. 403-413, ISSN 0024-3205

Frick, L. R.; Palumbo, M. L.; Zappia, M. P.; Brocco, M. A.; Cremaschi, G. A. & Genaro, A. M. (2008). Inhibitory effect of fluoxetine on lymphoma growth through the modulation of antitumor T-cell response by serotonin-dependent and independent mechanisms. *Biochemical Pharmacology*, Vol.75, pp. 1817-1826, ISSN 0006-2952

Frick, L. R.; Rapanelli, M.; Cremaschi, G. A. & Genaro, A. M. (2009). Fluoxetine directly counteracts the adverse effects of chronic stress on T cell immunity by compensatory and specific mechanisms. *Brain, Behavior, and Immunity*, Vol.23, pp. 36–40, ISSN 0889-1591

Genaro, A. M.; Edgar, V. A. & Sterin-Borda, L. (2000) Differential effects of fluoxetine on murine B-cell proliferation depending on the biochemical pathways triggered by distinct mitogens. *Biochemical Pharmacology*, Vol.60, pp. 1279-1283, ISSN 0006-2952

Guéguinou, N.; Bojados, M.; Jamon, M.; Derradji, H.; Baatout, S.; Tschirhart, E.; Frippiat, J-P. & Legrand-Frossi, C. (2011) Stress response and humoral immune system alterations related to chronic hypergravity in mice. *Psychoneuroendocrinology*, in press, ISSN 0306-4530

Gutiérrez, A.; Saracíbar, G.; Casis, L.; Echevarría, E.; Rodríguez, V. M.; Macarulla, M. T.; Abecia, L. C. & Portillo, M. P. (2002). Effects of fluoxetine administration on neuropeptide Y and orexins in obese Zucker rat hypothalamus. *Obesity Research*, Vol.10, pp. 532-540, ISSN 0306-7548

Grundmann, O.; LV, Y.; Kelber, O. & Butterweck, V. (2010) Mechanism of St. John's wort extract (STW3-VI) during chronic restraint stress is mediated by the interrelationship of the immune, oxidative defense, and neuroendocrine system. *Neuropharmacology*, Vol.58, pp. 767-773, ISSN 0028-3908

Hansen, F.; Oliveira, D. L.; Amaral, F. U. Í.; Guedes, F. S.; Schneider, T. J.; Tumelero, A. C.; Hansela, G. Schmidt, K. H.; Giacomini, A. C. V. V. & Torresa, F. V. (2011) Effects of chronic administration of tryptophan with or without concomitant fluoxetine in depression-related and anxiety-like behaviors on adult rat. *Neuroscience Letters*, Vol.499, pp. 59-63, ISSN 0304-3940

Hawley, D. M.; Lindström, K.; Wikelski, M. (2006) Experimentally increased social competition compromises humoral immune responses in house finches. *Hormones and Behavior*, Vol.49, pp. 417–424, ISSN 1095-6867

Irwin, M. R.; Levin, M. J.; Carrillo, C.; Olmstead, R.; Lucko, A.; Lang, N.; Caulfield, M. J.; Weinberg, A.; Chan, I. S.; Clair, J.; Smith, J. G.; Marchese, R. D.; Williams, H. M.; Beck, D. J.; McCook, P. T.; Johnson, G. & Oxman, M. N. (2011) Major depressive disorder and immunity to varicella-zoster virus in the elderly. *Brain, Behavior and Immunity*, Vol.25, No.4, pp. 759-766, ISSN 0889-1591

Jabbi, M.; Korf, J.; Ormel, J.; Kema, I. P. & Den Boer, J. A. (2008) Investigating the molecularb asis of major depressive disorder etiology: a functional convergent genetic approach. *Annals of the New York Academy of Sciences*, Vol.1148, pp. 42-56, ISSN 1749-6632

Janssen, D. G.; Caniato, R. N.; Verster, J. C. & Baune, B. T. (2010) A psychoneuroimmunological review on cytokines involved in antidepressant treatment response. *Human Psychopharmacology*, Vol.25, No.3, pp. 201-215, ISSN 1099-1077

Jazayeri, S.; Keshavarz, S. A.; Tehrani-Doost, M.; Djalali, M.; Osseini, M.; Amini, H.; Chamari, M. & Djazayery, A. (2010). Effects of eicosapentaenoic acid and fluoxetine on plasma cortisol, serum interleukin-1beta and interleukin-6 oncentrations in patients with major depressive disorder. *Psychiatry Research*, Vol.178, pp. 112-115, ISSN 0165-1781

Kendler, K. S.; Kessler, R. C.; Walters, E. E.; Maclean, C.; Nelae, M. C.; Hesth, A. C. & EAVES, L. J. (1995) Stressful life events, genetic liability, and onset of an episode of major depression in women. *The American Journal of Psychiatry*, Vol.152, No.6, pp. 833-842, ISSN 1535-7228

Kennedy, S. L.; Nickerson, M.; Campisi, J.; Johnson, J. D.; Smith, T. P.; Sharkey, C. & Fleshner, M. (2005) Splenic norepinephrine depletion following acute stress suppresses in vivo antibody response. *Journal of Neuroimmunology*, Vol.165, pp. 150-160, ISSN 0165-5728

Kessler, R. C. (1997) The effects of stressful life events on depression. *Annual Review of Psychology*, Vol.48, pp. 191-214, ISSN 0066-4308

Kronfol, Z. & House, J. D.; (1989) Lymphocyte mitogenesis, immunoglobulin and complement levels in depressed patients and normal controls. *Acta Psychiatrica Scandinavica*, Vol.80, pp. 142-147, ISSN 1600-0447

Kubera, M.; Symbirtsev, A.; Basta-Kaim, A.; Borycz, J.; Roman, A.; Papp, M. & Claesson, M. (1996) Effect of chronic treatment with imipramine on interleukin 1 and interleukin 2 production by splenocytes obtained from rats subjected to a chronic mild stress model of depression. *Polish Journal of Pharmacology*, Vol.48, No.5, pp. 503-506, ISSN 0301-0244

Kubera, M.; Simbirtsev, A.; Mathison, R. & Maes, M. (2000) Effects of repeated fluoxetine and citalopram administration on cytokinerelease in C57BL/6 mice. *Psychiatry Research*, Vol.96, pp. 255-266, ISSN 0165-1781

Kubera, M.; Kenis, G.; Bosmans, E.; Kajta, M.; Basta-Kaim, A.; Scharpe, S.; Budziszewska, B. & Maes, M. (2004). Stimulatory effect of antidepressants on the production of IL-6. *International Immunopharmacology*, Vol.4, pp. 185-192, ISSN 1567-5769

Kubera, M.; Basta-Kaim, A.; Budziszewska, B.; Rogóz, Z.; Skuza, G.; Lesiewicz, M.; Tetich, M.; Jaworska-Feil, L.; Maes, M. & Lason, W. (2006) Effect of amantadine and imipramine on immunological parameters of rats subjected to a forced swimming test. *The International Journal of Neuropsychopharmacology*, Vol.9, pp. 297-305, ISSN 1461-1457

Laudenslager, M. L. & Clarke, A. S. (2000) Antidepressant treatment during social challenge prior to 1 year of age affects immune and endocrine responses in adult macaques. *Psychiatry Research*, Vol.95, pp. 25-34, ISSN 0165-1781

Leonard, B. E. (2001) The immune system, depression and the action of antidepressants, *Progress in Neuro-Psychopharmacology and Biological Psychiatry*, Vol.25, pp. 767-780, ISSN 0278-5846

Lépine, J. P. & Briley, M. (2011) The increasing burden of depression. *Journal of Neuropsychiatric Disease and Treatment*, Vol.7, No.1, pp. 3-7, ISSN 1178-2021

Lichtman, J. H.; J. Bigger, T. Jr.; Blumenthal, J. A.; Frasure-Smith, N.; Kaufmann, P.; Lespérance, F.; Mark, D. B.; Sheps, D. S.; Taylor, B. & Froelicher, E. S. (2009) Depression and Coronary Heart Disease: Recommendations for Screening, Referral, and Treatment. *Focus*, Vol.7, No.3, pp. 406-413, ISSN 1663-0459

Lipp, M. E. N. (1994) *Stress, hipertensão arterial e qualidade de vida*. Papirus, Campinas, São Paulo.

Loskutov, L. V.; Idova, G. V. & Gevorgyan, M. M. (2007). Immune Response in Wistar Rats with High and Low Level of Situational Anxiety. *Bulletin of Experimental Biology and Medicine*, Vol.144, pp. 706-708, ISSN 1573-8221

Lucki, I. (1997) The forced swimming test as a model for core and component behavioral effects of antidepressant drugs. *Behaviroual Pharmacology*, Vol.8, pp.523–532, ISSN 1473-5849

Maes, M.; Meltzer, H. Y.; Bosmans, E.; Bergmans, R.; Vandoolaeghe, E.; Ranjan, R. & Desnyder, R. (1995). Increased plasma concentrations of interleukin-6, soluble interleukin-6, soluble interleukin-2 and transferrin receptor in major depression. *Journal of Affective Disorders*, Vol.34, pp. 301-309 ISSN 0165-0327

Miller, A. H. (2010) Depression and immunity: A role for T cells? *Brain, Behavior, and Immunity*, Vol.24, pp. 1-8, ISSN 0889-1591

Nishida, A.; Hisaoka, K.; Zensho, H.; Uchitomi, Y.; Morinobu, S. & Yamawaki, S. (2002). Antidepressant drugs and cytokines in mood disorders. *International Immunopharmacology*, Vol.2, pp. 1619–1626, ISSN 1567-5769

Nunes, S. O. V.; Reiche, E. M. V.; Morimoto, H. K.; Matsuo, T.; Itano, E. N.; Xavier, E. C. D.; Yamashita, C. M.; Vieira, V. R.; Menoli, A. V.; Silva, S. S.; Costa, F. B.; Reiche, F. V.; Silva, F. L. V. & Kaminami, M. S. (2002) Immune and hormonal activity in adults suffering from depression. *Brazilian Journal of Medical and Biological Research*, Vol.35, pp. 581-587, ISSN 1678-4510

Page, M. E.; Detke, M. J.; Kirby, A. D. L. G. & Lucki, I. (1999). Serotonergic mediation of the effects of fluoxetine, but not desipramine, in the rat forced swimming test. *Psychopharmacology*, Vol.147, pp. 162–167, ISSN 1432-2072

Pellegrino, T. C. & Bayer, B. M. (2002). Role of Central 5-HT2 Receptors in Fluoxetine-Induced Decreases in T Lymphocyte Activity. *Brain, Behavior, and Immunity*, Vol.16, pp. 87–103, ISSN 0889-1591

Pedersen, K. B.; Hoffman-Goetz, L. (2000) Exercise and the immune system: regulation, integration and adaptation. *Physiology Reviews*, Vol.80, No.3, pp. 1055-1081, ISSN 0066-4294

Pedreañez, A.; Arcaya, J. L.; Carrizo, E.; Rincón, J.; Viera, N.; Peña, C.; Vargas, R. & Mosquera, J. (2011) Experimental depression induces renal oxidative stress in rats. *Physiology & Behavior*, in press, ISSN 0031-9384

Piras, G.; Giorgi, O. & Corda, M. G. (2010) Effects of antidepressants on the performance in the forced swim test of two psychogenetically selected lines of rats that differ in coping strategies to aversive conditions. *Psychopharmacology*, Vol.211, pp. 403-414, ISSN 1432-2072

Porsolt, R.D.; Le Pichon, M.; Jalfre, M. (1977) Depression: a new animal model sensitive to antidepressant treatments. *Nature*, Vol.266, pp.730–732, ISSN 0028-0836

Post, R. M. (1992) Transduction of psychosocial stress into the neurobiology of recurrent affective disorder. *American Journal of Psychology*, Vol.149, No.8, pp. 999-1010, ISSN 0002-9556

Rammal, H.; Bouayed, J.; Falla, J.; Boujedaini, N. & Soulimani, R. (2010) The Impact of High Anxiety Level on Cellular and Humoral Immunity in Mice. *Neuroimmunomodulation*, Vol.17, pp. 1–8 ISSN 1021-7401

Reiche, E. M. V.; Nunes, S. O. V. & Marimoto, H. K. (2004) Stress, depression, the immune system, and cancer. *The Lancet Oncology*, Vol.5, pp. 617-625, ISSN 1470-2045

Robles, T. F.; Glaser, R. & Kiecolt-Glaser, J. K. (2005) A New Look at Chronic Stress, Depression, and Immunity. *Current Directions in Psychological Science*, Vol.14, No.2, pp. 111-115, ISSN 0963-7214

Rogóz, Z.; Kubera, M.; Rogóz, K.; Basta-Kaim, A. & Budziszewska, B. (2009) Effect of co-administration of fluoxetine and amantadine on immunoendocrine parameters in rats subjected to a forced swimming test. *Pharmacological Reports*, Vol.61, pp. 1050-1060, ISSN 1734-1140

Rosas-Ballina, M.; Olofsson, P. S.; Ochani, M.; Valdés-Ferrer, S. I.; Levine, Y. A.; Reardon, C.; Tusche, M. W.; Pavlov, V. A.; Andersson, U.; Chavan, S.; Mak, T. W. &, Tracey, K. J. (2011) Acetylcholine-synthesizing T cells relay neural signals in a vagus nerve circuit. *Science*, Vol.334, No.6052, pp. 98-101 ISSN 1095-9203

Roumestan, C.; Michel, A.; Bichon, F.; Portet, K.; Detoc, M.; Henriquet, C.; Jaffuel, D. & Mathieu, M. (2007). Anti-inflammatory properties of desipramine and fluoxetine. *Respiratory Research*, Vol.8, pp. 1-11, ISSN 1465-9921

Sacre, S.; Medghalchi, M.; Gregory, B.; Brennan, F. & Williams, R. (2010). Fluoxetine and Citalopram Exhibit Potent Antiinflammatory Activity in Human and Murine Models of Rheumatoid Arthritis and Inhibit Toll-like Receptors. *Arthritis and rheumatism*, Vol.62, pp. 683–693, ISSN 1529-0131

Schleifer SJ, Keller SE, Meyerson AT, Raskin MJ, Davis KL, Stein M. (1984) Lymphocyte function in major depressive disorder. *Archives of General Psychiatry*, Vol.41, No.5, pp.484-486 ISSN 0003-990x

Schleifer, S. J.; Keller, S. E.; Siris, S. G.; Davis, K. L. & Stein, M. (1985) Depression and immunity. Lymphocyte function in ambulatory depressed patients, hospitalized schizophrenic patients, and patients hospitalized for herniorrhaphy. *Archives of General Psychiatry*, Vol.43, pp. 129-133, ISSN 0003-990X

Schleifer, S. J.; Keller, S. E.; Meyerson, A. T.; Rashkin, M. J.; Davis, K. L.; Stein, M. (1996) Lymphocyte function in major depression disorder. *Archives of General Psychiatry*, Vol.41, pp. 484-486, ISSN 0003-990X

Seedat, S.; Scott, K. M.; Angermeyer, M. C.; Berglund, P.; Bromet, E. J.; Brugha, T. S.; Demyttenaere, K.; De Girolamo, G.; Haro, J. M.; Jin, R.; Karam, E. G.; Kovess-Masfety, V.; Levinson, D.; Medina-Mora, M. E.; Ono, Y.; Ormel, J.; Pennell, B. E.; Posada-Villa, J.; Sampson, N. A.; Williams, D. & Kessler, R. C. (2009) Cross-national associations between gender and mental disorders in the World Health Organization World Mental Health Surveys. *Archives of General Psychiatry*, Vol.66, No.7, pp. 785-795, ISSN 0003-990X

Segerstrom, S. C. & Miller, G. E. (2004) Psychological Stress and the Human Immune System: A Meta-Analytic Study of 30 Years of Inquiry. *Psychopharmacology Bulletin*, Vol.130, No.4, pp. 601–630, ISSN 0048-5764

Seidel, A.; Arolt, V.; Hunstiger, M.; Rink, L.; Behnisch, A. & Kirchner, H. (1995) Cytokine production and serum proteins in depression. *Scandinavian Journal of Immunology*, Vol.41, pp. 534–538, ISSN 1365-3083

Selye, H. A (1936) Syndrome produced by diversal nocuous agents. *Nature*, pp. 13-32, ISSN 0028-0836

Sluzewska, A.; Rybakowski, J. K.; Laciak, M.; Mackewicz, A.; Sobieska, M. & Wiktorowicz, K.; (1995) Interleukin-6 serum leves in depressed patients before and after treatment with fluoxetine. *Annals of the New York Academy of Sciences*, Vol.762, pp. 474-476, ISSN 1749-6632

Smith, R.S. (1991) The macrophage theory of depression. *Medical Hypotheses*, Vol.35, No.4, pp. 298-306, ISSN 0306-9877

Song, C.; Dinan, T. & Leonard, B. E. (1994) Changes in immunoglobulin, complement and acute phase protein concentrations in depressed patients and normal controls. *Journal of Affective Disorders*, Vol.49, pp. 211-219 ISSN 0165-0327

Stacciarini, J. M. R. & Tróccoli, B. T. (2004) Occupational stress and constructive thinking: health and job satisfaction. *Journal of Advanced Nursing*, Vol.46, No.5, pp. 480–487, ISSN 1365-2648

Stahl, S. M. (1997) *Psychopharmacology of Antidepressants*. Martin Dunitz, London, England

Stanojevic, S.; Dimitrijevic, M.; Kovacevic-Jovanovic, V.; Miletic, T.; Vujic, V.; Radulovic, J. (2003) Stress Applied During Primary Immunization Affects the Secondary Humoral Immune Response in the Rat: Involvement of Opioid Peptides. *Stress*, Vol.6, No.4, pp. 247–258, ISSN 1607-8888

Szuster-Ciesielska, A.; Słotwińska, M.; Stachura, A.; Marmurowska-Michałowska, H.; Dubas-Slemp, H.; Bojarska-Junak, A. & Kandefer-Szerszeń, M. (2008) Accelerated apoptosis of blood leukocytes and oxidative stress in blood of patients with major depression. *Progress in Neuro-psychopharmacology & Biological Psychiatry*, Vol.32, No.3, pp. 686-694 ISSN 0278-5846

Vismari, L.; Alves, G. J. & Palerm-Neto, J. (2008) Depressão, antidepressivos e sistema imune: um novo olhar sobre um velho problema. *Revista de Psiquiatria Clínica*, Vol.35, No.5, pp.196-204, ISSN 0101-6083

Waraich, P.; Goldner, E. M.; Somers, J. M. & Hsu, L. (2004) Prevalence and incidence studies of mood disorders: a systematic review of the literature. *Canadian Journal of Psychiatry*, Vol.49, No.2, pp. 124-138, ISSN 0703-7437

Wellman, P. J.; Jones, S. L. & Miller, D. K. (2003). Effects of preexposure to dexfenfluramine, phentermine, dexfenfluramine–phentermine, or fluoxetine on sibutramine-induced hypophagia in the adult rat. *Pharmacology Biochemistry and Behavior*, Vol.75, pp. 103-114 ISSN 0091-3057

Willner, P. (1992) Animal models of depression: an overview. *Pharmacology and Therapeutics*. Vol.45, pp. 425–455, ISSN 0163-7258

Wise, S. D. (1992). Clinical studies with fluoxetine in obesity. *American Journal of Clinical Nutrition*, Vol.55, pp. 181S-184S, ISSN 1938-3207

Zafir, A. & Banu, N. (2007). Antioxidant potential of fluoxetine in comparison to Curcuma longa in restraint-stressed rats. *European Journal of Pharmacology*, Vol.572, pp. 23–31, ISSN 0014-2999

Zivkovic, I.; Rakina, A.; Petrovic-Djergovic, D.; Miljkovic, B. & Micic, M. (2005a) The effects of chronic stress on thymus innervations in the adult rat. *Acta histochemica*, Vol.106, pp. 449-458, ISSN 0065-1281

Zivkovic, I.; Rakina, A.; Petrovic-Djergovic, D.; Miljkovic, B. & Micic, M. (2005b) Exposure to forced swim stress alters morphofunctional characteristics of the rat thymus. *Journal of Neuroimmunology*, Vol.160, pp. 77- 86, ISSN 0165-5728

2

Effects of Antidepressants on Inhibitory Avoidance in Mice: A Review

Concepción Vinader-Caerols, Andrés Parra and Santiago Monleón
Department of Psychobiology, University of Valencia
Spain

1. Introduction

Neither the biological basis of depression (Nemeroff & Vale, 2005; Kasper & McEwen, 2008) nor the precise mechanism of antidepressant efficacy are completely understood (Dudra-Jastrzebska et al., 2007). Indeed, antidepressants are widely prescribed for anxiety and disorders other than depression. For example, they are the drug therapy of choice for severe anxiety disorders such as agoraphobia, generalized anxiety disorder, social phobia, obsessive-compulsive disorder and post-traumatic stress disorder (Baldessarini, 2001). Antidepressants are also employed as a therapeutic tool in disorders such as drug addition (e.g. Schatzberg, 2000), enuresis (e.g. Humphreys & Reinberg, 2005) and chronic pain (e.g. Sindrup et al., 2005). This wide application of the effects of antidepressants and the heterogeneity of their mechanism of action suggest the existence of a common therapeutic mechanism among the disorders which these drugs are employed to treat.

A series of studies have associated major depression with significant atrophy within the hippocampus (Campbell et al., 2004; Paizanis et al., 2007). If the hippocampus plays a central role in learning and memory, alterations in this structure could well be related to the cognitive deficits observed during depressive episodes (Paizanis et al., 2007; Sahay & Hen, 2007). The cognitive impact of antidepressants (Amado-Boccara et al., 1995) and the association between depression and memory impairment (Castaneda et al., 2008) are better understood in the framework of an emerging hypothesis that suggests that the pathogenesis and treatment of depression are involved in the plasticity of neuronal pathways (Pittenger & Duman, 2008; Vaidya & Duman, 2001). This plasticity would seem to modify the strength of synapses in the neural pathway involved in depression.

Given that the strength of synapses is key to the neurobiology of memory (Hebb, 1949; Morris et al., 2003), it was proposed some years ago that memory impairment - understanding memory as the trace left in the nervous system not only by individual experiences but also by genetic and epigenetic phenomena - is central to the therapeutic action of antidepressants and other psychotropic medications (Parra, 2003). This idea is complementary to the concept that depression circuits learn to malfunction and retain the memory of said malfunctioning (Parra, 2003). A similar vision of the relationship between learning, memory and depression was upheld in a later publication by Stahl (2008), who argued that, in depression, neural circuits learn to become inefficient in a process so called "diabolical learning" (p. 229). In this context, antidepressants would modify this memory trace through a process of neural plasticity. Moreover, due to evolutionary economy, there would be similarities among the molecular changes induced by different causes of neural plasticity, including chronic treatment with antidepressants (Duman et al., 1999) or antipsychotics (Konradi & Heckers, 2001), long-term sensitization of the gill-withdrawal reflex of aplysia (Kandel, 2001), and delayed neural death after ischemic insult (Tsukahara et al., 1998). The similarities among these causes were discussed in a review by Parra (2003; in particular Fig. 1).

Different neurotransmission systems have been implicated in high brain functions such as learning and memory (Myhrer, 2003). Some of them are implicated in the mechanism of action of antidepressant drugs and could be responsible for the memory deficits observed with these drugs: the cholinergic system (Everitt & Robbins, 1997), the serotonergic system (Bert et al., 2008), the noradrenergic system (Hertz et al., 2004) and the histaminergic system (Passani et al., 2000). The effects of antidepressants on memory in animals may be attributable to a combination of their neuropharmacological properties, including anticholinergic, antihistaminergic, serotonergic and noradrenergic activity (Monleón et al., 2008).

We have previously reviewed studies of the effects of antidepressants on animal memory (Monleón et al., 2008). These studies provide several valuable insights into the effects of antidepressants on memory:

1. The memory impairment produced by several antidepressants is not confined to those with anticholinergic properties.
2. Although there are relatively few studies involving chronic antidepressant administration, they reveal an absence of tolerance, which is present regardless of the mechanism responsible for the therapeutic effects of antidepressants. This lack of tolerance suggests that the influence of antidepressants on memory is related to their therapeutic effects.
3. When the effects of antidepressants are assessed, in addition to their effects on mood and anxiety, those on cognitive processes, such as learning and memory, should also be considered.
4. The plethora of studies performed with aversive stimuli is understandable given the negative nature of depression. However, the scarcity of studies involving female subjects is less comprehensible and indeed inexcusable given that the incidence of depression is much higher among women than men.

A series of experiments on the effects of different antidepressants on memory in mice have been carried out in our laboratory. These experiments have already been previously, or will be published. Specifically these experiments were programmed to study:

- The effects of acute and chronic administration of several antidepressants (amitriptyline, maprotiline and fluoxetine) on inhibitory avoidance (IA) learning.
- The effects of antidepressants on learning and memory, dissociating them from those on activity, anxiety and analgesia, which can interfere with the performance of the IA response.
- The potential state-dependent learning (SDL) of antidepressants in the IA task. SDL is a useful behavioural model to explain the influence of drugs on memory, and more specifically for the study of memory-retrieval mechanisms (Arkhipov, 1999).

- The neurochemical substrates of IA learning in association with the neurochemical substrates of antidepressants. The cholinergic, histaminergic and serotonergic systems are involved in IA learning, and the effects of antidepressants on these systems can modulate the learning of this task.
- The possible sex differences in these effects of antidepressants.

An in-depth review of this body of work is presented herein. We will summarize and discuss the effects of the antidepressants amitriptyline, maprotiline and fluoxetine on an IA task in male and female mice, with reference to specific memory processes such as acquisition, consolidation and retrieval.

2. Behavioural procedures: Inhibitory avoidance learning and complementary tests

2.1 Inhibitory avoidance learning

Inhibitory avoidance (also called passive avoidance) is one of the most common procedures for evaluating memory in animals (e.g. Gold, 1986; Heise, 1981), as this task is learned in a single trial, which facilitates the timing of drug administration. This is crucial in discriminating the effects of a drug on different memory processes, such as acquisition, consolidation or retrieval (for a review of the usefulness of the IA procedure in memory studies, see Izquierdo & McGaugh, 2000).

The step-through version of IA conditioning was used in the experiments reviewed here (see Figure 1). The IA apparatus (Ugo Basile, Comerio-Varese, Italy), which was placed within an isolation box, consisted of a cage made of Perspex sheets and divided into two compartments (both 15 cm high x 9.5 cm wide x 16.5 cm long). The chambers are separated widthwise by a flat-box partition with an automatically-operated sliding door at floor level. The floor is made of stainless steel bars of 0.7 mm in diameter and situated 8 mm apart. The starting compartment is white and continuously illuminated by a light fixture fastened to the cage lid (24 V, 10 W, light intensity of 290 lux at floor level, measured with the Panlux Electronic2 photometer, manufactured by GOSSEN, Nürnberg, Germany), whereas the "shock" compartment is comprised of black Perspex panels and is kept in darkness at all times.

The procedure was completed in two phases: training and test.

- Training began with a 90 sec period of adaptation to the light compartment before the door to the other compartment was opened. This door was then opened for a maximum of 300 sec, and if the animal entered the dark compartment it received an inescapable footshock of 0.3-0.7 mA that was delivered for 5-10 sec (0.3 mA and 5 sec were the more frequently used values).
- During the test, mice were placed once again in the light compartment of the apparatus and the procedure used in the training phase was repeated, but without the shock. The time taken to enter the dark compartment, defined as latency, was automatically measured in tenths of a second and recorded manually at the end of each phase. Crossing latencies longer than 300 sec in the test phase resulted in the trial being terminated and a latency of 300 sec recorded.

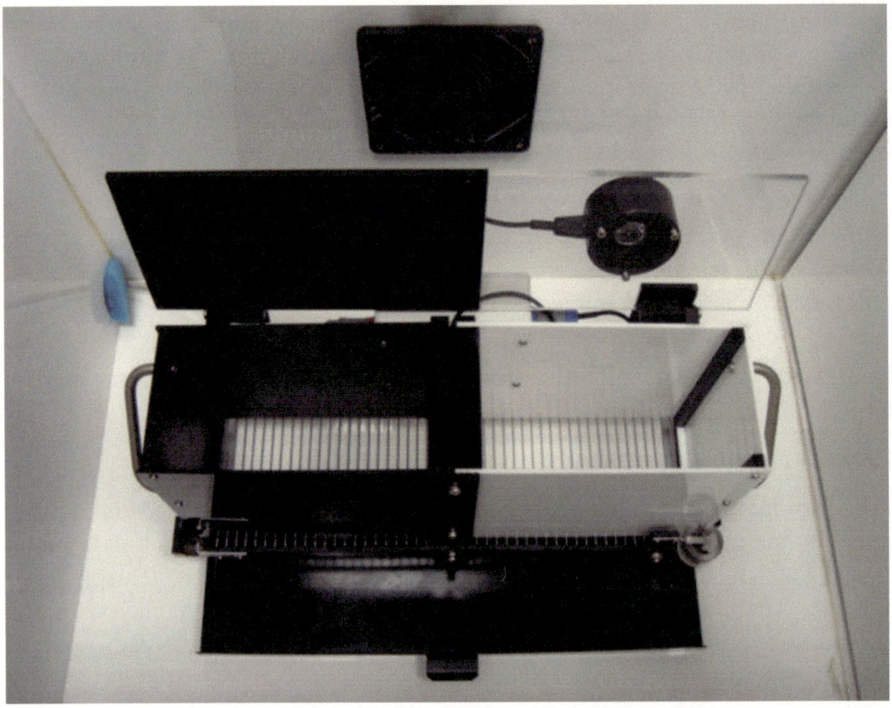

Fig. 1. Inhibitory avoidance apparatus. A step-through version of inhibitory avoidance conditioning for mice, placed inside an isolation box. The two compartments are separated widthwise by a flat-box partition.

Tests were always carried out during the dark phase of the light/dark cycle, after 7-10 days of acclimatization to the animal facility. The training-test interval was 24 hours, or 4, 7 or 21 days (according to the drug administered and the administration schedule). Latencies that were longer in the test than in the training phase were considered IA.

2.2 Complementary tests

The effects of antidepressants on locomotor activity (e.g. Mitchell et al., 2006), anxiety (e.g. Hascoët et al., 2000) and analgesia (e.g. Duric & McCarson, 2006) can interfere with the performance of subjects in the IA task (McGaugh & Izquierdo, 2000). Thus, it was important for the purpose of this investigation to dissociate the effects of the drugs on learning and memory from those on activity, anxiety and analgesia (McGaugh, 1989). In order to clarify the effects of antidepressants on IA learning, the following complementary tests were used:

- Two actimeters. In one of the actimeters (ACTIMET from Cibertec S.A., Madrid, Spain) the horizontal activity was measured using an infrared photocell system. The photocell line was located 2.5 cm above the floor. Each photocell box measured 8.5 x 17 x 35 cm and had sixteen photocells located along its long side (see Figure 2). The animals' behaviour was continuously recorded and accumulated every minute for five minutes.

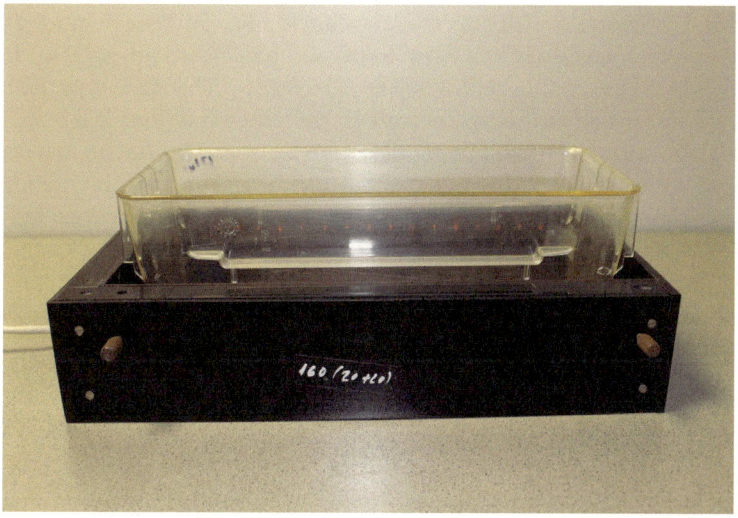

Fig. 2. Complementary tests: Actimeter. This apparatus registers the spontaneous locomotor activity of the animals by means of an infrared photocell system.

The second actimeter (Actisystem II with 'DAS 16' software from Panlab S.L., Barcelona, Spain) registered the spontaneous locomotor activity as a function of the variations produced by mouse' movements on the standard frequency (484 kHz) of the electromagnetic field of the sensory unit (35 x 35 cm^2). Frequency variations were transformed into voltage changes, which, in turn, were converted into impulses that were collected by a counter when they reached a certain level (see Figure 3). The locomotor activity of the animals was monitored for five minutes.

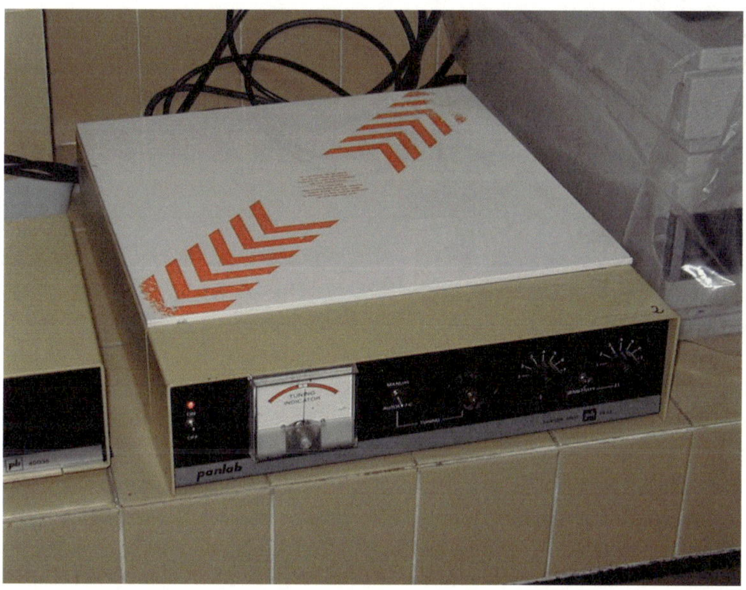

Fig. 3. Complementary tests: Sensor unit of the actimeter. This unit registers the variations of the oscillation frequency in the electromagnetic field produced by the mouse' movements.

- An elevated plus-maze (Cibertec S.A., Madrid, Spain) (see Figure 4). This maze consisted of two open arms (30 x 5 cm^2 each) and two closed arms (30 x 15 x 5 cm^3 each) which all fed into a common central square (5 x 5 cm^2). The maze was made of Plexiglas (black floor and walls) and was elevated 45 cm above the floor level. Sessions lasted 5 min and began with the subject being placed in an open arm (facing the central square). All sessions were videotaped with a standard VHS system for subsequent analysis. The maze was cleaned after each subject. The number of entries into open and closed arms (arm entry is defined as all four paws entering an arm) was scored by a trained observer who was unaware of the treatment applied. This provided a measurement of anxiety, the percentage of open arm entries [(open/open + closed) X 100], and a measurement of activity (number of closed arm entries). These measurements were based on former studies: File (2001), Lister (1987), and Rodgers & Johnson (1995).

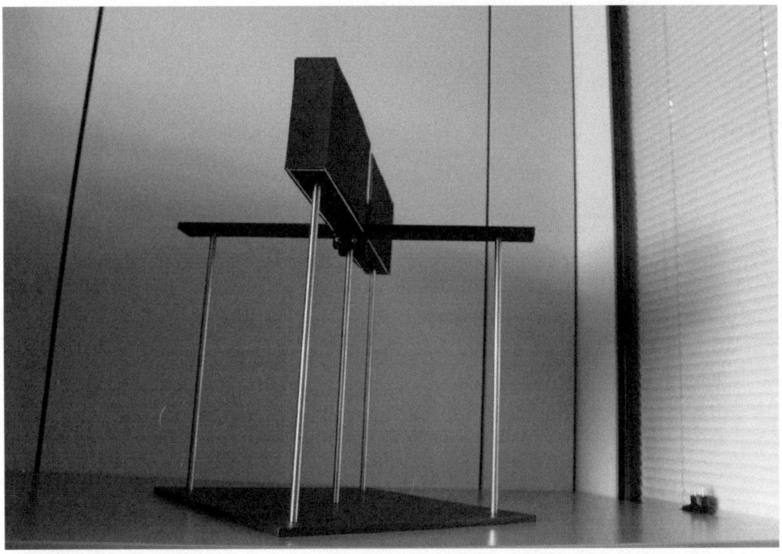

Fig. 4. Complementary tests: Elevated plus-maze for mice. This test measures anxiety and activity.

- A prototype of analgesia (Cibertec S.A., Madrid, Spain) (see Figure 5). This apparatus consisted of a translucent Perspex box of the same dimensions as those of one side of the avoidance apparatus, with a similar floor to the IA apparatus and a constant current source with increasing output steps of 0.059 mA. Subjects were individually introduced into the test box and allowed a 2 min adaptation period. Subsequently, the animal received a 5 sec shock of 0.059 mA, increasing proportionately by 0.059 mA every 10 sec. The test was interrupted when the subject removed all four paws from the grid for the first time during the shock (this was done while the test was underway; and is a different criterion to that of jump threshold, which was determined on viewing the recorded sessions). The highest shock delivered was 0.77 mA. Results were represented as flinch and jump thresholds in milliamperes. Flinch threshold was defined as the lowest shock level that elicited a detectable response, and jump threshold as the lowest shock level that elicited simultaneous removal of three paws from the grid. All tests were videotaped with a standard VHS system and later assessed.

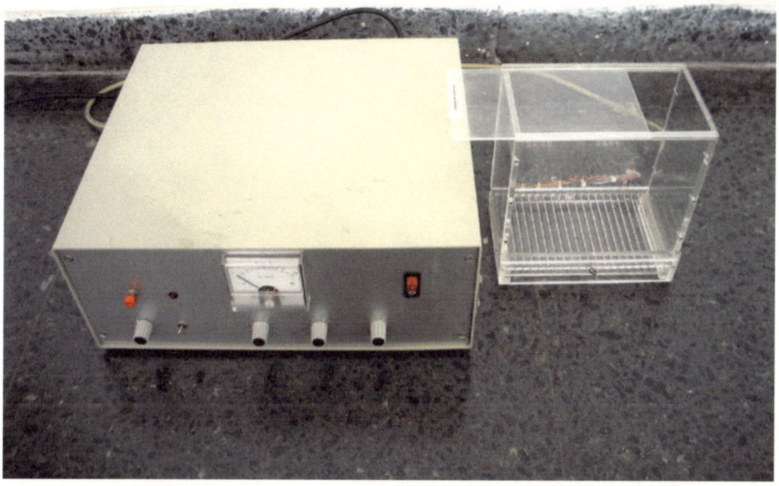

Fig. 5. Complementary tests: Prototype of analgesia. This test measures flinch and jump thresholds.

- A Morris water maze (Cibertec S.A., Madrid, Spain) (see Figure 6). This test was employed in order to evaluate the effects of maprotiline on spatial learning. The maze consisted of a circular pool made of black Plexiglas (1 m diameter and 30 cm high), based on that described by Morris (1984) but adapted for mice (Lamberty & Gower, 1990). The maze was filled with water to a depth of 15 cm and maintained at 24 ± 1 °C. A small platform (6 x 6 cm) was submerged 1 cm below the surface of the water in the target quadrant. Several extramaze cues, including laboratory equipment and posters, were available around the pool. During the acquisition phase mice performed 4 trials per day for 4 consecutive days. After an inter-trial interval of 30 sec the trial began by placing the mouse on the platform for 30 sec. Mice were then placed in the water with their noses pointing towards the wall at one of the three starting points in a random manner. During this phase animals were allowed 60 sec to find the hidden platform. If unable to do so, they were led to it by the experimenter. Animals were allowed to stay on the platform for 30 sec, regardless of whether they had found it independently or after guidance. Starting positions were chosen at random from the three possible sites around the pool's perimeter, which were situated in each of the quadrants not occupied by the platform. The starting positions were determined so that two successive trials never began from the same position. In a retention phase (probe trial) carried out on the fifth day the platform was removed and mice were allowed to swim for 100 sec after starting in the opposite quadrant to that in which was the platform during acquisition. A video-camera recorded the probe trials. The measures obtained were escape latency (time to reach the submerged platform) during the acquisition trials and search time in each quadrant during the probe trial. The drug was administered 30 min before each experimental session. The use of this test was occasional in our research and complementary to the IA learning.

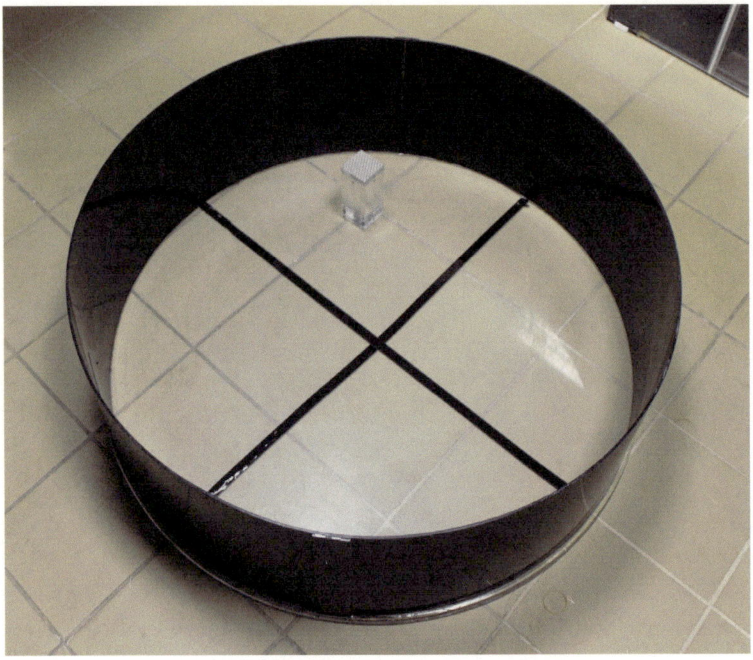

Fig. 6. Morris water maze for mice. This test evaluates spatial learning.

3. Antidepressant and complementary drugs

The following antidepressant drugs were used in these experiments:

- Amitriptyline hydrochloride (Sigma-Aldrich Química, Madrid, Spain). This tricyclic antidepressant is a mixed serotonergic and noradrenergic uptake inhibitor with a strong anticholinergic and antihistaminergic effect (Richelson, 2003). Amitriptyline is one of the most-studied antidepressants with regard to effects on cognitive functions, including memory and tends to be the standard against which newer compounds are compared (Thompson, 1991). Among currently available antidepressants, amitriptyline is the most potent in blocking muscarinic cholinergic receptors (Frazer, 1997; Owens et al., 1997, Richelson, 2001; Stahl, 1998). The effects of acute administration of amitriptyline on IA were evaluated at doses of 2.5, 5, 7.5, 10, 15, 20 and 30 mg/kg. Chronic administration of the highest dose was also evaluated.
- Maprotiline hydrochloride (Ciba-Geigy A.G., Basel, Switzerland). This is a tetracyclic antidepressant prescribed largely for the elderly (Gareri et al., 2000). It selectively inhibits norepinephrine reuptake and has a high antihistaminergic activity, a modest anticholinergic activity and a low serotonin reuptake inhibitory effect (Gareri et al., 2000; Harvey et al., 2000; Pinder et al., 1977; Redrobe & Bourin, 1997; Richelson & Nelson, 1984). This compound has fewer side effects than classic tricyclic antidepressants (Grüter & Pöldinger, 1982), but what it does have in common is the impairment of memory (Gareri et al., 2000). The effects of acute administration of Maprotiline on IA were evaluated at doses of 2.5, 5, 10, 15, 20 and 25 mg/kg. The 5, 10 and 20 mg/kg doses were also evaluated after chronic administration and the effects of the 15, 20 and 25 mg/kg doses on spatial learning were evaluated after subchronic administration.

- Fluoxetine hydrochloride (Eli Lilly, Indianapolis, U.S.A.). This is a selective serotonin reuptake inhibitor with little affinity for muscarinic, histaminic H1, serotonergic 5-HT1 or 5-HT2, or noradrenergic alpha 1 or alpha 2 receptors (Beasley et al., 1992; Stark et al., 1985). The effects of acute administration of fluoxetine on IA were evaluated at doses of 5, 10, 15 and 20 mg/kg. Chronic administration of the highest dose was also analysed.

The following complementary drugs were also used in some of the experiments:

- Piracetam (Sigma-Aldrich Química, Madrid, Spain), whose mechanism of action is still unclear but which appears to be a non-specific activator of neuronal excitability (Gouliaev & Senning, 1994). A 100 mg/kg dose of piracetam was evaluated in the IA procedure after both acute and chronic administration and in combination with amitriptyline (100 mg/kg dose of piracetam and 30 mg/kg of amitriptyline).
- Oxotremorine sesquifumarate (Sigma-Aldrich Química, Madrid, Spain), a centrally acting muscarinic cholinergic agonist (Introini-Collison & Baratti, 1992). The effects of acute administration of oxotremorine on IA were evaluated at doses of 0.05 and 0.1 mg/kg and in combination with amitriptyline (0.05 mg/kg dose of oxotremorine and 5, 10 or 15 mg/kg of amitriptyline; 0.1 mg/kg dose of oxotremorine and 5, 7.5 or 10 mg/kg of amitriptyline).
- Physostigmine salicylate (Sigma-Aldrich Química, Madrid, Spain), a centrally acting anticholinesterase (Boccia et al., 2003). The effects of acute administration of physostigmine on IA were evaluated at doses of 0.15, 0.3 and 0.6 mg/kg, and each of these doses were also combined with 5 mg/kg of amitriptyline.
- L-Histidine monohydrochloride monohydrate (Sigma–Aldrich Química, Madrid, Spain), a precursor of histamine (Prell et al., 1996), was evaluated in the IA procedure, given alone (250, 500 and 1000 mg/kg) and in combination with amitriptyline (1000 mg/kg of l-histidine and 2.5 or 10 mg/kg of amitriptyline).
- Pyrilamine maleate (Sigma–Aldrich Química, Madrid, Spain), a histamine H1 postsynaptic receptor antagonist (Yanai et al., 1990), was administered alone (5, 10 and 20 mg/kg) and with amitriptyline (20 mg/kg of pyrilamine and 2.5, 5, or 10 mg/kg of amitriptyline) in order to study their effects on IA.

All drugs were diluted in physiological saline and intraperitoneally injected at a volume of 0.01 ml/g body weight. Doses were calculated as the weight of the base. Control groups received the same volume of physiological saline.

4. Results

4.1 Amitriptyline

Table 1 summarizes the results and some procedural details of the experiments carried out with amitriptyline. They are grouped below in seven categories: 1) Effects of acute administration of amitriptyline on IA; 2) Effects of chronic administration of amitriptyline on IA; 3) Modulation of the acute and chronic effects of amitriptyline by piracetam; 4) Modulation of the acute effects of amitriptyline by the cholinergic system; 5) Modulation of the acute effects of amitriptyline by the serotonergic system; 6) Modulation of the acute effects of amitriptyline by the histaminergic system; 7) Study of potential state-dependent learning.

Strain	Sex	Doses (mg/kg)	Tr.	Administration	Learning	Activity	Anxiety	SDL	Reference
OF1	M	7.5, 15, 30	A	Post-training	–				Everss et al., 1999
CD1	M	7.5, 15, 30	A	Post-training	–	– (15, 30)	0		Parra et al., 2002
CD1	F	15	A	Post-training	0	–	0		Parra et al., 2002
CD1	F	7.5, 30	A	Post-training	–	– (30)	0		Parra et al., 2002
CD1	M, F	2.5	A	Pre-training	0				Parra et al., 2009
CD1	M	5	A	Pre-training	0				Parra et al., 2009
CD1	F	5	A	Pre-training	–				Parra et al., 2009
CD1	M, F	10, 20	A	Pre-training	–				Parra et al., 2009
CD1	M	20	A	Pre-training	–				González-Pardo et al., 2008
CD1	M, F	2.5, 5, 10	A	Pre-training	0				Parra et al., 2010
CD1	M, F	10	A	Pre-training	–				Ferrer-Añó, 2008
CD1	M, F	5, 7.5, 10, 15, 20, 30	A	Pre-training	–				Urquiza, 2007
CD1	M, F	30	A	Post-training	0				Urquiza, 2007
CD1	M, F	30	A	Post-training	–				Everss et al., 2005
CD1	M	30	C	Pre-training	–				Parra et al., 2006
CD1	F	30	C	Pre-training	0				Parra et al., 2006
CD1	M, F	30	C	Post-training	0	0	0		Parra et al., 2006
CD1	M, F	30	C	Pre-training and Post-training	–	0	0		Everss et al., 2005
CD1	M, F	30	A	Pre-training	–			0 a	Arenas et al., 2006
CD1	M	30	A	Pre-test	0			0 a	Arenas et al., 2006
CD1	F	30	A	Pre-test	–			0 a	Arenas et al., 2006
CD1	M, F	30	A	Pre-training and Pre-test	–			0 a	Arenas et al., 2006

Abbreviations: Tr. = Treatment; SDL = state dependent learning; M = male; F = female; A = Acute administration; SC = Subchronic administration (5 days); C = Chronic administration (21 days); 0 = No effect; – = impairment; + = improvement; a = memorization deficit; b = memorization deficit and performance facilitation.

Table 1. Effects of different doses of amitriptyline on IA learning, activity, anxiety and SDL in mice.

1. Effects of acute administration of amitriptyline on memory acquisition/consolidation in male OF1 mice (Everss et al., 1999) and CD1 mice of both sexes (Parra et al., 2002). Three doses of this tricyclic antidepressant (7.5, 15 and 30 mg/kg) were administered immediately after IA training. Subjects were tested for avoidance twenty four hours later. Amitriptyline impaired IA consolidation at doses of 7.5, 15 and 30 mg/kg in OF1 and CD1 males, and at doses of 7.5 and 30 mg/kg in CD1 females. The sex differences observed were limited to a slightly stronger effect of amitriptyline on IA in males than in females. These results indicate that acute amitriptyline administration produces retrograde amnesia in a IA task, which does not seem to be mediated by anxiolytic effects: when CD1 mice explored an elevated plus-maze during a five-minute period forty-five minutes after injection amitriptyline had no effect on anxiety (percentage of open arm entries) and induced a dose-dependent impairment of activity (number of closed arm entries), which did not affect IA, as the drug was administered after training (see conclusions regarding pharmacokinetic rationale).
   Another series of experiments were performed to evaluate the effects of acute pre-training (5, 7.5, 10, 15, 20 and 30 mg/kg) and post-training (30 mg/kg) administration of amitriptyline on IA learning (Urquiza, 2007). Results showed that only acute pre-training administration produced an impairment of learning. The dose-response relationship of the effect of amitriptyline on IA (Parra et al., 2009) was also evaluated at doses of 2.5, 5, 10 and 20 mg/kg, which were administered before the training session. Results showed a clear dose-dependent impairment of amitriptyline on IA in both male and female mice. However, the 2.5 mg/kg dose had no effect on either sex, 5 mg/kg had a significant effect only on females, and 10 and 20 mg/kg produced similar significant effects in both sexes. A study evaluating changes in the brain metabolism induced by training in IA and acute administration of amitriptyline also showed an impairing effect of 20 mg/kg of this drug tested in male mice (González-Pardo et al., 2008).
2. Effects of 21-day chronic administration of amitriptyline (30 mg/kg) on the acquisition and consolidation of an IA task in male and female CD1 mice. It was also investigated whether amitriptyline, when administered after consolidation of this task, blocked memory retrieval (Parra et al., 2006). Amitriptyline given before the training phase blocked learning of IA in males, and a similar tendency was observed in females. However, when the drug was administered between training and test phases it did not affect conditioning. Anxiety and spontaneous motor activity in the elevated plus maze were also assessed in the same subjects, but no effects of amitriptyline were observed. Thus, the impairing effects of amitriptyline on IA would seem to be independent of its actions on anxiety and locomotor activity.
3. Modulation of the acute and chronic effects of amitriptyline on IA by piracetam in male and female CD1 mice (Everss et al., 2005). The purpose was to study the effects of amitriptyline on animal cognition in relation to some characteristics of its therapeutic effects. Two experiments were run. In Experiment 1, mice underwent an IA training phase sixty minutes after acute piracetam (100 mg/kg) or physiological saline administration. Immediately after the behavioural task, they received a single injection of the tricyclic antidepressant amitriptyline (30 mg/kg) or physiological saline. Twenty four hours later, subjects were tested for avoidance. In Experiment 2, the same doses of amitriptyline and piracetam were chronically administered. Mice underwent the IA training phase on the

22nd day, and the test phase a further 24 h later. Forty-five minutes after the test, subjects were allowed to explore the elevated plus-maze for five minutes in order to assess whether the effects of amitriptyline on avoidance performance reflected general behavioural changes. The following results were obtained:

a. Acute and chronic amitriptyline impaired IA in male and female mice.
b. Piracetam counteracted the effect of acutely administered amitriptyline on IA.
c. Piracetam counteracted the effects of chronically administered amitriptyline in males but not in females in the same learning task. These effects did not seem to be mediated by non-specific drug effects on spontaneous motor activity or anxiety.

4. Modulation of the acute effects of amitriptyline on IA by the cholinergic system in male and female CD1 mice (Monleón et al., 2009; Urquiza, 2007). The amnesic effect produced by amitriptyline (5, 10 or 15 mg/kg) was not completely counteracted by the agonist cholinergic oxotremorine (0.05, 0.1 mg/kg), but a tendency in that direction was observed. However the amnesic effect produced by 5 mg/kg of amitriptyline was counteracted by several doses of the agonist cholinergic physostigmine (0.15, 0.3 and 0.6 mg/kg). In this way, physostigmine counteracted the impairing effects of amitriptyline on IA to a greater degree than oxotremorine. These differences in the effects of the two cholinergic agonists could be due to them possessing different mechanisms of action. Oxotremorine is a ligand present at all five of the muscarinic receptor subtypes (Choi et al., 1973), while physostigmine is a potent cholinesterase inhibitor (Taylor, 2001) that enhances the levels of acetylcholine, which eventually interacts with both the muscarinic and nicotinic receptor subtypes. These results demonstrate that the IA impairment produced by amitriptyline in both male and female mice is mediated, at least partially, by the cholinergic system.
5. Modulation of the acute effects of amitriptyline on IA by the serotonergic system in male and female CD1 mice (Parra et al., 2010). A combination of 2.5 mg/kg of amitriptyline with fluoxetine (10, 15 or 20 mg/kg), a selective serotonin reuptake inhibitor, revealed that the joint administration of amitriptyline 2.5 mg/kg and fluoxetine 15 mg/kg had a clear impairing effect on IA. These results highlight the involvement of the serotonergic system in the effects of amitriptyline.
6. Modulation of the acute effects of amitriptyline on IA by the histaminergic system in male and female CD1 mice (Ferrer-Añó, 2008). Amitriptyline (10 mg/kg) produced amnesic effects that were not modified in mice treated with this drug and a histaminergic precursor, L-histidine (1000 mg/kg), or a H1 antagonist, pyrilamine (20 mg/kg). L-histidine (250, 500, or 1000 mg/kg) was also administered alone and did not produce any effect on IA. No effect was produced by pyrilamine (5, 10, or 20 mg/kg) when administered alone. Neither of the two kinds of manipulation of the histamine neurotransmitter system (favouring the synthesis of histamine or blocking its action on postsynaptic receptors) had an effect on IA. Furthermore, when administered in combination with amitriptyline, these drugs did not modify the impairing effect of the antidepressant on that memory task. Given that amitriptyline has antihistaminergic properties and that the results were not modified by histaminergic manipulation, it would appear that the histaminergic system is not involved in the behaviour studied.
7. Study of potential state-dependent learning. To study the effects of the antidepressants on memory we carried out some experiments to investigate whether amitriptyline (30 mg/kg), maprotiline (25 mg/kg) and fluoxetine (15 mg/kg) produce state-dependent

learning (SDL) in the IA task in male and female CD1 mice (Arenas et al., 2006). SDL is a phenomenon in which the retrieval of newly acquired information is possible if the subject is in the same physiological state as during the encoding phase. Independent groups were used for each pharmacological treatment and for each sex using a 2 X 2 experimental design. The groups were: physiological saline before training and test phases (SS); physiological saline before training and amitriptyline before phase test (SA); amitriptyline before training and physiological saline before test phase (AS); amitriptyline before training and test phases (AA). The interval between phases was of 24 h. SDL was not detected, and results with amitriptyline can be interpreted as representing a memorization deficit (the groups that received a drug before training did not show increased test latencies, independently of the treatment administered prior to the test session; see Overton, 1974). In addition, males showed a slightly higher deterioration in their performance than females.

4.2 Maprotiline

Table 2 summarizes the results and some procedural details of the experiments carried out with maprotiline. They are grouped below in four categories: 1) Effects of acute and chronic administration of maprotiline on IA; 2) Effects of maprotiline on learning, anxiety, activity and analgesia; 3) Effects of subchronic administration of maprotiline on spatial learning; 4) Study of potential state-dependent learning.

1. Effects of acute and chronic administration of maprotiline (5, 10 or 20 mg/kg) on IA in male OF1 mice (Parra et al., 2000). Acute administration before training did not affect training phase latencies but did impair performance in the test at doses of 5 and 20 mg/kg. When given after training, the drug did not modify test latencies at any of the doses used. Chronic administration for 21 days (interrupted 24 h before training) also shortened latencies in the test, but not in training. An experiment was performed in naive animals to evaluate the acute effects of maprotiline on analgesia at the doses stated. No analgesic effect of the drug was observed. Considered as a whole, these results indicate that acute maprotiline produces anterograde amnesia, and that tolerance does not appear after 21 days of treatment.
2. Effects of a wide range of doses of maprotiline (2.5, 5, 10, 15, 20 and 25 mg/kg) on learning, anxiety, activity and analgesia in male and female CD1 mice (Vinader-Caerols et al., 2006). IA learning was complemented with measures of anxiety and locomotor activity, which were assessed in the same animals in an elevated plus-maze. A study of the acute effects of maprotiline (15, 20 and 25 mg/kg) on analgesia was carried out in naive animals of both sexes. Maprotiline impaired IA at doses of 15, 20 and 25 mg/kg. The highest dose produced an anxiolytic effect in females, and 20 and 25 mg/kg both reduced locomotor activity. Analgesia was observed with the highest dose. The IA impairment produced by maprotiline seemed to be independent of the drug's influence on anxiety, was not shadowed by an instrumental performance deficit and, at least in the case of the highest dose, appeared to be influenced by the drug's effects on analgesia. It can be hypothesised that acquisition is the memory process principally affected by maprotiline, and in particular stimuli processing. The lack of sex differences in the effects of maprotiline on IA supports the generalization of data previously reported exclusively in males.

Strain	Sex	Doses (mg/kg)	Tr.	Administration	Learning	Activity	Anxiety	Analgesia	SDL	Reference
OF1	M	5, 20	A	Pre-training	-					Parra et al., 2000
OF1	M	10	A	Pre-training	0					Parra et al., 2000
OF1	M	5, 10, 20	A	Post-training	0					Parra et al., 2000
OF1	M	5, 10, 20	A	Pre-test analgesia				0		Parra et al., 2000
CD1	M, F	2.5, 5, 10	A	Pre-training	0	0	0			Vinader-Caerols et al., 2006
CD1	M, F	15	A	Pre-training	–	0	0			Vinader-Caerols et al., 2006
CD1	M, F	20	A	Pre-training	–	–	0			Vinader-Caerols et al., 2006
CD1	M	25	A	Pre-training	–	–	0			Vinader-Caerols et al., 2006
CD1	F	25	A	Pre-training	–	–	+			Vinader-Caerols et al., 2006
CD1	M, F	15, 20	A	Pre-test analgesia				0		Vinader-Caerols et al., 2006
CD1	M, F	25	A	Pre-test analgesia				+		Vinader-Caerols et al., 2006
CD1	M	15, 25	SC	Pre-training	- SL					Vinader-Caerols et al., 2002
CD1	M	20	SC	Pre-training	0 SL					Vinader-Caerols et al., 2002
CD1	F	15, 20, 25	SC	Pre-training	0 SL					Vinader-Caerols et al., 2002
CD1	M, F	15, 20, 25	SC	Pre-actimeter		–				Vinader-Caerols et al., 2002
OF1	M	5, 20	C	Pre-training	–					Parra et al., 2000
OF1	M	10	C	Pre-training	0					Parra et al., 2000
CD1	M, F	25	A	Pre-training	–				0 b	Arenas et al., 2006
CD1	M	25	A	Pre-test	+				0 b	Arenas et al., 2006
CD1	F	25	A	Pre-test	0				0 b	Arenas et al., 2006
CD1	M, F	25	A	Pre-training and Pre-test	0				0 b	Arenas et al., 2006

Abbreviations: Tr. = Treatment; SDL = state dependent learning; M = male; F = female; A = Acute administration; SC = Subchronic administration (5 days); C = Chronic administration (21 days); 0 = No effect; – = impairment; + = improvement; SL= spatial learning; a = memorization deficit; b = memorization deficit and performance facilitation.

Table 2. Effects of different doses of maprotiline on inhibitory avoidance learning, activity, anxiety and SDL in mice.

3. Effects of subchronic administration of maprotiline (15, 20 and 25 mg/kg) on spatial learning and general activity in male and female CD1 mice in the Morris water maze (Vinader-Caerols et al., 2002). In the acquisition phase, maprotiline (15 and 25 mg/kg) impaired learning in males but not in females. Sex differences were not found in the control group in this phase. In the retention phase, all three doses of maprotiline rectified the sex differences observed in the control group. In the general activity test, all three doses of maprotiline decreased activity and removed the sex differences found in the control group. This sexual dimorphism in the effects of maprotiline on spatial learning is in accordance with the findings of studies of the effects of antidepressants and antipsychotics on different learning tasks in mice. When this dimorphism is present, the drug effect is observed only in males or, if present in males and females, is stronger in the former.
4. Study of potential SDL with maprotiline (25 mg/kg) following the same procedure as that used for amitriptyline (Arenas et al., 2006). The results were interpreted as simultaneous memorization deficit and performance facilitation due to motor impairment. Similarly to that observed with amitriptyline, males treated with maprotiline showed a slightly higher deterioration than females in their performance.

4.3 Fluoxetine

Table 3 summarizes the results and some procedural details of the experiments with fluoxetine. They are grouped below in three categories: 1) Effects of acute administration of fluoxetine on IA; 2) Effects of chronic administration of fluoxetine on IA; 3) Study of potential state-dependent learning.

1. Effects of acute administration of fluoxetine (5, 10 and 20 mg/kg) on memory consolidation in male and female OF1 mice (Monleón et al., 2001). The drug was administered immediately after the training session and there was a four-day interval between sessions. The results confirmed IA learning in all the treatment groups. Fluoxetine did not impair memory consolidation in any of the subjects; even the animals treated with the highest dose showed significantly increased response latencies of IA compared with those treated with the lowest dose or saline. As the drug was administered immediately after the training session these results cannot be attributed to unspecific effects, which occur when drugs are administered before the training session (McGaugh, 1989). Sex differences in this task were observed, with females performing better. However, the drug's effects were not sexually dimorphic: sex differences were observed in control animals and they remained with every dose of fluoxetine. Analysis of the locomotor activity of the animals did not reveal any significant differences between the treatment groups. In another experiment, acute doses of fluoxetine (10, 15 and 20 mg/kg) were tested in male and female CD1 mice (Parra et al., 2010). The drug was administered 30 min before the training phase and the test phase was carried out 24 h later. Acquisition and consolidation phases of IA not were impaired by fluoxetine. In addition, the analysis of fluoxetine revealed that females exhibited longer test latencies than males, irrespectively of the pharmacological treatment they had received. The very minor sex differences detected in the present study are in accordance with existing evidence in the literature which suggest that differences observed in the effects of psychotropic medication on the memory of mice are generally stronger among males while IA tends to be more pronounced in females.

Strain	Sex	Doses (mg/kg)	Tr.	Administration	Learning	Activity	SDL	Reference
OF1	M, F	5, 10	A	Post-training	0	0		Monleón et al., 2001
OF1	M, F	20	A	Post-training	+	0		Monleón et al., 2001
CD1	M, F	10, 15, 20	A	Pre-training	0			Parra et al., 2010
CD1	M	20	C	Pre-training	–	0		Monleón et al., 2002
CD1	F	20	C	Pre-training	0	0		Monleón et al., 2002
CD1	M, F	20	C	Post-training	0			Monleón et al., 2002
CD1	M, F	15	A	Pre-training	0		0	Arenas et al., 2006
CD1	M	15	A	Pre-test	0		0	Arenas et al., 2006
CD1	F	15	A	Pre-test	+		0	Arenas et al., 2006
CD1	M, F	15	A	Pre-training and pre-test	0		0	Arenas et al., 2006

Abbreviations: Tr. = Treatment; SDL = state dependent learning; M = male; F = female; A = Acute administration; SC = Subchronic administration (5 days); C = Chronic administration (21 days); 0 = No effect; – = impairment; + = improvement; a = memorization deficit; b = memorization deficit and performance facilitation.

Table 3. Effects of different doses of fluoxetine on inhibitory avoidance learning, activity and SDL in mice.

2. Effects of chronic administration of fluoxetine (20 mg/kg) on IA in male and female CD1 mice (Monleón et al., 2002). In Experiment 1, the drug was administered for 21 days before the training session, whereas in Experiment 2, other subjects were subjected to the same treatment schedule, only that it began 24 h after the training session. The comparison of test versus training latencies revealed a deterioration of memory after pre-training administration of fluoxetine (Experiment 1) in males but not females. Sex differences in this task were also observed in Experiment 1, with females showing a better performance. Sex differences were evident in controls as well as in treated animals. The locomotor activity of the animals was also analysed in Experiment 1 and showed no statistically significant differences in this measure between treated and non-treated groups. Due to the absence of sex differences in the effects of fluoxetine on this measure, the sex differences observed in the effects of the drug on IA cannot have been attributable to non-specific effects on locomotor activity. The lack of an effect of post-training administration of fluoxetine (Experiment 2) constitutes additional support for the idea that the effect on IA observed in Experiment 1 was specifically related to learning and memory. In summary, we can affirm that fluoxetine impairs IA in chronic pre-training but not in post-training administration.
3. Study of potential SDL with fluoxetine (15 mg/kg), following the same procedure as that employed for amitriptyline and maprotiline (Arenas et al., 2006). Fluoxetine did not produce any deteriorating effect on conditioning.

5. Conclusions

In order to construct a global perspective, the results discussed in this review can be summarised as follows:

- In general, acute pre-training administration of amitriptyline and maprotiline impairs the acquisition of IA at a wide range of doses, while fluoxetine does not produce any effect.
- Acute post-training administration produces ambiguous results. Amitriptyline can have an undermining effect or an absence of effects. Maprotiline does not exert any effects and fluoxetine only produces an improvement of memory consolidation at a high dose.
- Chronic treatment has an effect on pre-training administration of amitriptyline and fluoxetine. Males are more affected than females with these antidepressants, with an impairment of the acquisition of IA being observed at high doses. Maprotiline, which in chronic administration was tested only pre-training, showed a biphasic effect: the lowest and the highest doses impair the acquisition of the IA but not the intermediate dose.
- Maprotiline and amitriptyline at high doses reduce locomotor activity. With respect to instrumental performance, the decrease in activity observed does not appear to influence the performance of animals in the test phase of IA learning, as they cross the compartment in less time than controls. This is contrary to what would be expected (i.e., that if performance of certain animals is affected, they would show longer test latencies). Furthermore, there is a pharmacokinetic reason for ruling out a locomotor effect of these drugs in the avoidance test phase, as the interval between injection of the drug and the behavioural test was sufficient for the drug to have been eliminated. Therefore, the IA impairment produced by maprotiline and amitriptyline is not shadowed by their effects on activity. Fluoxetine is the only drug which does not produce any effects on locomotor activity.
- The effects on anxiety were tested with maprotiline and amitriptyline and only the highest dose of maprotiline produced an anxiogenic effect in female subjects. The same dose of maprotiline also produced an analgesic effect in both male and female mice. The effects of this dose on IA learning could be shadowed by its effects on anxiety and analgesia, and so this is not a suitable dose to be used in the study of maprotiline and IA memory in mice.
- SDL is a useful behavioural model to explain the influence of drugs on memory, and more specifically for the study of memory-retrieval mechanisms (Arkhipov, 1999). SDL is employed to refer to behavioural responses learnt while animals are under the influence of a centrally acting drug, as thereafter animals perform most efficiently only when the same drug condition is re-established (Overton, 1974, 1984). The antidepressants tested affect the acquisition/consolidation but not the retrieval process in IA learning. In conclusion, our study shows that the effects of the antidepressants amitriptyline, maprotiline and fluoxetine are not state-dependent: the drugs' actions on IA learning affect acquisition/consolidation but not the retrieval process. Nevertheless, there are some differences between the three antidepressants. Amitriptyline produces a memorization deficit in the IA task, while maprotiline exerts a less obvious effect on the consolidation of memory due to its interference with motor effects, and fluoxetine has no impairing effects on learning. We believe that the differences observed in the effects of these three

antidepressants on IA memory can be explained by their distinct action on the cholinergic system; i.e., the higher the anticholinergic effect, the greater the memory impairment. The results reported here were obtained under acute treatment, and therefore should not be considered a model of clinical treatment, since antidepressants are chronically administered when applied for therapeutic purposes. However, these findings and those of similar studies contribute to a better understanding of the effects of antidepressants on memory processes, which is crucial for improving their prescription in humans.

- The neurotransmitters histamine, acetylcholine and serotonin have been related with the acquisition and consolidation of memory in IA tasks (Babar et al., 2002; Eidi et al., 2003). The amnesic effect produced by amitriptyline in our laboratory was not confined to the cholinergic system (Monleón et al., 2009; Urquiza, 2007). In fact, the serotonergic system was also involved (Parra et al., 2010), as the joint administration of amitriptyline and fluoxetine at doses which did not have an effect when given alone had a clear impairing effect. We believe this represents a synergistic effect of both drugs, which confirms the implication of the serotonergic system in the impairing effects of amitriptyline on IA in mice. The histaminergic system does not seem to be implicated in this impairing effect of amitriptyline (Ferrer-Añó, 2008).
- The use of both male and female subjects is especially relevant in animal studies of disorders in which sex differences have been described in human beings. In fact, epidemiological studies have shown that the lifetime prevalence of major depressive disorder in women (21.3%) is almost twice that in men (12.7%), and this ratio has been documented in different countries and ethnic groups (Noble, 2005). These sex differences have been observed in the prevalence of mental disorders as well as in responses to treatment (Frackiewicz et al., 2000). Sex differences in control subjects were observed in some experiments carried out in our laboratory, with females exhibiting longer latencies than males in the test phase, thus indicating a more effective IA learning in females. We have also detected sex differences in the effects of amitriptyline, maprotiline and fluoxetine on IA learning. When this dimorphism is present, the drug effect is generally stronger in males than in females.
- Most preclinical trials are carried out with males only due to a supposedly higher variability among females, not confirmed by data from our laboratory (Parra et al., 1999). This is a somewhat inappropriate policy given that women consume more psychotropic medication than men (Cafferata et al., 1983). Furthermore, there are important reasons for evaluating the impact of antidepressants on both male and female subjects:
  a. Gender differences in the epidemiology of depression, which is more common in women than in men (American Psychiatric Association, 1994; Kornstein, 1997).
  b. Gender differences in the efficacy of some antidepressants, such as maprotiline and fluoxetine (Martényi et al., 2001).
  c. Differences in pharmacokinetics and pharmacodynamics between men and women have been reported for several drugs, including antidepressants (Frackiewicz et al., 2000; Gandhi et al., 2004).

6. Acknowledgements

The authors wish to thank the Spanish "Ministerio de Ciencia y Tecnología" and the European Regional Development Fund (ERDF) (Grant, BSO2003-07163), the Spanish

"Ministerio de Ciencia e Innovación" (PSI2008-06116) and the "Universitat de València" (UV-AE-07-564) for funding the work reviewed herein (P.I.: Andrés Parra). Ongoing research is funded by the Spanish "Ministerio de Ciencia e Innovación" (PSI2008-06116; P.I.: Andrés Parra) and "Generalitat Valenciana" (Prometeo/2011/048; P.I.: Alicia Salvador). They also wish to thank Mr. Brian Normanly for his editorial assistance and Encarna Rama Galdón and Marta Arsenal Castillo for their help with the figures.

7. References

Amado-Boccara, I.; Gougoulis, N.; Poirier, M.F.; Galinowski, A. & Lo^o, H. (1995). Effects of antidepressants on cognitive functions: A review. *Neuroscience & Biobehavioral Reviews*, Vol.19, pp. 479-493.

American Psychiatric Association (1994). *DSM IV-Diagnostic and Statistical Manual of Mental Disorders. Fourth ed.* American Psychiatric Association, Washington D.C.

Arenas, M.C.; Vinader-Caerols, C.; Monleón, S.; Martos, A.J.; Everss, E.; Ferrer-Añó, A. & Parra, A. (2006). Are the effects of the antidepressants amitriptyline, maprotiline, and fluoxetine on inhibitory avoidance state-dependent? *Behavioural Brain Research*, Vol.166, pp. 150-158.

Arkhipov, V.I. (1999). Memory dissociation: the approach to the study of retrieval process. *Behavioural Brain Research*, Vol.106, pp. 39–46.

Babar, E.; Melik, E.; Ozgunen, T.; Kaya, M. & Polat, S. (2002). Effects of excitotoxic median raphe lesions on scopolamine-induced working memory deficits in inhibitory avoidance. *International Journal of Neuroscience*, Vol.112, pp. 525-35.

Baldessarini, R.J. (2001). Drugs and the treatment of psychiatric disorders: depression and anxiety disorders, In: *Goodman & Gilman's The pharmacological basis of therapeutics, 10th edition*, J.G. Hardman, L.E. Limbird & A.G. Gilman, (Eds.), pp. 447-483, McGraw-Hill, New York.

Bert, B.; Fink, H.; Rothe, J.; Walstab, J. & Bönisch, H. (2008). Learning and memory in 5-HT(1A)-receptor mutant mice. *Behavioural Brain Research*, Vol.195, pp. 78-85.

Beasley, C.M.; Masica, D.N. & Potvin, J.H. (1992). Fluoxetine: a review of receptor and functional effects and their clinical implications. *Psychopharmacology*, Vol.107, pp. 1-10.

Boccia, M.M.; Blake, M.G.; Acosta, G.B. & Baratti, C.M. (2003). Atropine, an anticholinergic drug, impairs memory retrieval of a high consolidated avoidance response in mice. *Neuroscience Letters*, Vol.345, pp. 97-100.

Cafferata, G.L.; Kasper, J. & Bernstein, A. (1983). Family roles, structure and stressors in relation to sex differences in obtaining psychotropic drugs. *Journal of Health & Social Behavior*, Vol.24, pp. 132–143.

Campbell, S.; Marriott, M.; Nahmias, C. & MacQueen, G.M. (2004). Lower hippocampal volume in patients suffering from depression: a meta-analysis. *American Journal of Psychiatry*, Vol.161, pp. 598-607.

Castaneda, A.E.; Tuulio-Henriksson, A.; Marttunen, M.; Suvisaari, J. & Lönnqvist, J. (2008). A review on cognitive impairments in depressive and anxiety disorders with a focus on young adults. *Journal of Affective Disorders*, Vol.106, pp. 1-27.

Choi, R.L.; Roch, M. & Jenden, D.J. (1973). A regional study of acetylcholine turnover in rat brain and the effects of oxotremorine. *Proceedings of the Western Pharmacology Society*, Vol.16, pp. 188-190.

Dudra-Jastrzebska, M.; Andres-Mach, M.M.; Łuszczki, J.J. & Czuczwar, S.J. (2007). Mood disorders in patients with epilepsy. *Pharmacological Reports*, Vol.59, pp. 369-378.

Duman, R.S.; Malberg, J. & Thome, J. (1999). Neural plasticity to stress and antidepressant treatment. *Biological Psychiatry*, Vol.46, pp. 1181-1191.

Duric, V. & McCarson, K.E. (2006). Effects of analgesic or antidepressant drugs on pain- or stress-evoked hippocampal and spinal neurokinin-1 receptor and brain-derived neurotrophic factor gene expression in the rat. *Journal of Pharmacology and Experimental Therapeutics*, Vol.319, pp. 1235-1243.

Eidi, M.; Zarrindast, M.R.; Eidi, A.; Oryan, S. & Parivar, K. (2003). Effects of histamine and cholinergic systems on memory retention of passive avoidance learning in rats. *European Journal of Pharmacology*, Vol.465, pp. 91-96.

Everitt, B.J. & Robbins, T.W. (1997). Central cholinergic systems and cognition. *Annual Review of Psychology*, Vol.48, pp. 649-684.

Everss, E.; Arenas, M.C.; Vinader-Caerols, C.; Monleón, S. & Parra, A. (1999). Effects of amitriptyline on memory consolidation in male and female mice. *Medical Science Research*, Vol.27, pp. 237-239.

Everss, E.; Arenas, M.C.; Vinader-Caerols, C.; Monleón, S. & Parra, A. (2005). Piracetam counteracts the effects of amitriptyline on inhibitory avoidance in CD1 mice. *Behavioural Brain Research*, Vol.159, pp. 235-242.

Ferrer-Añó, A. (2008). *Estudio de la mediación del sistema histaminérgico en el efecto producido por la amitriptilina sobre la evitación inhibitoria en ratones*. Doctoral Thesis, University of Valencia, Spain.

File, S.E. (2001). Factors controlling measures of anxiety and responses to novelty in the mouse. *Behavioural Brain Research*, Vol.125, pp. 151-157.

Frackiewicz, E.J.; Sramek, J.J. & Cutler, N.R. (2000). Gender differences in depression and antidepressant pharmacokinetics and adverse events. *The Annals of Pharmacotherapy*, Vol.34, pp. 80-88.

Frazer, A. (1997). Pharmacology of antidepressants. *Journal of Clinical Psychopharmacology*, Vol.17(suppl 1), pp. 2S-18S.

Gandhi, M.; Aweeka, F.; Greenblatt, R.M. & Blaschke, T.F. (2004). Sex differences in pharmacokinetics and pharmacodynamics. *Annual Review of Pharmacology and Toxicology*, Vol.44, pp. 499–523.

Gareri, P.; Falconi, U.; de Fazio, P. & de Sarro, G. (2000). Conventional and new antidepressant drugs in the elderly. *Progress in Neurobiology*, Vol.61, pp. 353-396.

Gold, P.E. (1986). The use of avoidance training in studies of modulation of memory storage. *Behavioral and Neural Biology*, Vol.46, pp. 87-98.

González-Pardo, H.; Conejo, N.M.; Arias, J.L.; Monleón, S.; Vinader-Caerols, C. & Parra, A. (2008). Changes in brain oxidative metabolism induced by inhibitory avoidance learning and acute administration of amitriptyline. *Pharmacology Biochemistry and Behavior*, Vol.89, pp. 456-462.

Gouliaev, A.H. & Senning, A. (1994). Piracetam and other structurally related nootropics. *Brain Research Reviews*, Vol.19, pp. 180-222.

Grüter, W. & Pöldinger, W. (1982). Maprotiline. *Modern Problems of Pharmacopsychiatry*, Vol.18, pp. 17-48.

Harvey, A.T.; Rudolph, R.L. & Preskorn, S.H. (2000). Evidence of the dual mechanisms of action of venlafaxine. *Archives of General Psychiatry*, Vol.57, pp. 503-509.

Hascoët, M.; Bourin, M.; Colombel, M.C.; Fiocco, A.J. & Baker, G.B. (2000). Anxiolytic-like effects of antidepressants after acute administration in a four-plate test in mice. *Pharmacology Biochemistry and Behavior*, Vol.65, pp. 339-344.

Hebb, D.O. (1949). *The organization of behavior*. John Wiley & Sons, Inc., New York.

Heise, G.A. (1981). Learning and memory facilitators: Experimental definition and current status. *Trends in Pharmacological Sciences*, Vol.2, pp. 158-160.

Hertz, L.; Chen, Y.; Gibbs, M.E.; Zang, P. & Peng, L. (2004). Astrocytic adrenoceptors: a major drug target in neurological and psychiatric disorders? *Current Drug Targets - CNS & Neurological Disorders*, Vol.3, pp. 239-267.

Humphreys, M.R. & Reinberg, Y.E. (2005). Contemporary and emerging drug treatments for urinary incontinence in children. *Pediatric Drugs*, Vol.7, 151-162.

Introini-Collison, I.B. & Baratti, C.M. (1992). Memory-modulatory effects of centrally acting noradrenergic drugs: possible involvement of brain cholinergic mechanisms. *Behavioral and Neural Biology*, Vol.57, pp. 248-255.

Izquierdo, I. & McGaugh, J.L. (2000). Behavioural pharmacology and its contribution to the molecular basis of memory consolidation. *Behavioural Pharmacology*, Vol.11, pp. 517-534.

Kandel, E.R. (2001). The molecular biology of memory storage: a dialogue between genes and synapses. *Science*, Vol.294, pp. 1030-1038.

Kasper, S. & McEwen, B.S. (2008). Neurobiological and clinical effects of the antidepressant tianeptine. *CNS Drugs*, Vol.22, pp. 15-26.

Konradi, C. & Heckers, S. (2001). Antipsychotic drugs and neuroplasticity: insights into the treatment and neurobiology of schizophrenia. *Biological Psychiatry*, Vol.50, pp. 729-742.

Kornstein, S. (1997). Gender differences in depression: implications for treatment. *Journal of Clinical Psychiatry*, Vol.58, pp. 2–18.

Lamberty, Y. & Gower, A.J. (1990). Age-related changes in spontaneous behavior and learning in NMRI mice from maturity to middle age. *Physiology and Behavior*, Vol. 47, pp. 1137-1144.

Lister, R.G. (1987). The use of a plus-maze to measure anxiety in the mouse. *Psychopharmacology*, Vol.92, pp. 180-185.

McGaugh, J.L. (1989). Dissociating learning and performance: Drug and hormone enhancement of memory storage. *Brain Research Bulletin*, Vol.23, pp. 339-345.

McGaugh, J.L. & Izquierdo, I. (2000). The contribution of pharmacology to research on the mechanisms of memory formation. *Trends in Pharmacological Sciences*, Vol.21, pp. 208-210.

Martényi, F.; Dossenbach, M.; Mraz, K. & Metcalfe, S. (2001). Gender differences in the efficacy of fluoxetine and maprotiline in depressed patients: a double-blind trial of antidepressants with serotonergic or norepinephrine reuptake inhibition profile. *European Neuropsychopharmacology*, Vol.11, pp. 227–232.

Mitchell, H.A.; Ahern, T.H.; Liles, L.C.; Javors, M.A. & Weinshenker, D. (2006). The effects of norepinephrine transporter inactivation on locomotor activity in mice. *Biological Psychiatry*, Vol.60, pp. 1046-1052.

Monleón, S.; Casino, A.; Vinader-Caerols, C. & Arenas MC. (2001). Acute effects of fluoxetine on inhibitory avoidance consolidation in male and female OF1 mice. *Neuroscience Research Communications*, Vol.28, pp. 123-130.

Monleón, S.; Urquiza, A.; Arenas, M.C.; Vinader-Caerols, C. & Parra, A. (2002). Chronic administration of fluoxetine impairs inhibitory avoidance in male but not female mice. *Behavioural Brain Research*, Vol.136, pp. 483-488.

Monleón, S.; Vinader-Caerols, C.; Arenas, M.C. & Parra, A. (2008). Antidepressant drugs and memory: insights from animal studies. *European Neuropsychopharmacology*, Vol.18, pp. 235-248.

Monleón, S.; Urquiza, A.; Vinader-Caerols, C. & Parra, A. (2009). Effects of oxotremorine and physostigmine on the inhibitory avoidance impairment produced by amitriptyline in male and female mice. *Behavioural Brain Research*, Vol.205, pp. 367-371.

Morris, R.G. (1984). Development of a water-maze procedure for studying spatial leaming in the rat. *Journal of Neuroscience Methods*, Vol.11, pp. 47-60.

Morris, R.G.; Moser, E.I.; Riedel, G.; Martin, S.J.; Sandin, J.; Day, M. & O'Carroll, C. (2003). Elements of a neurobiological theory of the hippocampus: the role of activity-dependent synaptic plasticity in memory. *Philosophical Transactions of the Royal Society of London. Series B, Biological Sciences*, Vol.358, pp. 773-786.

Myhrer, T. (2003). Neurotransmitter systems involved in learning and memory in the rat: a meta-analysis based on studies of four behavioral tasks. *Brain Research Reviews*, Vol.41, pp. 268-287.

Nemeroff, C.B. & Vale, W.W. (2005). The neurobiology of depression: inroads to treatment and new drug discovery. *Journal of Clinical Psychiatry*, Vol.66: 5-13.

Noble, R.E. (2005). Depression in women. *Metabolism*, Vol.54, pp. 49-52.

Overton, D.A. (1974). Experimental methods for the study of state-dependent learning. *Federation Proceedings*, Vol.54, 1800-1813.

Overton, D.A. (1984). State dependent learning and drug discriminations. In: *Handbook of Psychopharmacology*, L.L. Iversen, S.D. Iversen & S.H. Snyder, (Eds.), pp. 59-127, Plenum Press, New York.

Owens, M.J.; Morgan, W.N.; Plott, S.J. & Nemeroff, C.B. (1997). Neurotransmitter receptor and transporter binding profile of antidepressants and their metabolites. *Journal of Pharmacology and Experimental Therapeutics*, Vol.283, pp. 1305-1322.

Paizanis, E.; Hamon, M. & Lanfumey, L. (2007). Hippocampal neurogenesis, depressive disorders, and antidepressant therapy. *Neural Plasticity*, Vol.2007, pp. 73754-73760.

Parra, A. (2003). A common role for psychotropic medications: memory impairment. *Medical Hypotheses*, Vol.60, pp. 133-142.

Parra, A.; Arenas, M.C.; Monleón, S.; Vinader-Caerols, C. & Simón, V.M. (1999). Sex differences in the effects of neuroleptics on escape-avoidance behavior in mice: a review. *Pharmacology Biochemistry and Behavior*, Vol.64, pp. 813-820.

Parra, A.; Monleón, S.; Arenas, M.C. & Vinader-Caerols, C. (2000). Effects of acute and chronic maprotiline administration on inhibitory avoidance in male mice. *Behavioural Brain Research*, Vol.109, pp. 1-7.

Parra, A.; Everss, E.; Monleón, S.; Vinader-Caerols, C. & Arenas, M.C. (2002). Effects of acute amitriptyline administration on memory, anxiety and activity in male and female mice. *Neuroscience Research Communications*, Vol.31, pp. 135-144.

Parra, A.; Everss, E.; Arenas, M.C.; Vinader-Caerols, C. & Monleón, S. (2006). Amitriptyline administered after consolidation of inhibitory avoidance does not affect memory retrieval. *Psicothema*, Vol.18, pp. 514-518.

Parra, A.; Vinader-Caerols, C.; Ferrer-Añó, A.; Urquiza, A. & Monleón, S. (2009). The effect of amitriptyline on inhibitory avoidance in mice is dose-dependent. *Psicothema,* Vol.21, pp. 528-530.

Parra, A.; Ferrer-Añó, A.; Fuentes, C.; Monleón, S. & Vinader-Caerols, C. (2010). Effects of co-administration of amitriptyline and fluoxetine on inhibitory avoidance in mice. *Behavioural Brain Research,* Vol.214, pp. 343-348.

Passani, M.B.; Bacciottini, L.; Mannaioni, P.F. & Blandina, P. (2000). Central histaminergic system and cognition. *Neuroscience & Biobehavioral Reviews,* Vol.24, pp. 107-113.

Pinder, R.M.; Brogden, R.N.; Speight, T.M. & Avery, G.S. (1977). Maprotiline, a review of its pharmacological properties and therapeutic efficacy in mental depressive states. *Drugs,* Vol.13, pp. 321–352.

Pittenger, C. & Duman, R.S. (2008). Stress, depression, and neuroplasticity: a convergence of mechanisms. *Neuropsychopharmacology,* Vol.33, pp. 88-109.

Prell, G.D.; Hough, L.B.; Khandelwal, J. & Green, J.P. (1996). Lack of a precursor-product relationship between histamine and its metabolites in brain after histidine loading. *Journal of Neurochemistry,* Vol.67, pp. 1938–1944.

Redrobe, J.P. & Bourin, M. (1997). Partial role of 5-HT2 and 5-HT3 receptors in the activity of antidepressants in the mouse forced swimming test. *European Journal of Pharmacology,* Vol.325, pp. 129-135.

Richelson, E. & Nelson, A. (1984). Antagonism by antidepressants of neurotransmitter receptors of normal human brain in vitro. *Journal of Pharmacology and Experimental Therapeutics,* Vol.230, pp. 94–102.

Richelson, E. (2001). Pharmacology of antidepressants. *Mayo Clinic Proceedings,* Vol.76, pp. 511-527.

Richelson, E. (2003). Interactions of antidepressants with neurotrasmitter transpoters and receptors and their clinical relevance. *Journal of Clinical Psychiatry,* Vol.64, pp. 5-12.

Rodgers, R.J. & Johnson, N.J. (1995). Factor analysis of spatiotemporal and ethological measures in the murine elevated plus-maze test of anxiety. *Pharmacology Biochemistry and Behavior,* Vol.52, pp. 297-303.

Sahay, A. & Hen, R. (2007). Adult hippocampal neurogenesis in depression. *Nature Neuroscience,* Vol.10, pp. 1110-1115.

Schatzberg, A.F. (2000). New indications for antidepressants. *Journal of Clinical Psychiatry,* Vol.61, pp. 9-17.

Sindrup, S.H.; Otto, M.; Finnerup, N.B. & Jensen, T.S. (2005). Antidepressants in the treatment of neuropathic pain. *Basic & Clinical Pharmacology & Toxicology,* Vol.96, pp. 399-409.

Stahl, S.M. (1998). Basic psychopharmacology of antidepressants. Part 1: Antidepressants have seven distinct mechanism of action. *Journal of Clinical Psychiatry,* Vol.59, pp. 5-14.

Stahl, S.M. (2008). *Stahl's essential psychopharmacology. Neuroscientific basis and practical aplications. 3rd edition,* Cambridge University Press, New York.

Stark, P.; Fuller, R.W. & Wong, D.T. (1985). The pharmacologic profile of fluoxetine. *Journal of Clinical Psychiatry,* Vol.46, pp. 7-13.

Taylor, P. (2001). Anticholinesterase agents, In: *Goodman & Gilman's The pharmacological basis of therapeutics, 10th edition,* J.G. Hardman, L.E. Limbird & A.G. Gilman, (Eds.), pp. 175-191, McGraw-Hill, New York.

Thompson, P.J. (1991). Antidepressants and memory: a review. *Human Psychopharmacology: Clinical and Experimental*, Vol.6, pp. 79-90.

Tsukahara, T.; Iihara, K.; Hashimoto, N.; Nishijima, T. & Taniguchi, T. (1998). Increases in levels of brain-derived neurotrophic factor mRNA and its promoters after transient forebrain ischemia in the rat brain. *Neurochemistry International*, Vol.33, pp. 201-207.

Urquiza, A. (2007). *Estudio de la intervención del sistema colinérgico en el efecto producido por la amitriptilina en una tarea de evitación inhibitoria en ratones machos y hembras*. Doctoral Thesis, University of Valencia, Spain.

Vaidya, V.A. & Duman, R.S. (2001). Depresssion-emerging insights from neurobiology. *British Medical Bulletin*, Vol.57, pp. 61-79.

Vinader-Caerols, C.; Ferrer-Añó, A.; Arenas, M.C.; Monleón, S. & Parra, A. (2002). La maprotilina anula las diferencias entre ratones machos y hembras en el laberinto de agua de Morris. *Psicothema*, Vol.14, pp. 823-827.

Vinader-Caerols, C.; Martos, A.J.; Monleón, S.; Arenas, M.C. & Parra, A. (2006). Acute effects of maprotiline on learning, anxiety, activity and analgesia in male and female mice. *Acta Neurobiologiae Experimentalis*, Vol.66, pp. 23-31.

Yanai, K.; Yagi, N.; Watanabe, T.; Itoh, M.; Ishiwata, K.; Ido, T. & Matsuzawa, T. (1990). Specific binding of [3H]pyrilamine to histamine H1 receptors in guinea pig brain in vivo: determination of binding parameters by a kinetic four-compartment model. *Journal of Neurochemistry*, Vol 55, pp. 409-420.

3

Participation of the Monoaminergic System in the Antidepressant-Like Actions of Estrogens: A Review in Preclinical Studies

Carolina López-Rubalcava[1], Nelly Maritza Vega-Rivera[1,2], Nayeli Páez-Martínez[3] and Erika Estrada-Camarena[2*]
[1]*Departamento de Farmacobiología, Cinvestav-IPN,*
[2]*Laboratorio de Neuropsicofarmacología,*
Instituto Nacional de Psiquiatria Ramón de la Fuente,
[3]*Sección de Graduados, Escuela Superior de Medicina IPN*
Mexico

1. Introduction

1.1 Estrogen receptors – Classification and distribution

Estrogens are steroid hormones produced by gonads that bind to different receptor types and mediate numerous actions, like growth, development, cognition, neuroprotection and participate in mood regulation (Margeat *et al.*, 2003; Vasudevan & Pfaff, 2007). The classic estrogen receptors (ER) are: ERα and ERβ. These receptors are ligand-activated transcription factors (Kuiper & Gustafsson, 1997) with nuclear and non-nuclear distribution (Monje & Boland, 2001; Weiser *et al.*, 2008). In ovariectomized rats, ERβ and ERα are co-localized in various brain regions, including the bed nucleus of the stria terminalis, the medial and cortical amygdaloid nuclei, the preoptic area, the lateral habenula, the periacueductal gray, the locus coeruleus, the hippocampus and the brain cortex (Shughrue *et al.*, 1997). In these last two structures, ERβ is more abundant than ERα. Other structures that contain only ERβ are the olfactory bulb, the ventral tegmental area, the zona incerta, the cerebellum, the pineal gland and some hypothalamic nuclei (such as the supraoptic, the paraventricular, the supraquiasmatic and the tuberal nuclei). By contrast, brain areas with solely ERα are the ventromedial hypothalamic nuclei and the subfornical organ (Shughrue *et al.*, 1997).

Several reports have described two membrane estrogen receptors unrelated to ERα and ERβ: an orphan receptor coupled to G proteins called GPR30 (Filardo *et al.*, 2002) and another, named ER-X, that posses characteristics of tyrosine-kynase activity (Toran-Allerand, 2004). GPR30 is a seven transmembrane ER that binds estrogens with high affinity and acts independently of ERα and ERβ to stimulate adenyl cyclase and phopholipase C via Gαs proteins, which in turn, generates classic second messengers such as the cyclic

* Corresponding author

adenosine monophosphate (cAMP), inositol trisphosphate and Ca+ and induces the release of the epidermal growth factor (Filardo *et al.*, 2002). On the other hand, the ER-X is a plasma membrane ER enriched in a caveolar-like microdomain that is expressed during development and after ischemic brain injury (Toran-Allerand *et al.*, 2005). ER-X mediates 17α-estradiol and 17 β-estradiol (E2) activation of MAPK/ERK in development neocortical explants, after ischemic injury and in animal models of Alzheimer's disease and Down's syndrome. These characteristics could explain estrogen's rapid actions in the central nervous system.

2. Monoamines and depression

One of the earliest theories in the biology of depression is the monoaminergic hypothesis that proposed a dysfunction of the serotonegic/catecholaminergic function that leads to depression. The neurotransmitters serotonin (5-HT), dopamine (DA) and noradrenaline (NA) (NA) are localized in limbic brain regions involved in the regulation of mood, cognition and anxiety, among others. This theory was proposed in the early 50s, with the observation that reserpine, a drug with antihypertensive activity and that inhibits catecholamine vesiculation, induced signs of depression (Lopez-Muñoz & Alamo, 2009). On the other hand, drugs that facilitate monoamine release were found to be antidepressant. At present, serotonin transporters, noradrenaline transporters and the monoamine oxidase enzyme (MAO) are targets of antidepressant therapy, all of which increase the serotonergic and/or noradrenaline tone through an inhibition of monoamine reuptake or inhibition of monoamine catabolism (MAO inhibition) (Kalia, 2005; Lopez-Muñoz & Alamo, 2009; Osterlund, 2009).

Although the pharmacological and biochemical effects of antidepressant drugs occur rapidly (within minutes), in clinical practice the antidepressants drugs produce their therapeutic actions after at least 10 to 14 days after treatment initiation. This suggests that antidepressants act via a delayed postsynaptic receptor-mediated event (Kalia, 2005). It is hypothesized that the delayed time of onset for antidepressant drugs is due to the feedback mechanism of the somatodendritic 5-HT1A receptor. In this case, increased release of serotonin by acute administration of antidepressants such as the selective serotonin reuptake inhibitors (SSRIs) leads to a dose-dependent inhibition of 5-HT neuronal firing rate (Osterlund, 2009) due to the activation of the presynaptic 5-HT1A receptors, followed by inhibition of neuronal firing and terminal serotonin release. Chronic administration of reuptake inhibitors leads to desensitization of the presynaptic 5-HT1A autoreceptors and thereby restores serotonergic firing and terminal serotonin release (Krishnan & Nestler, 2008). The observed desensitization of presynaptic 5-HT1A autoreceptors is in line with the time course for therapeutic onset of reuptake inhibitors (Maletic *et al.*, 2007; Osterlund, 2009).

Similarly to serotonergic receptors, it has been reported that chronic antidepressant treatments caused subsensitivity of the noradrenergic receptor–coupled adenylate cyclase system in the brain (Vetulani *et al.*, 1976). This work shifted the emphasis from acute presynaptic (α2-adrenergic receptors) to delayed postsynaptic receptor-mediated events in the mode of action of antidepressants. The delayed desensitization of the noradrenergic β-adrenoceptor- coupled adenylate-cylase system in the brain is an action that is common to almost all antidepressant treatments (Kalia, 2005).

3. Depression in women: Role of estrogens

In women, changes in the incidence of mental illnesses (particularly in major depressive disorder) can be found in three important periods of their reproductive life span. These periods are characterized by drastic hormonal oscilations (Girdler & Klatzkin, 2007; Payne *et al.*, 2007). For example, a correlation was found between the onset of depressive and anxiety symptoms and the rapid decrease of progesterone and allopregnanolone levels during the late lutheal phase of the menstrual cycle in vulnerable women (Halbreich & Kahn, 2001; Backstrom *et al.*, 2003); by contrast, when a gradual reduction in progesterone concentrations occurs, a reduction of depression, anxiety, food cravings, mood swings and cramps is observed (Contreras *et al.*, 2006). In addition, a positive correlation between the abrupt fall of hormones levels and post-partum depression has been established (Jensvold, 1996). Hence, some reports indicate that hormones such as estradiol are a useful therapy to relief the postpartum depression symptoms (Soares *et al.*, 2001).

The most characterized endocrine period where hormonal fluctuations influence depressive states is the perimenopause transition. Several reports indicate that follicular stimulating and luteinizing hormones and estradiol oscillations are correlated with the onset or worsening of depression symptoms during early perimenopause (Halbreich & Kahn, 2001; Pae *et al.*, 2009), when major depressive disorder incidence is 3-5 times higher than the male matched population of the same aged (Riecher-Rossler & Geyter, 2007). Several longitudinal studies that followed women across the menopausal transition indicate that the risk for significant depressive symptoms increases during the menopausal transition and then decreases in the early postmenopause (Soares & Zitek, 2008) and in the last years of menopause its incidence is comparable to that shown by men (Payne *et al.*, 2007; Riecher-Rossler & Geyter, 2007). Also, epidemiological studies showed that women vulnerable to hormonal fluctuations, who suffer premenstrual dysphoric disorders, are susceptible to develop post-partum- and perimenopausal-depression (Richards *et al.*, 2006; Payne *et al.*, 2007). The sum of all these depressive episodes results in a long term deficient quality of life due to many years of poor mental health.

Other studies that have shown the participation of estrogens in the etiology of depression are the following: a prospective study showed that women with a lifetime history of depression had high levels of follicle-stimulating and luteinizing hormones levels, but low estradiol concentrations (Harlow *et al.*, 2003). In this case, authors concluded that a lifetime history of major depression may be associated with an early decline of ovarian function, a situation that characterizes menopause transition (Harlow *et al.*, 2003). On the other hand, in a similar study, women with no history of depression, had increased levels of FSH and LH and increased variability of estradiol that were significantly associated with depressive symptoms (Freeman *et al.*, 2006). In fact, it was proposed that the unstable and irregular pattern of hormone production during perimenopausal transition, in susceptible women, may increase vulnerability to mood disorders (Sherwin & Henry, 2008; Rocca *et al.*, 2010).

In addition, it has been reported that in depressive women, high levels of FSH correlate with the severity of depression and the intensity of menopausal symptoms (Rajewska & Rybakowski, 2003). Interestingly, these women presented a transient decreased response to the stimulation of the serotonergic system with D-fenfluramine, suggesting hypoactivity of the serotonergic system during depression (Rajewska & Rybakowski, 2003). Therefore, the impact of hormone oscillations during perimenopause transition may affect the serotonergic system function and increase vulnerability to develop depression.

4. Antidepressant like actions of estrogens in clinical and preclinical studies

4.1 Effects of estrogens in clinical studies

The participation of estrogens in the etiology of depression is evident when they are used as part of the pharmacotherapy of depression associated to perimenopause. Clinical research has found clear antidepressant effects of various estrogens when given alone (Schmidt *et al.*, 2000; Soares *et al.*, 2001) or in combination with classic antidepressants (Soares *et al.*, 2001; Morgan *et al.*, 2005). However, an equal amount of reports have failed to find antidepressant effects of estrogens administered alone (Coope, 1975; Saletu *et al.*, 1995; Morrison *et al.*, 2004) or a lack of further benefit from that produced by an antidepressant treatment (Shapira *et al.*, 1985; Amsterdam *et al.*, 1999). The nature of such differences is unknown; however, factors, including age, type of compounds, depression scales, duration of treatment, type of depression, endocrine stage and time after cessation of menses, may be responsible for these differences.

For example, in a double-blind placebo-controlled study of 34 perimenopausal women with major depressive disorder or minor depression, 3 weeks of estradiol monotherapy resulted in significant improvement (Schmidt *et al.*, 2000). Furthermore, in another placebo controlled double-blind study of perimenopausal women, 17 β-estradiol delivered transdermally was also efficacious (Soares *et al.*, 2001). An open study also showed that in women with major depressive disorder, estradiol either as monotherapy or added to an SSRI antidepressant was effective after 6 weeks of treatment (Rasgon *et al.*, 2002). However, studies in which menopausal women with or without depression diagnosis were included, estrogens were ineffective to reduce depressive symptoms (Coope, 1975; Strickler *et al.*, 1977).

On the other hand, two out of four studies of varying designs suggest that estrogen may improve responsiveness to antidepressants. A randomized, controlled, multicenter trial of fluoxetine in geriatric depression found that women who were incidentally taking estrogen improved better on fluoxetine than placebo, whereas those who were not taking estrogen showed no difference between fluoxetine and placebo (Schneider *et al.*, 1997). On the negative side, a recent retrospective study found no difference in the proportion of responders to fluoxetine between women who took estrogen replacement therapy and women who did not (Amsterdam *et al.*, 1999). Finally, another study failed to show efficacy for estrogen augmentation of imipramine in either pre- or postmenopausal women with treatment-resistant depression (Shapira *et al.*, 1985). Some examples of estrogens used as therapy for depression alone or in combination with antidepressants or other hormones are illustrated in table 1 and table 2.

4.2 Antidepressant-like effects of estrogens on basic research

In basic research, animal models of experimental depression have been extensively used in the development of novel therapeutic compounds and for the understanding of the neural substrates underlying depressive behavior (Holmes, 2003; Cryan *et al.*, 2005; Markou *et al.*, 2009). Thus, using animal models for the screening of compounds with antidepressant-like properties, estrogens have antidepressant-like effects. For example, it was found that 7 days of estradiol treatment reduces the immobility behavior in gonadectomized mice in the tail suspension test, suggesting an antidepressant-like action (Bernardi *et al.*, 1989).

Other studies have been performed in rats and mice using the forced swimming test (FST) which has been primarily developed as a test for screening the efficacy of novel antidepressants (López-Rubalcava *et al.*, 2009). It is noticeable that antidepressant-like actions of estrogenic compounds have been detected after acute (1 injection) and chronic treatments (7-14 days) if they are administered close to the time of ovaries elimination, i. e. either immediately or few weeks after estrogens decline. For example, the administration of estradiol benzoate for 7 or 14 days, induces antidepressant-like effects in the FST (Okada *et al.*, 1997; Rachman *et al.*, 1998). Besides, the antidepressant-like action of estrogenic compounds like 17β-estradiol (E2), 17α-ethinyl-estradiol (EE2) and diarylpropionitrile (DPN, an agonist to estrogen receptors type β) was also observed after an acute treatment (Estrada-Camarena *et al.*, 2003; Walf *et al.*, 2004). Interestingly, a selective estrogen receptor modulator, raloxifene, was only effective after 7 days of treatment; whereas tamoxifen, or the ERα agonist, 4,4',4''-(4-Propyl-[1H]-pyrazole-1,3,5-triyl)trisphenol (PPT) were ineffective in the FST after an acute or chronic treatment (table 3). Hence, the antidepressant-like effect of compounds with estrogenic activity depends on the type of compound and on the length of the treatment, suggesting that different mechanisms are involved. In addition, the antidepressant-like effect of estrogens also seems to depend on the time of estrogen restitution after the ovariectomy (OVX) as well as on the age of the animals. In this sense, if the restitution with E2 in young animals is initiated after three weeks post-OVX, but not five or more weeks, antidepressant-like effects are observed (Estrada-Camarena *et al.*, 2011). In contrast, if middle age rats (around 12 months old) are ovariectomized, the antidepressant-like effect of E2 is restricted to one week post-OVX (unpublished data).

5. Actions of estrogens on monoaminergic systems

5.1 Evidence of estrogens interactions with the serotonegic system

In vitro and in vivo studies, with non-stressed animals, have analyzed estrogens' effects on the serotonergic system. For example, in ovariectomized rats, acute and chronic estradiol treatment resulted in increased serotonin levels in specific brain areas such as the dorsal raphe nucleus and hippocampus (Lubbers *et al.*, 2010). Similar results were found in the hypothalamus of guinea pigs (Lu *et al.*, 1999) and in the dorsal raphe nucleus of nonhuman primates (Lu & Bethea, 2002). Furthermore, human studies reported increased serotonin levels in postmenopausal women receiving hormone replacement therapy with estrogens (Blum *et al.*, 1996) and suggest that estradiol enhances 5-HT synthesis in serotonergic neurons (O'Keane *et al.*, 1991).

Estrogens effects on serotonin levels could be related with an increase on tryptophan hydroxylase activity (Donner & Handa, 2009). Thus, in rat´s dorsal raphe nucleus, it has been shown that the tryptophan hydroxylase enzyme expression is directly modulated by estrogens (McEwen, 1999; Donner & Handa, 2009). Furthermore, inmunohistochemical studies revealed the existence of ER-β mRNA in neurons of the dorsal raphe nucleus (McEwen, 1999). Therefore, it is suggested that estrogens might modulate the enzyme's activity or synthesis through ER-β, and consequently have an impact on serotonin levels (McEwen, 1999; Donner & Handa, 2009).

Another site of action through which estrogens can influence serotonin levels is the serotonin transporter (SERT). Studies in monkeys showed that E2 and the selective modulators of estrogen receptors, raloxifene and arzoxifene, increased tryptophan hydroxylase mRNA expression and decreased SERT's mRNA expression (Bethea *et al.*, 2002; Smith *et al.*, 2004). Interestingly, in the FST, raloxifene induced antidepressant-like effects similar to SSRIs such as fluoxetine (Estrada-Camarena *et al.*, 2003; Estrada-Camarena *et al.*, 2010). Studies in rats, analyzing different brain areas, indicate that acute or chronic treatment with estradiol benzoate decreased the number of ^{3}[H] paroxetine binding sites (Mendelson *et al.*, 1993). These results are in agreement with in vitro studies that reported that some estrogenic compounds interact with the serotonin transporter in membranes obtained from cerebral cortex, hippocampus, hypothalamus and striatum (Chang & Chang, 1999).

Reference	Study population	Estrogenic compound	Findings
(Lopez-Jaramillo *et al.*, 1996)	Post-menopausal women	Conjugate equine estrogens, oral	E>placebo ↓ Beck scale
(Soares *et al.*, 2001)	Perimenopausal women with depression (40-45 years old)	17 β-estradiol path	E>placebo ↓ MADRS y BKMI scales
(Montgomery *et al.*, 1987)	Peri, postmenopausal and hysterectomized women without depression (44-50 years old)	17 β-estradiol with or without testosterone	E o E+T > placebo in perimenopausic interview and SRD30
(Strickler *et al.*, 1977)	Perimenopausal and hysterectomized women with unipolar and bipolar depression or healthy (35-66 years old)	Conjugate equine estrogens, oral	E=placebo MMPI y 16PF scales
(Coope, 1975)	Menopausal, hysterectomized and oophorectomized women with depression (40-61 years old)	Conjugate equine estrogens, oral	E=placebo
(Bukulmez *et al.*, 2001)	Postmenopausal women without depression (45-60 years old)	Equine estrogens + medroxyprogesterone or Tibolone, oral	E+MHP o E+tibolone>placebo ↓ Beck scale
(Schmidt *et al.*, 2000)	Perimenopausal women with depression	17 β-estradiol patch	E>placebo

Table 1. Effect of estrogens as antidepressants in clinical practice

Reference	Study population	Antidepressant	Type of estrogen	Results
(Shapira *et al.*, 1985)	Pre and postmenopausal women with depression treatment resistant (26-74 years old)	Imipramine 200 mg/day/3 months	Conjugate equine estrogens, oral 1.25-3.75 mg/day/month	E+imipramine = placebo+imipramine Hamilton and Becker scales
(Amsterdam *et al.*, 1999)	Pre and postmenopausal women with depression with or without treatment with estrogens alone or in combination with progesterone (<45 a > 45)	Fluoxetine 20 mg/day/3 months	Conjugate equine estrogens, oral 0.625 mg/day/3 months with or without progesterone	E+fluoxetine= placebo+fluoxetine Hamilton scale
(Schneider *et al.*, 1997)	postmenopausal women with depression	Fluoxetine	ERT Estrogens 1.5 month	E+FLX >E+placebo, placebo+FLX y placebo+placebo
(Schneider *et al.*, 2001)	postmenopausal women with depression > 60 years old	Sertraline	Conjugate equine estrogones oral (0.625 mg/day) /3 months	E+SERT improves of quality of life
(Soares *et al.*, 2001)	Peri and post-menopausal women with depression	Citalopram 20-40 mg/day/2 months	17 β-estradiol (100 μg/day/1 month + CIT/2 months	E+CIT> E+placebo ↓ MADRS scale
(Joffe *et al.*, 2001)	Peri and post-menopausal women with depression	Mirtazepine 30-45 mg/day 2 months	estrogens+MIRT	E+MIRT ↓ Hamilton scale

Table 2. Effect of estrogens combination with antidepressant drugs in the treatment of depression

Estrogenic compound	Behavioral effect	Test	References
Agonist with more activity on ERα			
Propyl-pyrazol-triol (PPT) 17α-estradiol 17α-Ethynyl-estradiol	- - + Low doses - High doses	FST FST FST FST	(Estrada-Camarena *et al.*, 2003; Walf *et al.*, 2004; Walf & Frye, 2007)
Agonist with more activity on ERβ			
Diaryl-propionitrile (DPN) Cumestrol	+ +	FST FST	(Walf *et al.*, 2004; Walf & Frye, 2007)
Agonist of GPR30			
G1	+	TST	(Dennis *et al.*, 2009)
Agonist of ERα and ERβ			
17 β-Estradiol* Estradiol benzoate * Diethyl-stilbestrol Estradiol valerate	+ +/- - +	FST FST, TST FST CMS	(Bernardi *et al.*, 1989; Okada *et al.*, 1997; Rachman *et al.*, 1998; Galea *et al.*, 2002; Estrada-Camarena *et al.*, 2003; Dalla *et al.*, 2005; Romano-Torres & Fernandez-Guasti, 2010)
Selective estrogen receptor modulators of ERα and ERβ			
Raloxifene Tamoxifen	+ -	FST FST	(Estrada-Camarena *et al.*, 2010; Walf & Frye, 2010)
Antagonist of ERα and ERβ			
RU 58668 ICI 182780	- -	FST FST	(Estrada-Camarena *et al.*, 2006b; López-Rubalcava *et al.*, 2007)
Phytoestrogens			
Pomegranate (Estradiol, estrone, estriol, cumestrol, genistien)	+	FST	(Mori-Okamoto *et al.*, 2004)

FST=Forced swimming test; TST= tail suspension test; CMS = chronic mild stress. +: decrease of anhedonia or immobility behavior; - : no change of anhedonia or immobility behavior

Table 3. Effect of different types of estrogenic compounds in ovariectomized female rodents tested in different animal models for the screening of antidepressant-drugs.

As for the action of estrogens on serotonergic receptors, an interaction with 5-HT1A, 5-HT1B 5-HT2A/2C and 5-HT3 receptors has been demonstrated (Osterlund & Hurd, 1998; Raap *et al.*, 2000; Hiroi & Neumaier, 2009). In general, it is proposed that estrogens produce a desensitization of 5-HT1A receptors (Lu & Bethea, 2002) which is associated with decreased Gi protein coupled receptors (Mize & Alper, 2000; Raap *et al.*, 2000; Lu & Bethea, 2002). Moreover, another mechanism of action involves the phosphorylation of 5-HT1A receptor via activation of protein kinase-A; this effect is proposed to be mediated through the activation of an estrogen membrane receptor (Mize & Alper, 2002).

Recently, our laboratory found that E2 requires the presence of 5-HT since its depletion or the selective destruction of the presynaptic terminal, partially blocked E2's antidepressant-like effects (López-Rubalcava *et al.*, 2005). Furtheremore, the antidepressant-like actions of E2 and EE2, alone or in combination with fluoxetine require the activation of 5-HT1A receptors, since the selective 5-HT1A antagonist, WAY100635 blocked the antidepressant-like effect induced by these estrogens (Estrada-Camarena *et al.*, 2006a; Estrada-Camarena *et al.*, 2006b). In support of this proposal, the administration of the specific 5-HT1A post-synaptic receptor antagonist MM-77, canceled E2 antidepressant-like effects in the FST (López-Rubalcava *et al.*, 2005).

Results suggest that estrogenic actions on the serotonergic system require estrogen receptor activation. For example, our research group found that RU58688, an estrogen receptor antagonist, blocks E2 antidepressant-like effects in the FST (Estrada-Camarena *et al.*, 2006b); while the desensitization of postsynaptic 5-HT1A receptors located in the hippocampus of the rat requires the participation of a membrane estrogen receptor (Mize *et al.*, 2001). Recently, it was demonstrated that the membrane estrogen receptor GPR30, is involved in 5-HT1A receptor desensitization in the hypothalamus of the rat (Rossi *et al.*, 2010). Taken together, these data may explain why the blockade of ER and 5-HT1A receptor cancels E2 antidepressant-like effects.

In conclusion, it can be proposed that the antidepressant-like effects of E2 are due to its effects on the serotonergic system at both, a pre-and post-synaptic terminals. Thus, in the presynaptic neuron, estrogens are likely to stimulate the activity of the enzyme tryptophan hydroxylase and at the same time inhibit the SERT, this would lead to an increased in the availability of 5-HT in the synaptic cleft. On the postsynaptic site, 5-HT1A and possibly 5-HT2A receptors contribute to trigger signaling cascades that would allowed the modulation of other neurotransmitter systems and processes as complex as the modulation of neuronal plasticity (Fig. 1).

5.2 Evidence of the interaction of estrogens with the noradrenergic system

Several reports, including electrophysiological records (Wagner *et al.*, 2001) and ligand binding studies (Wilkinson & Herdon, 1982) have shown that estrogens can also modulate noradrenergic neurotransmission in the central nervous system (CNS). Several studies reported that estrogenic compounds can influence noradrenergic neurotransmission through an interaction with the noradrenergic transporter and the MAO or tyrosine hydroxylase enzymes. For example, in vitro studies have shown that E2, EE2, DES and some catechol-estrogens such as 2-hydroxy-EE2 (2-OH-EE2) and 2-hydroxy-E1 (2-OHE) inhibit NA reuptake sites in synaptosomes from the cerebral cortex and hypothalamus of rats that resulted in increased levels of NA in the synaptic cleft (Ghraf *et al.*, 1983). In line with these findings, acute E2 administration to ovariectomized rats decreased NA reuptake rate in the hypothalamus (Hiemke *et al.*, 1985) and increases mRNA levels of tyrosine hydroxylase in the locus coeruleus (Serova *et al.*, 2002). Finally, it has been reported that estrogens increased NA concentration by inhibiting MAO-A activity (Holschneider *et al.*, 1998). These data collectively suggest that estrogens interact with the noradrenergic system through the modulation of NA release, as well as in processes of synthesis and elimination of the neurotransmitter. Thus, E2 given to ovariectomized female rats increased the firing rate of noradrenergic neurons that project to the preoptic area and to the anterior hypothalamus (Kaba *et al.*, 1983). Similarly to some antidepressant drugs, such as desipramine (noradrenergic reuptake inhibitor), E2 decreased mRNA expression and density of α2 receptors (Karkanias *et al.*, 1997); it has been reported that chronic treatment with E2 reduces β adrenergic receptors response (Carlberg & Fregly, 1986).

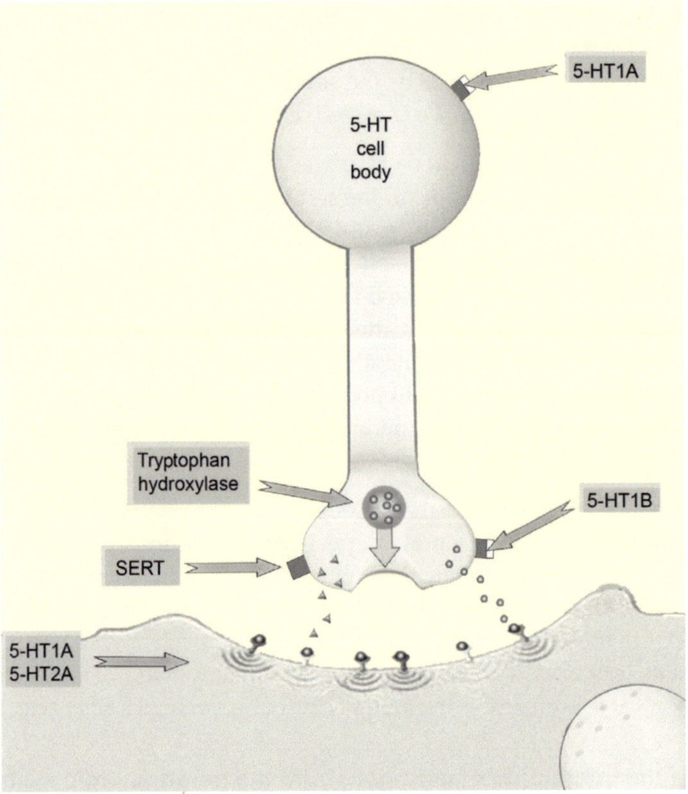

Fig. 1. Esquematic representation of proposed mechanism of action of estradiol's antidepressant-like actions on the serotonergic system in the forced swimming test (an animal model of depression). First, estradiol increases the activity of tryptophan hydroxylase and inhibits the serotonin transporter to induce an increase in serotonin levels in the synaptic clef. Second, estradiol could also induce a desensitization of 5-HT1A and 5-HT1B presynaptic receptors and modulate serotonin release and firing of serotonergic neurons; as a consequence, the increase of serotonin in the synaptic clef may activate 5-HT1A and 5-HT2A postsynaptic receptors and promote the activation of signal transduction pathways. SERT= serotonin transporter.

On the same research line, it has been suggested that EE2 interaction with the noradrenergic system may be mediated through α2 adrenergic receptors, since idazoxan, a selective antagonist of these receptors, is able to block the antidepressant-like effect of EE2 (López-Rubalcava *et al.*, 2007). In addition to these studies, recently we have found that the DSP4, a neurotoxin that selectively destroys noradrenergic nerve terminals in the locus coeruleus was able to blocked the antidepressant-like effects induced by EE2 in the FST (López-Rubalcava *et al.*, 2007). Together, these findings suggest that estrogen may facilitate the noradrenergic transmission by: 1) increasing NA synthesis, 2) by reducing NA reuptake, and by improving NA availability, or 3) through a mechanism involving both proposals.

5.3 Evidence of estrogens interactions with the dopaminergic system

The finding that some estrogens increase the activity of tyrosine-hydroxylase enzymes and inhibit the MAO-A activity may lead to the speculation that an increase in dopaminergic activity could mediate the antidepressant-like effect of estrogens. To our knowledge, there is no direct correlation between brain levels of dopamine or its metabolites and the antidepressant-like effect of these steroids. However, some preclinical reports indicates that agonist to ERα increase dopamine and DOPAC (dopamine metabolite) levels in the hippocampus and the frontal cortex (Lubbers *et al.*, 2010), areas involved in the effect of several antidepressant drugs. In fact, bupropion, a catecholamine enhancer, produces antidepressant-like actions in preclinical models (Reneric & Lucki, 1998; Dhir & Kulkarni, 2008; Bourin *et al.*, 2009).

Evidences in non-stressed animals also support the effect of estrogens on the dopaminergic system. For example, ovariectomy induces a decrease in D1 and D2 receptors density (Bosse & DiPaolo, 1996) which is reverse by 17β-estradiol chronic treatment (Bosse & DiPaolo, 1996; Landry *et al.*, 2002). In acute treatment, estradiol does not alter D2 receptors density but induces changes in the proportion of high to low affinity sites (Levesque & Di Paolo, 1993). In relation to the dopamine transporter (DAT), it has been shown that ovariectomy increases the DAT in the striatum, and this increase was reverted by estradiol chronic treatment (Attali *et al.*, 1997).

It has been reported that D1 and D2 receptor blockade may contribute to reduce negative effects derived from the Hypothalamus-Pituitary-adrenal axis (HPA) activation during stress response (Sullivan & Dufresne, 2006; Belda & Armario, 2009). For example, the administration of dopamine agonists in different brain areas resulted in the increase of plasma corticosterone levels (Ikemoto & Goeders, 1998), whereas the administration of antagonists to D1 and D2 receptors reduces the increase in plasma ACTH and corticosterone concentrations induced by stress (Belda & Armario, 2009). Thus, it is suggested that dopamine receptors are involved in the regulation of the stress response (Belda & Armario, 2009).

In addition, in transgenic mice with functional alterations of the HPA axis, the antidepressant treatment with FLX or amitryptiline corrected the increased binding on D1 and D2 receptors in the striatum and decreased dopamine transporter levels (Cyr *et al.*, 2001). Therefore, if estrogens are able to modulate dopamine receptors and DAT, it is possible that these effects contribute to explain their antidepressant-like effect. Supporting this assumption, a recent report in ovariectomized rats shows that chronic administration of SCH 23390 (D1 antagonist) plus E2 induces robust antidepressant-like actions in the FST (Fedotova & Ordyan, 2011). Additionally, in an experiment performed in male mice it was found that the blockage of D1 or

D2 receptors cancelled the antidepressant-like action of the acute administration of E2 (Dhir & Kulkarni, 2008). Consequently, the information about the specific participation of dopaminergic receptors in the antidepressant-like action of estrogens is yet controversial and need further exploration in order to establish any conclusion.

6. Proposed mechanism of action in the antidepressant-like effects of estrogens

As mentioned earlier, estrogens increases the activity of enzymes involved in the synthesis of 5-HT (tryptophan hydroxylase) and catecholamines (tyrosine hydroxylase and dopamine β-hydroxylase) at the same time that posses the ability to inhibit or decrease the activity of the serotonin and noradrenaline transporters in several brain areas. Interestingly, at the presynaptic terminal, estrogens can also activate the 5-HT1A/5-HT1B and α2-adrenoceptor that regulates the discharge and release of both NA and 5-HT. Together, these effects may contribute to increase the levels of monoamines in the synaptic clef and promote the activation of post-synaptic receptors such as 5-HT2A and β-adrenergic receptors as well as the activation or deactivation of several signal transduction pathways such as cAMP-PKA and IP3-PKC, among others. These signal transduction pathways may contribute to the activation of transcription factors like CREB and promote neuroplastic remodeling and/or neuroprotection processes (Bethea *et al.*, 2009) that could be effective in the development of strategies to cope with stress. Additionally, it has been reported that E2 administration decreases the activity of monoamine oxidase enzymes activity (type A and B) (involved in the degradation monoamines) in several areas of brain (Gundlah *et al.*, 2002).

Recently, it was shown that the monoaminergic neurotransmission is sensitive to modulation of estrogenic compounds, in this sense, the effects of estrogens on monoamine levels may be dependent of the type of estrogen receptor used; thus, ERα or ERβ agonists increases the levels of NA in the frontal cortex and hippocampus; similarly, ERα agonist increase the levels of the metabolites of NA and dopamine, 3-methoxy-4-hydroxyphenylglycol (MHPG) and DOPAC in hippocampus or frontal cortex; and ERβ agonist increase the levels of 5-HIIA in amygdala, hippocampus and ventral tegmental area (Lubbers *et al.*, 2010). It was shown that that the effects of estrogens on cathecolaminergic biosynthetic enzymes are due to the activation of estrogens receptors α and the serotonergic enzyme stimulation has been related with the activation of ER β (Donner & Handa, 2009; Serova *et al.*, 2010). Therefore, it is possible to considerer that the modulation of serotonergic and noradrenergic activity depends in part of the activation of ER. Based on this evidence, it seems possible that ERα are more related with the modulation of the catecholaminergic system, while ERβ with the serotonergic one; notwithstanding future studies are needed to confirm this hypothesis.

It is important to mention that participation of estrogens' membrane receptors in the modulation of monoamines activity needs to be further investigated. For example, it has been shown that the desensitization of 5-HT1A receptor induced by 17 β-estradiol in oxytocin cells of hypothalamus is independent of the activation of ERβ and may involve only the membrane estrogen receptor GPR30 (Rossi *et al.*, 2010); while the desensitization of the same receptors in the ACTH cells are depend of both GPR30 and ERβ (Rossi *et al.*, 2010). This evidence shows the complexity in the relationship between estrogens and monoamines.

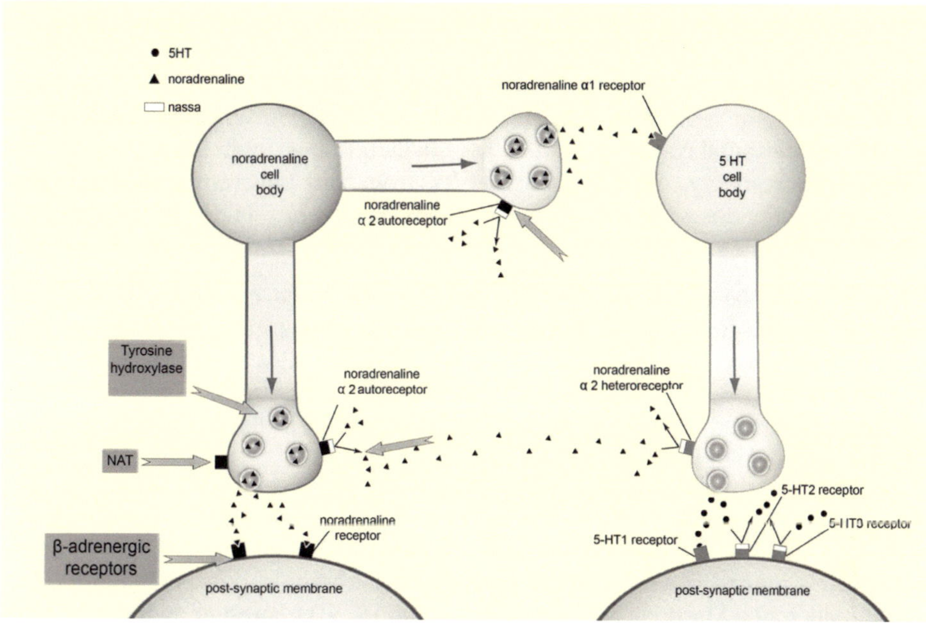

Fig. 2. Esquematic representation proposed for the mechanism of action of ethynyl estradiol's antidepressant-like actions on the noradrenergic and serotonergic systems in the forced swimming test (an animal model of depression). Ethynyl-estradiol increases tyrosine hydroxylase activity and simultaneously inhibits the noradrenergic transporter, facilitating the release of noradrenaline. Increases in NA concentration promote α2-autoadrenoceptors desensitization. In addition, estrogens activate α2-adrenoceptors located on the serotonergic terminals and, therefore, contribute to regulate serotonin release. NAT= Noradrenergic Transporter

7. Possible implications of estrogens actions on the modulation of monoamines activity

The modulation of noradrenergic and serotonergic systems by estrogens could have important physiological implications in the regulation of stress response. It has been reported that corticotrophin releasing factor (CRF) stimulates locus coeruleus activity under stressful situations and this is associated with a heightened arousal (Valentino & Van Bockstaele, 2008; Bangasser *et al.*, 2010). In this case, there is direct evidence that CRF genes expression is regulated by estrogens and that estradiol reduces plasma ACTH and blood pressure increases induced by restrain stress (Bangasser *et al.*, 2010). These responses occurred simultaneously to a differential modulation of cathecolamine biosynthetic enzymes gene expression in the nucleus of the solitary tract and the locus coeruleus (Serova *et al.*, 2005).

Recently, it was reported that an animal model of depression, the FST, increased corticosterone and estrogen plasma concentrations in adult females rats (Martinez-Mota *et al.*, 2011), suggesting that estrogens function as a compensatory mechanism against stress-response. Furthermore, estradiol administration prevented the increase in the percentage of discharge of the locus coeruleus induced by the FST in ovariectomized rats. As a result, it is possible to considerer that estrogens modulation of the noradrenergic system results in an increase expression of coping behaviors in the FST and in the regulation of HPA function. In addition, it has been reported that stress induced by the FST reduces 5-HT levels in the amygdala and lateral septum in male rats (Kirby *et al.*, 1995), while in females, 5-HT is reduced in the prefrontal cortex and in the hypothalamus, but not in the amygdala (Dalla *et al.*, 2005). Interestingly, unpublished results from our laboratory showed that E2 administration, previous to the FST, prevented the decline of 5-HT concentration in some brain areas during the FST and at the same time E2 induces an antidepressant-like effect.

Therefore it could be suggested that estrogenic compounds contribute to increase the serotonergic activity and simultaneously decrease noradrenergic activity, improving the behavioral strategies to cope with acute stressful situations. Also these protective actions of estrogens have been shown using animal models of chronic stress; in this case, estradiol administration reversed chronic stress-induced sensitization in the paraventricular nucleus and central amygdala of female rats (Gerrits *et al.*, 2006).

8. Acknowledgments

Authors wish to thank Mr. Raúl Cardoso for figure elaboration and Isabel Beltrán Villalobos and José Juan Cruz Martínez for technical assistance. The present work was partially supported by the following Grants: Conacyt-104654 for E E-C and Conacyt-155255 for C L-R.

9. References

Amsterdam, J., Garcia-Espana, F., Fawcett, J., Quitkin, F., Reimherr, F., Rosenbaum, J.&Beasley, C. (1999). Fluoxetine efficacy in menopausal women with and without estrogen replacement. *J Affect Disord* 55, 11-17. URL:http://www.ncbi.nlm.nih.gov/entrez/query.fcgi?cmd=Retrieve&db=PubMed&dopt=Citation&list_uids=10512601

Attali, G., Weizman, A., Gil-Ad, I.&Rehavi, M. (1997). Opposite modulatory effects of ovarian hormones on rat brain dopamine and serotonin transporters. *Brain Res* 756, 153-159. URL:http://www.ncbi.nlm.nih.gov/entrez/query.fcgi?cmd=Retrieve&db=PubMed&dopt=Citation&list_uids=9187326

Backstrom, T., Andreen, L., Birzniece, V., Bjorn, I., Johansson, I. M., Nordenstam-Haghjo, M., Nyberg, S., Sundstrom-Poromaa, I., Wahlstrom, G., Wang, M.&Zhu, D. (2003). The role of hormones and hormonal treatments in premenstrual syndrome. *CNS Drugs* 17, 325-342. URL:http://www.ncbi.nlm.nih.gov/entrez/query.fcgi?cmd=Retrieve&db=PubMed&dopt=Citation&list_uids=12665391

Bangasser, D. A., Curtis, A., Reyes, B. A., Bethea, T. T., Parastatidis, I., Ischiropoulos, H., Van Bockstaele, E. J.&Valentino, R. J. (2010). Sex differences in corticotropin-releasing factor receptor signaling and trafficking: potential role in female vulnerability to stress-related psychopathology. *Mol Psychiatry* 15, 877, 896-904. URL:http://www.ncbi.nlm.nih.gov/entrez/query.fcgi?cmd=Retrieve&db=PubMed&dopt=Citation&list_uids=20548297

Belda, X.&Armario, A. (2009). Dopamine D1 and D2 dopamine receptors regulate immobilization stress-induced activation of the hypothalamus-pituitary-adrenal axis. *Psychopharmacology (Berl)* 206, 355-365. URL:http://www.ncbi.nlm.nih.gov/entrez/query.fcgi?cmd=Retrieve&db=PubMed&dopt=Citation&list_uids=19621214

Bernardi, M., Vergoni, A. V., Sandrini, M., Tagliavini, S.&Bertolini, A. (1989). Influence of ovariectomy, estradiol and progesterone on the behavior of mice in an experimental model of depression. *Physiol Behav* 45, 1067-1068. URL:http://www.ncbi.nlm.nih.gov/entrez/query.fcgi?cmd=Retrieve&db=PubMed&dopt=Citation&list_uids=2780868

Bethea, C. L., Mirkes, S. J., Su, A.&Michelson, D. (2002). Effects of oral estrogen, raloxifene and arzoxifene on gene expression in serotonin neurons of macaques. *Psychoneuroendocrinology* 27, 431-445. URL:http://www.ncbi.nlm.nih.gov/entrez/query.fcgi?cmd=Retrieve&db=PubMed&dopt=Citation&list_uids=11911997

Bethea, C. L., Reddy, A. P., Tokuyama, Y., Henderson, J. A.&Lima, F. B. (2009). Protective actions of ovarian hormones in the serotonin system of macaques. *Front Neuroendocrinol* 30, 212-238. URL:http://www.ncbi.nlm.nih.gov/entrez/query.fcgi?cmd=Retrieve&db=PubMed&dopt=Citation&list_uids=19394356

Blum, I., Vered, Y., Lifshitz, A., Harel, D., Blum, M., Nordenberg, Y., Harsat, A., Sulkes, J., Gabbay, U.&Graff, E. (1996). The effect of estrogen replacement therapy on plasma serotonin and catecholamines of postmenopausal women. *Isr J Med Sci* 32, 1158-1162. URL:http://www.ncbi.nlm.nih.gov/entrez/query.fcgi?cmd=Retrieve&db=PubMed&dopt=Citation&list_uids=9007144

Bosse, R.&DiPaolo, T. (1996). The modulation of brain dopamine and GABAA receptors by estradiol: a clue for CNS changes occurring at menopause. *Cell Mol Neurobiol* 16, 199-212. URL:http://www.ncbi.nlm.nih.gov/entrez/query.fcgi?cmd=Retrieve&db=PubMed&dopt=Citation&list_uids=8743969

Bourin, M., Chenu, F., Prica, C.&Hascoet, M. (2009). Augmentation effect of combination therapy of aripiprazole and antidepressants on forced swimming test in mice. *Psychopharmacology (Berl)* 206, 97-107. URL:http://www.ncbi.nlm.nih.gov/entrez/query.fcgi?cmd=Retrieve&db=PubMed&dopt=Citation&list_uids=19517098

Bukulmez, O., Al, A., Gurdal, H., Yarali, H., Ulug, B.&Gurgan, T. (2001). Short-term effects of three continuous hormone replacement therapy regimens on platelet tritiated imipramine binding and mood scores: a prospective randomized trial. *Fertil Steril* 75, 737-743. URL:http://www.ncbi.nlm.nih.gov/entrez/query.fcgi?cmd=Retrieve&db=PubMed&dopt=Citation&list_uids=11287028

Carlberg, K. A.&Fregly, M. J. (1986). Catecholamine excretion and beta-adrenergic responsiveness in estrogen-treated rats. *Pharmacology* 32, 147-156. URL:http://www.ncbi.nlm.nih.gov/entrez/query.fcgi?cmd=Retrieve&db=PubMed&dopt=Citation&list_uids=3008199

Contreras, C. M., Azamar-Arizmendi, G., Saavedra, M.&Hernandez-Lozano, M. (2006). A five-day gradual reduction regimen of chlormadinone reduces premenstrual anxiety and depression: a pilot study. *Arch Med Res* 37, 907-913. URL:http://www.ncbi.nlm.nih.gov/entrez/query.fcgi?cmd=Retrieve&db=PubMed&dopt=Citation&list_uids=16971235

Coope, J. (1975). The post-hysterectomy syndrome. *Nurs Times* 71, 1285-1286. . http://www.ncbi.nlm.nih.gov/entrez/query.fcgi?cmd=Retrieve&db=PubMed&dopt=Citation&list_uids=1144136

Cryan, J. F., Valentino, R. J.&Lucki, I. (2005). Assessing substrates underlying the behavioral effects of antidepressants using the modified rat forced swimming test. *Neurosci Biobehav Rev* 29, 547-569. URL:http://www.ncbi.nlm.nih.gov/entrez/query.fcgi?cmd=Retrieve&db=PubMed&dopt=Citation&list_uids=15893822

Cyr, M., Morissette, M., Barden, N., Beaulieu, S., Rochford, J.&Di Paolo, T. (2001). Dopaminergic activity in transgenic mice underexpressing glucocorticoid receptors: effect of antidepressants. *Neuroscience* 102, 151-158. URL:http://www.ncbi.nlm.nih.gov/entrez/query.fcgi?cmd=Retrieve&db=PubMed&dopt=Citation&list_uids=11226678

Chang, A. S.&Chang, S. M. (1999). Nongenomic steroidal modulation of high-affinity serotonin transport. *Biochim Biophys Acta* 1417, 157-166. URL:http://www.ncbi.nlm.nih.gov/entrez/query.fcgi?cmd=Retrieve&db=PubMed&dopt=Citation&list_uids=10076044

Dalla, C., Antoniou, K., Drossopoulou, G., Xagoraris, M., Kokras, N., Sfikakis, A.&Papadopoulou-Daifoti, Z. (2005). Chronic mild stress impact: are females more vulnerable? *Neuroscience* 135, 703-714. URL:http://www.ncbi.nlm.nih.gov/entrez/query.fcgi?cmd=Retrieve&db=PubMed&dopt=Citation&list_uids=16125862

Dennis, M. K., Burai, R., Ramesh, C., Petrie, W. K., Alcon, S. N., Nayak, T. K., Bologa, C. G., Leitao, A., Brailoiu, E., Deliu, E., Dun, N. J., Sklar, L. A., Hathaway, H. J., Arterburn, J. B., Oprea, T. I.&Prossnitz, E. R. (2009). In vivo effects of a GPR30 antagonist. *Nat Chem Biol* 5, 421-427. URL:http://www.ncbi.nlm.nih.gov/entrez/query.fcgi?cmd=Retrieve&db=PubMed&dopt=Citation&list_uids=19430488

Dhir, A.&Kulkarni, S. K. (2008). Possible involvement of sigma-1 receptors in the anti-immobility action of bupropion, a dopamine reuptake inhibitor. *Fundam Clin Pharmacol* 22, 387-394. URL:http://www.ncbi.nlm.nih.gov/entrez/query.fcgi?cmd=Retrieve&db=PubMed&dopt=Citation&list_uids=18705749

Donner, N.&Handa, R. J. (2009). Estrogen receptor beta regulates the expression of tryptophan-hydroxylase 2 mRNA within serotonergic neurons of the rat dorsal raphe nuclei. *Neuroscience* 163, 705-718. URL:http://www.ncbi.nlm.nih.gov/entrez/query.fcgi?cmd=Retrieve&db=PubMed&dopt=Citation&list_uids=19559077

Estrada-Camarena, E., Fernandez-Guasti, A.&Lopez-Rubalcava, C. (2003). Antidepressant-like effect of different estrogenic compounds in the forced swimming test. *Neuropsychopharmacology* 28, 830-838.

http://www.ncbi.nlm.nih.gov/entrez/query.fcgi?cmd=Retrieve&db=PubMed&dopt=Citation&list_uids=12637949

Estrada-Camarena, E., Fernandez-Guasti, A.&Lopez-Rubalcava, C. (2006a). Participation of the 5-HT1A receptor in the antidepressant-like effect of estrogens in the forced swimming test. *Neuropsychopharmacology* 31, 247-255. URL:http://www.ncbi.nlm.nih.gov/entrez/query.fcgi?cmd=Retrieve&db=PubMed&dopt=Citation&list_uids=16012533

Estrada-Camarena, E., Lopez-Rubalcava, C.&Fernandez-Guasti, A. (2006b). Facilitating antidepressant-like actions of estrogens are mediated by 5-HT1A and estrogen receptors in the rat forced swimming test. *Psychoneuroendocrinology* 31, 905-914. URL:http://www.ncbi.nlm.nih.gov/entrez/query.fcgi?cmd=Retrieve&db=PubMed&dopt=Citation&list_uids=16843610

Estrada-Camarena, E., Lopez-Rubalcava, C., Hernandez-Aragon, A., Mejia-Mauries, S.&Picazo, O. (2011). Long-term ovariectomy modulates the antidepressant-like action of estrogens, but not of antidepressants. *J Psychopharmacol.* URL:http://www.ncbi.nlm.nih.gov/entrez/query.fcgi?cmd=Retrieve&db=PubMed&dopt=Citation&list_uids=21890587

Estrada-Camarena, E., Lopez-Rubalcava, C., Vega-Rivera, N., Recamier-Carballo, S.&Fernandez-Guasti, A. (2010). Antidepressant effects of estrogens: a basic approximation. *Behav Pharmacol* 21, 451-464. URL:http://www.ncbi.nlm.nih.gov/entrez/query.fcgi?cmd=Retrieve&db=PubMed&dopt=Citation&list_uids=20700047

Fedotova, J.&Ordyan, N. (2011). Involvement of D1 receptors in depression-like behavior of ovariectomized rats. *Acta Physiol Hung* 98, 165-176. URL:http://www.ncbi.nlm.nih.gov/entrez/query.fcgi?cmd=Retrieve&db=PubMed&dopt=Citation&list_uids=21616775

Filardo, E. J., Quinn, J. A., Frackelton, A. R., Jr.&Bland, K. I. (2002). Estrogen action via the G protein-coupled receptor, GPR30: stimulation of adenylyl cyclase and cAMP-mediated attenuation of the epidermal growth factor receptor-to-MAPK signaling axis. *Mol Endocrinol* 16, 70-84. URL:http://www.ncbi.nlm.nih.gov/entrez/query.fcgi?cmd=Retrieve&db=PubMed&dopt=Citation&list_uids=11773440

Freeman, E. W., Sammel, M. D., Lin, H.&Nelson, D. B. (2006). Associations of hormones and menopausal status with depressed mood in women with no history of depression. *Arch Gen Psychiatry* 63, 375-382. URL:http://www.ncbi.nlm.nih.gov/entrez/query.fcgi?cmd=Retrieve&db=PubMed&dopt=Citation&list_uids=16585466

Galea, L. A., Lee, T. T., Kostaras, X., Sidhu, J. A.&Barr, A. M. (2002). High levels of estradiol impair spatial performance in the Morris water maze and increase 'depressive-like' behaviors in the female meadow vole. *Physiol Behav* 77, 217-225. URL:http://www.ncbi.nlm.nih.gov/entrez/query.fcgi?cmd=Retrieve&db=PubMed&dopt=Citation&list_uids=12419397

Gerrits, M., Bakker, P. L., Koch, T.&Ter Horst, G. J. (2006). Stress-induced sensitization of the limbic system in ovariectomized rats is partly restored by cyclic 17beta-estradiol administration. *Eur J Neurosci* 23, 1747-1756.

URL:http://www.ncbi.nlm.nih.gov/entrez/query.fcgi?cmd=Retrieve&db=PubMed&dopt=Citation&list_uids=16623831

Ghraf, R., Michel, M., Hiemke, C.&Knuppen, R. (1983). Competition by monophenolic estrogens and catecholestrogens for high-affinity uptake of [3H](-)-norepinephrine into synaptosomes from rat cerebral cortex and hypothalamus. *Brain Res* 277, 163-168. URL:http://www.ncbi.nlm.nih.gov/entrez/query.fcgi?cmd=Retrieve&db=PubMed&dopt=Citation&list_uids=6315138

Girdler, S. S.&Klatzkin, R. (2007). Neurosteroids in the context of stress: implications for depressive disorders. *Pharmacol Ther* 116, 125-139. URL:http://www.ncbi.nlm.nih.gov/entrez/query.fcgi?cmd=Retrieve&db=PubMed&dopt=Citation&list_uids=17597217

Gundlah, C., Lu, N. Z.&Bethea, C. L. (2002). Ovarian steroid regulation of monoamine oxidase-A and -B mRNAs in the macaque dorsal raphe and hypothalamic nuclei. *Psychopharmacology (Berl)* 160, 271-282. URL:http://www.ncbi.nlm.nih.gov/entrez/query.fcgi?cmd=Retrieve&db=PubMed&dopt=Citation&list_uids=11889496

Halbreich, U.&Kahn, L. S. (2001). Role of estrogen in the aetiology and treatment of mood disorders. *CNS Drugs* 15, 797-817. URL:http://www.ncbi.nlm.nih.gov/entrez/query.fcgi?cmd=Retrieve&db=PubMed&dopt=Citation&list_uids=11602005

Harlow, B. L., Wise, L. A., Otto, M. W., Soares, C. N.&Cohen, L. S. (2003). Depression and its influence on reproductive endocrine and menstrual cycle markers associated with perimenopause: the Harvard Study of Moods and Cycles. *Arch Gen Psychiatry* 60, 29-36. URL:http://www.ncbi.nlm.nih.gov/entrez/query.fcgi?cmd=Retrieve&db=PubMed&dopt=Citation&list_uids=12511170

Hiemke, C., Bruder, D., Poetz, B.&Ghraf, R. (1985). Sex-specific effects of estradiol on hypothalamic noradrenaline turnover in gonadectomized rats. *Exp Brain Res* 59, 68-72. URL:http://www.ncbi.nlm.nih.gov/entrez/query.fcgi?cmd=Retrieve&db=PubMed&dopt=Citation&list_uids=4018199

Hiroi, R.&Neumaier, J. F. (2009). Estrogen decreases 5-HT1B autoreceptor mRNA in selective subregion of rat dorsal raphe nucleus: inverse association between gene expression and anxiety behavior in the open field. *Neuroscience* 158, 456-464. URL:http://www.ncbi.nlm.nih.gov/entrez/query.fcgi?cmd=Retrieve&db=PubMed&dopt=Citation&list_uids=19049819

Holmes, P. V. (2003). Rodent models of depression: reexamining validity without anthropomorphic inference. *Crit Rev Neurobiol* 15, 143-174. URL:http://www.ncbi.nlm.nih.gov/entrez/query.fcgi?cmd=Retrieve&db=PubMed&dopt=Citation&list_uids=14977368

Holschneider, D. P., Kumazawa, T., Chen, K.&Shih, J. C. (1998). Tissue-specific effects of estrogen on monoamine oxidase A and B in the rat. *Life Sci* 63, 155-160. URL:http://www.ncbi.nlm.nih.gov/entrez/query.fcgi?cmd=Retrieve&db=PubMed&dopt=Citation&list_uids=9698044

Ikemoto, S.&Goeders, N. E. (1998). Microinjections of dopamine agonists and cocaine elevate plasma corticosterone: dissociation effects among the ventral and dorsal striatum and medial prefrontal cortex. *Brain Res* 814, 171-178. URL:http://www.ncbi.nlm.nih.gov/entrez/query.fcgi?cmd=Retrieve&db=PubMed&dopt=Citation&list_uids=9838097

Jensvold, M. (1996). Non-pregnant reproductive-age women. Part II: exogenous sex steroid hormones and psychopharmacology. In: *Psychopharmacology and woman: Sex, gender and hormones*, Jensvold, M., Halbreich, U.&Hamilton, J. (eds), pp 170-190. URL: Washington, DC: American Psychiatric Press.

Joffe, H., Groninger, H., Soares, C. N., Nonacs, R.&Cohen, L. S. (2001). An open trial of mirtazapine in menopausal women with depression unresponsive to estrogen replacement therapy. *J Womens Health Gend Based Med* 10, 999-1004. URL:http://www.ncbi.nlm.nih.gov/entrez/query.fcgi?cmd=Retrieve&db=PubMed&dopt=Citation&list_uids=11788110

Kaba, H., Saito, H., Otsuka, K., Seto, K.&Kawakami, M. (1983). Effects of estrogen on the excitability of neurons projecting from the noradrenergic A1 region to the preoptic and anterior hypothalamic area. *Brain Res* 274, 156-159. URL:http://www.ncbi.nlm.nih.gov/entrez/query.fcgi?cmd=Retrieve&db=PubMed&dopt=Citation&list_uids=6412965

Kalia, M. (2005). Neurobiological basis of depression: an update. *Metabolism* 54, 24-27. URL:http://www.ncbi.nlm.nih.gov/entrez/query.fcgi?cmd=Retrieve&db=PubMed&dopt=Citation&list_uids=15877309

Karkanias, G. B., Li, C. S.&Etgen, A. M. (1997). Estradiol reduction of alpha 2-adrenoceptor binding in female rat cortex is correlated with decreases in alpha 2A/D-adrenoceptor messenger RNA. *Neuroscience* 81, 593-597. URL:http://www.ncbi.nlm.nih.gov/entrez/query.fcgi?cmd=Retrieve&db=PubMed&dopt=Citation&list_uids=9316013

Kirby, L. G., Allen, A. R.&Lucki, I. (1995). Regional differences in the effects of forced swimming on extracellular levels of 5-hydroxytryptamine and 5-hydroxyindoleacetic acid. *Brain Res* 682, 189-196. URL:http://www.ncbi.nlm.nih.gov/entrez/query.fcgi?cmd=Retrieve&db=PubMed&dopt=Citation&list_uids=7552310

Krishnan, V.&Nestler, E. J. (2008). The molecular neurobiology of depression. *Nature* 455, 894-902. URL:http://www.ncbi.nlm.nih.gov/entrez/query.fcgi?cmd=Retrieve&db=PubMed&dopt=Citation&list_uids=18923511

Kuiper, G. G.&Gustafsson, J. A. (1997). The novel estrogen receptor-beta subtype: potential role in the cell- and promoter-specific actions of estrogens and anti-estrogens. *FEBS Lett* 410, 87-90. URL:http://www.ncbi.nlm.nih.gov/entrez/query.fcgi?cmd=Retrieve&db=PubMed&dopt=Citation&list_uids=9247129

Landry, M., Levesque, D.&Di Paolo, T. (2002). Estrogenic properties of raloxifene, but not tamoxifen, on D2 and D3 dopamine receptors in the rat forebrain. *Neuroendocrinology* 76, 214-222. URL:http://www.ncbi.nlm.nih.gov/entrez/query.fcgi?cmd=Retrieve&db=PubMed&dopt=Citation&list_uids=12411738

Levesque, D.&Di Paolo, T. (1993). Modulation by estradiol and progesterone of the GTP effect on striatal D-2 dopamine receptors. *Biochem Pharmacol* 45, 723-733. URL:http://www.ncbi.nlm.nih.gov/entrez/query.fcgi?cmd=Retrieve&db=PubMed&dopt=Citation&list_uids=8095140

Lopez-Jaramillo, P., Teran, E., Molina, G., Rivera, J.&Lozano, A. (1996). Oestrogens and depression. *Lancet* 348, 135-136. URL:http://www.ncbi.nlm.nih.gov/entrez/query.fcgi?cmd=Retrieve&db=PubMed&dopt=Citation&list_uids=8676707

Lopez-Muñoz, F.&Alamo, C. (2009). Monoaminergic neurotransmission: the history of the discovery of antidepressants from 1950s until today. *Curr Pharm Des* 15, 1563-1586. URL:http://www.ncbi.nlm.nih.gov/entrez/query.fcgi?cmd=Retrieve&db=PubMed&dopt=Citation&list_uids=19442174

López-Rubalcava, C., Oikawa-Sala, J., Chávez-Álvarez, K.&Estrada-Camarena, E. (2005) Analysis of the participation of the serotonergic system in the antidepressant-like action of 17beta -estradiol in the forced swimming test (fst): presynaptic or postsynaptic actions. In: *Society for Neuroscience*, p No. 567.512. Washington, DC.

López-Rubalcava, C., Vega Rivera, N., Cruz-Martínez, J. J. &Estrada-Camarena, E. (2007) Participation of both estrogen and alpha2-adrenergic receptors, in the antidepressant-like actions of ethynil-estradiol in rats tested in the forced swimming test. In: *12th Biennial meeting of the European Behavioral Pharmacology Society*.

López-Rubalcva, C., Mostalac-Preciado, C.&Estrada-Camarena, E. (2009). The rat forced swimming test: an animal model for the study of the antidepressant drugs. In: *Models of Neuropharmacology*, Rocha, L. & Granados, V. (eds): Transworld Res Network.

Lu, N. Z.&Bethea, C. L. (2002). Ovarian steroid regulation of 5-HT1A receptor binding and G protein activation in female monkeys. *Neuropsychopharmacology* 27, 12-24. URL:http://www.ncbi.nlm.nih.gov/entrez/query.fcgi?cmd=Retrieve&db=PubMed&dopt=Citation&list_uids=12062903

Lu, N. Z., Shlaes, T. A., Gundlah, C., Dziennis, S. E., Lyle, R. E.&Bethea, C. L. (1999). Ovarian steroid action on tryptophan hydroxylase protein and serotonin compared to localization of ovarian steroid receptors in midbrain of guinea pigs. *Endocrine* 11, 257-267. URL:http://www.ncbi.nlm.nih.gov/entrez/query.fcgi?cmd=Retrieve&db=PubMed&dopt=Citation&list_uids=10786822

Lubbers, L. S., Zafian, P. T., Gautreaux, C., Gordon, M., Alves, S. E., Correa, L., Lorrain, D. S., Hickey, G. J.&Luine, V. (2010). Estrogen receptor (ER) subtype agonists alter monoamine levels in the female rat brain. *J Steroid Biochem Mol Biol* 122, 310-317. URL:http://www.ncbi.nlm.nih.gov/entrez/query.fcgi?cmd=Retrieve&db=PubMed&dopt=Citation&list_uids=20800684

Maletic, V., Robinson, M., Oakes, T., Iyengar, S., Ball, S. G.&Russell, J. (2007). Neurobiology of depression: an integrated view of key findings. *Int J Clin Pract* 61, 2030-2040. URL:http://www.ncbi.nlm.nih.gov/entrez/query.fcgi?cmd=Retrieve&db=PubMed&dopt=Citation&list_uids=17944926

Margeat, E., Bourdoncle, A., Margueron, R., Poujol, N., Cavailles, V.&Royer, C. (2003). Ligands differentially modulate the protein interactions of the human estrogen receptors alpha and beta. *J Mol Biol* 326, 77-92.
URL:http://www.ncbi.nlm.nih.gov/entrez/query.fcgi?cmd=Retrieve&db=PubMed&dopt=Citation&list_uids=12547192

Markou, A., Chiamulera, C., Geyer, M. A., Tricklebank, M.&Steckler, T. (2009). Removing obstacles in neuroscience drug discovery: the future path for animal models. *Neuropsychopharmacology* 34, 74-89.
URL:http://www.ncbi.nlm.nih.gov/entrez/query.fcgi?cmd=Retrieve&db=PubMed&dopt=Citation&list_uids=18830240

Martinez-Mota, L., Ulloa, R. E., Herrera-Perez, J., Chavira, R.&Fernandez-Guasti, A. (2011). Sex and age differences in the impact of the forced swimming test on the levels of steroid hormones. *Physiol Behav* 104, 900-905.
URL:http://www.ncbi.nlm.nih.gov/entrez/query.fcgi?cmd=Retrieve&db=PubMed&dopt=Citation&list_uids=21658399

McEwen, B. S. (1999). Clinical review 108: The molecular and neuroanatomical basis for estrogen effects in the central nervous system. *J Clin Endocrinol Metab* 84, 1790-1797.
URL:http://www.ncbi.nlm.nih.gov/entrez/query.fcgi?cmd=Retrieve&db=PubMed&dopt=Citation&list_uids=10372665

Mendelson, S. D., McKittrick, C. R.&McEwen, B. S. (1993). Autoradiographic analyses of the effects of estradiol benzoate on [3H]paroxetine binding in the cerebral cortex and dorsal hippocampus of gonadectomized male and female rats. *Brain Res* 601, 299-302.
URL:http://www.ncbi.nlm.nih.gov/entrez/query.fcgi?cmd=Retrieve&db=PubMed&dopt=Citation&list_uids=8431776

Mize, A. L.&Alper, R. H. (2000). Acute and long-term effects of 17beta-estradiol on G(i/o) coupled neurotransmitter receptor function in the female rat brain as assessed by agonist-stimulated [35S]GTPgammaS binding. *Brain Res* 859, 326-333.
URL:http://www.ncbi.nlm.nih.gov/entrez/query.fcgi?cmd=Retrieve&db=PubMed&dopt=Citation&list_uids=10719081

Mize, A. L.&Alper, R. H. (2002). Rapid uncoupling of serotonin-1A receptors in rat hippocampus by 17beta-estradiol in vitro requires protein kinases A and C. *Neuroendocrinology* 76, 339-347.
URL:http://www.ncbi.nlm.nih.gov/entrez/query.fcgi?cmd=Retrieve&db=PubMed&dopt=Citation&list_uids=12566941

Mize, A. L., Poisner, A. M.&Alper, R. H. (2001). Estrogens act in rat hippocampus and frontal cortex to produce rapid, receptor-mediated decreases in serotonin 5-HT(1A) receptor function. *Neuroendocrinology* 73, 166-174.
URL:http://www.ncbi.nlm.nih.gov/entrez/query.fcgi?cmd=Retrieve&db=PubMed&dopt=Citation&list_uids=11307035

Monje, P.&Boland, R. (2001). Subcellular distribution of native estrogen receptor alpha and beta isoforms in rabbit uterus and ovary. *J Cell Biochem* 82, 467-479.
URL:http://www.ncbi.nlm.nih.gov/entrez/query.fcgi?cmd=Retrieve&db=PubMed&dopt=Citation&list_uids=11500923

Montgomery, J. C., Appleby, L., Brincat, M., Versi, E., Tapp, A., Fenwick, P. B.&Studd, J. W. (1987). Effect of oestrogen and testosterone implants on psychological disorders in the climacteric. *Lancet* 1, 297-299. URL:http://www.ncbi.nlm.nih.gov/entrez/query.fcgi?cmd=Retrieve&db=PubMed&dopt=Citation&list_uids=2880114

Morgan, M. L., Cook, I. A., Rapkin, A. J.&Leuchter, A. F. (2005). Estrogen augmentation of antidepressants in perimenopausal depression: a pilot study. *J Clin Psychiatry* 66, 774-780. URL:http://www.ncbi.nlm.nih.gov/entrez/query.fcgi?cmd=Retrieve&db=PubMed&dopt=Citation&list_uids=15960574

Mori-Okamoto, J., Otawara-Hamamoto, Y., Yamato, H.&Yoshimura, H. (2004). Pomegranate extract improves a depressive state and bone properties in menopausal syndrome model ovariectomized mice. *J Ethnopharmacol* 92, 93-101. http://www.ncbi.nlm.nih.gov/entrez/query.fcgi?cmd=Retrieve&db=PubMed&dopt=Citation&list_uids=15099854

Morrison, M. F., Kallan, M. J., Ten Have, T., Katz, I., Tweedy, K.&Battistini, M. (2004). Lack of efficacy of estradiol for depression in postmenopausal women: a randomized, controlled trial. *Biol Psychiatry* 55, 406-412. http://www.ncbi.nlm.nih.gov/entrez/query.fcgi?cmd=Retrieve&db=PubMed&dopt=Citation&list_uids=14960294

O'Keane, V., O'Hanlon, M., Webb, M.&Dinan, T. (1991). d-fenfluramine/prolactin response throughout the menstrual cycle: evidence for an oestrogen-induced alteration. *Clin Endocrinol (Oxf)* 34, 289-292. URL:http://www.ncbi.nlm.nih.gov/entrez/query.fcgi?cmd=Retrieve&db=PubMed&dopt=Citation&list_uids=1879060

Okada, M., Hayashi, N., Kometani, M., Nakao, K.&Inukai, T. (1997). Influences of ovariectomy and continuous replacement of 17beta-estradiol on the tail skin temperature and behavior in the forced swimming test in rats. *Jpn J Pharmacol* 73, 93-96. URL:http://www.ncbi.nlm.nih.gov/entrez/query.fcgi?cmd=Retrieve&db=PubMed&dopt=Citation&list_uids=9032138

Osterlund, M. K. (2009). Underlying mechanisms mediating the antidepressant effects of estrogens. *Biochim Biophys Acta* 1800, 1136-1144. URL:http://www.ncbi.nlm.nih.gov/entrez/query.fcgi?cmd=Retrieve&db=PubMed&dopt=Citation&list_uids=19900508

Osterlund, M. K.&Hurd, Y. L. (1998). Acute 17 beta-estradiol treatment down-regulates serotonin 5HT1A receptor mRNA expression in the limbic system of female rats. *Brain Res Mol Brain Res* 55, 169-172. URL:http://www.ncbi.nlm.nih.gov/entrez/query.fcgi?cmd=Retrieve&db=PubMed&dopt=Citation&list_uids=9645972

Pae, C. U., Tharwani, H., Marks, D. M., Masand, P. S.&Patkar, A. A. (2009). Atypical depression: a comprehensive review. *CNS Drugs* 23, 1023-1037. URL:http://www.ncbi.nlm.nih.gov/entrez/query.fcgi?cmd=Retrieve&db=PubMed&dopt=Citation&list_uids=19958040

Payne, J. L., Roy, P. S., Murphy-Eberenz, K., Weismann, M. M., Swartz, K. L., McInnis, M. G., Nwulia, E., Mondimore, F. M., MacKinnon, D. F., Miller, E. B., Nurnberger, J. I.,

Levinson, D. F., DePaulo, J. R., Jr.&Potash, J. B. (2007). Reproductive cycle-associated mood symptoms in women with major depression and bipolar disorder. *J Affect Disord* 99, 221-229.
URL:http://www.ncbi.nlm.nih.gov/entrez/query.fcgi?cmd=Retrieve&db=PubMed&dopt=Citation&list_uids=17011632

Raap, D. K., DonCarlos, L., Garcia, F., Muma, N. A., Wolf, W. A., Battaglia, G.&Van de Kar, L. D. (2000). Estrogen desensitizes 5-HT(1A) receptors and reduces levels of G(z), G(i1) and G(i3) proteins in the hypothalamus. *Neuropharmacology* 39, 1823-1832.
URL:http://www.ncbi.nlm.nih.gov/entrez/query.fcgi?cmd=Retrieve&db=PubMed&dopt=Citation&list_uids=10884563

Rachman, I. M., Unnerstall, J. R., Pfaff, D. W.&Cohen, R. S. (1998). Estrogen alters behavior and forebrain c-fos expression in ovariectomized rats subjected to the forced swim test. *Proc Natl Acad Sci U S A* 95, 13941-13946.
URL:http://www.ncbi.nlm.nih.gov/entrez/query.fcgi?cmd=Retrieve&db=PubMed&dopt=Citation&list_uids=9811905

Rajewska, J.&Rybakowski, J. K. (2003). Depression in premenopausal women: gonadal hormones and serotonergic system assessed by D-fenfluramine challenge test. *Prog Neuropsychopharmacol Biol Psychiatry* 27, 705-709.
URL:http://www.ncbi.nlm.nih.gov/entrez/query.fcgi?cmd=Retrieve&db=PubMed&dopt=Citation&list_uids=12787860

Rasgon, N. L., Altshuler, L. L., Fairbanks, L. A., Dunkin, J. J., Davtyan, C., Elman, S.&Rapkin, A. J. (2002). Estrogen replacement therapy in the treatment of major depressive disorder in perimenopausal women. *J Clin Psychiatry* 63 Suppl 7, 45-48.
URL:http://www.ncbi.nlm.nih.gov/entrez/query.fcgi?cmd=Retrieve&db=PubMed&dopt=Citation&list_uids=11995778

Reneric, J. P.&Lucki, I. (1998). Antidepressant behavioral effects by dual inhibition of monoamine reuptake in the rat forced swimming test. *Psychopharmacology (Berl)* 136, 190-197.
URL:http://www.ncbi.nlm.nih.gov/entrez/query.fcgi?cmd=Retrieve&db=PubMed&dopt=Citation&list_uids=9551776

Richards, M., Rubinow, D. R., Daly, R. C.&Schmidt, P. J. (2006). Premenstrual symptoms and perimenopausal depression. *Am J Psychiatry* 163, 133-137.
URL:http://www.ncbi.nlm.nih.gov/entrez/query.fcgi?cmd=Retrieve&db=PubMed&dopt=Citation&list_uids=16390900

Riecher-Rossler, A.&Geyter, C. (2007). The forthcoming role of treatment with oestrogens in mental health. *Swiss Med Wkly* 137, 565-572.

Rocca, W. A., Grossardt, B. R.&Shuster, L. T. (2010). Oophorectomy, menopause, estrogen, and cognitive aging: the timing hypothesis. *Neurodegener Dis* 7, 163-166.
URL:http://www.ncbi.nlm.nih.gov/entrez/query.fcgi?cmd=Retrieve&db=PubMed&dopt=Citation&list_uids=20197698

Romano-Torres, M.&Fernandez-Guasti, A. (2010). Estradiol valerate elicits antidepressant-like effects in middle-aged female rats under chronic mild stress. *Behav Pharmacol* 21, 104-111.
URL:http://www.ncbi.nlm.nih.gov/entrez/query.fcgi?cmd=Retrieve&db=PubMed&dopt=Citation&list_uids=20168212

Rossi, D. V., Dai, Y., Thomas, P., Carrasco, G. A., DonCarlos, L. L., Muma, N. A.&Li, Q. (2010). Estradiol-induced desensitization of 5-HT1A receptor signaling in the paraventricular nucleus of the hypothalamus is independent of estrogen receptor-beta. *Psychoneuroendocrinology* 35, 1023-1033. URL:http://www.ncbi.nlm.nih.gov/entrez/query.fcgi?cmd=Retrieve&db=PubMed&dopt=Citation&list_uids=20138435

Saletu, B., Brandstatter, N., Metka, M., Stamenkovic, M., Anderer, P., Semlitsch, H. V., Heytmanek, G., Huber, J., Grunberger, J., Linzmayer, L.&et al. (1995). Double-blind, placebo-controlled, hormonal, syndromal and EEG mapping studies with transdermal oestradiol therapy in menopausal depression. *Psychopharmacology (Berl)* 122, 321-329. URL:http://www.ncbi.nlm.nih.gov/entrez/query.fcgi?cmd=Retrieve&db=PubMed&dopt=Citation&list_uids=8657828

Schmidt, P. J., Nieman, L., Danaceau, M. A., Tobin, M. B., Roca, C. A., Murphy, J. H.&Rubinow, D. R. (2000). Estrogen replacement in perimenopause-related depression: a preliminary report. *Am J Obstet Gynecol* 183, 414-420. URL:http://www.ncbi.nlm.nih.gov/entrez/query.fcgi?cmd=Retrieve&db=PubMed&dopt=Citation&list_uids=10942479

Schneider, L. S., Small, G. W.&Clary, C. M. (2001). Estrogen replacement therapy and antidepressant response to sertraline in older depressed women. *Am J Geriatr Psychiatry* 9, 393-399. URL:http://www.ncbi.nlm.nih.gov/entrez/query.fcgi?cmd=Retrieve&db=PubMed&dopt=Citation&list_uids=11739065

Schneider, L. S., Small, G. W., Hamilton, S. H., Bystritsky, A., Nemeroff, C. B.&Meyers, B. S. (1997). Estrogen replacement and response to fluoxetine in a multicenter geriatric depression trial. Fluoxetine Collaborative Study Group. *Am J Geriatr Psychiatry* 5, 97-106. URL:http://www.ncbi.nlm.nih.gov/entrez/query.fcgi?cmd=Retrieve&db=PubMed&dopt=Citation&list_uids=9106373

Serova, L., Rivkin, M., Nakashima, A.&Sabban, E. L. (2002). Estradiol stimulates gene expression of norepinephrine biosynthetic enzymes in rat locus coeruleus. *Neuroendocrinology* 75, 193-200. URL:http://www.ncbi.nlm.nih.gov/entrez/query.fcgi?cmd=Retrieve&db=PubMed&dopt=Citation&list_uids=11914591

Serova, L. I., Harris, H. A., Maharjan, S.&Sabban, E. L. (2010). Modulation of responses to stress by estradiol benzoate and selective estrogen receptor agonists. *J Endocrinol* 205, 253-262. URL:http://www.ncbi.nlm.nih.gov/entrez/query.fcgi?cmd=Retrieve&db=PubMed&dopt=Citation&list_uids=20348154

Serova, L. I., Maharjan, S.&Sabban, E. L. (2005). Estrogen modifies stress response of catecholamine biosynthetic enzyme genes and cardiovascular system in ovariectomized female rats. *Neuroscience* 132, 249-259. URL:http://www.ncbi.nlm.nih.gov/entrez/query.fcgi?cmd=Retrieve&db=PubMed&dopt=Citation&list_uids=15802180

Shapira, B., Oppenheim, G., Zohar, J., Segal, M., Malach, D.&Belmaker, R. H. (1985). Lack of efficacy of estrogen supplementation to imipramine in resistant female depressives. *Biol Psychiatry* 20, 576-579. URL:http://www.ncbi.nlm.nih.gov/entrez/query.fcgi?cmd=Retrieve&db=PubMed&dopt=Citation&list_uids=2985131

Sherwin, B. B.&Henry, J. F. (2008). Brain aging modulates the neuroprotective effects of estrogen on selective aspects of cognition in women: a critical review. *Front Neuroendocrinol* 29, 88-113. URL:http://www.ncbi.nlm.nih.gov/entrez/query.fcgi?cmd=Retrieve&db=PubMed&dopt=Citation&list_uids=17980408

Shughrue, P. J., Lane, M. V.&Merchenthaler, I. (1997). Comparative distribution of estrogen receptor-alpha and -beta mRNA in the rat central nervous system. *J Comp Neurol* 388, 507-525. URL:http://www.ncbi.nlm.nih.gov/entrez/query.fcgi?cmd=Retrieve&db=PubMed&dopt=Citation&list_uids=9388012

Smith, L. J., Henderson, J. A., Abell, C. W.&Bethea, C. L. (2004). Effects of ovarian steroids and raloxifene on proteins that synthesize, transport, and degrade serotonin in the raphe region of macaques. *Neuropsychopharmacology* 29, 2035-2045. URL:http://www.ncbi.nlm.nih.gov/entrez/query.fcgi?cmd=Retrieve&db=PubMed&dopt=Citation&list_uids=15199371

Soares, C. N., Almeida, O. P., Joffe, H.&Cohen, L. S. (2001). Efficacy of estradiol for the treatment of depressive disorders in perimenopausal women: a double-blind, randomized, placebo-controlled trial. *Arch Gen Psychiatry* 58, 529-534. URL:http://www.ncbi.nlm.nih.gov/entrez/query.fcgi?cmd=Retrieve&db=PubMed&dopt=Citation&list_uids=11386980

Soares, C. N.&Zitek, B. (2008). Reproductive hormone sensitivity and risk for depression across the female life cycle: a continuum of vulnerability? *J Psychiatry Neurosci* 33, 331-343. URL:http://www.ncbi.nlm.nih.gov/entrez/query.fcgi?cmd=Retrieve&db=PubMed&dopt=Citation&list_uids=18592034

Strickler, R. C., Borth, R.&Woodlever, C. A. (1977). The climacteric syndrome: an estrogen replacement dilemma. *Can Med Assoc J* 116, 586-587. http://www.ncbi.nlm.nih.gov/entrez/query.fcgi?cmd=Retrieve&db=PubMed&dopt=Citation&list_uids=204404

Sullivan, R. M.&Dufresne, M. M. (2006). Mesocortical dopamine and HPA axis regulation: role of laterality and early environment. *Brain Res* 1076, 49-59. URL: http://www.ncbi.nlm.nih.gov/entrez/query.fcgi?cmd=Retrieve&db=PubMed&dopt=Citation&list_uids=16483551

Toran-Allerand, C. D. (2004). Minireview: A plethora of estrogen receptors in the brain: where will it end? *Endocrinology* 145, 1069-1074. URL:http://www.ncbi.nlm.nih.gov/entrez/query.fcgi?cmd=Retrieve&db=PubMed&dopt=Citation&list_uids=14670986

Toran-Allerand, C. D., Tinnikov, A. A., Singh, R. J.&Nethrapalli, I. S. (2005). 17alpha-estradiol: a brain-active estrogen? *Endocrinology* 146, 3843-3850. URL:http://www.ncbi.nlm.nih.gov/entrez/query.fcgi?cmd=Retrieve&db=PubMed&dopt=Citation&list_uids=15947006

Valentino, R. J.&Van Bockstaele, E. (2008). Convergent regulation of locus coeruleus activity as an adaptive response to stress. *Eur J Pharmacol* 583, 194-203. URL:http://www.ncbi.nlm.nih.gov/entrez/query.fcgi?cmd=Retrieve&db=PubMed&dopt=Citation&list_uids=18255055

Vasudevan, N.&Pfaff, D. W. (2007). Membrane-initiated actions of estrogens in neuroendocrinology: emerging principles. *Endocr Rev* 28, 1-19. URL:http://www.ncbi.nlm.nih.gov/entrez/query.fcgi?cmd=Retrieve&db=PubMed&dopt=Citation&list_uids=17018839

Vetulani, J., Stawarz, R. J., Dingell, J. V.&Sulser, F. (1976). A possible common mechanism of action of antidepressant treatments: reduction in the sensitivity of the noradrenergic cyclic AMP gererating system in the rat limbic forebrain. *Naunyn Schmiedebergs Arch Pharmacol* 293, 109-114. URL:http://www.ncbi.nlm.nih.gov/entrez/query.fcgi?cmd=Retrieve&db=PubMed&dopt=Citation&list_uids=183150

Wagner, E. J., Ronnekleiv, O. K.&Kelly, M. J. (2001). The noradrenergic inhibition of an apamin-sensitive, small-conductance Ca2+-activated K+ channel in hypothalamic gamma-aminobutyric acid neurons: pharmacology, estrogen sensitivity, and relevance to the control of the reproductive axis. *J Pharmacol Exp Ther* 299, 21-30. URL:http://www.ncbi.nlm.nih.gov/entrez/query.fcgi?cmd=Retrieve&db=PubMed&dopt=Citation&list_uids=11561059

Walf, A. A.&Frye, C. A. (2007). Administration of estrogen receptor beta-specific selective estrogen receptor modulators to the hippocampus decrease anxiety and depressive behavior of ovariectomized rats. *Pharmacol Biochem Behav* 86, 407-414. http://www.ncbi.nlm.nih.gov/entrez/query.fcgi?cmd=Retrieve&db=PubMed&dopt=Citation&list_uids=16916539

Walf, A. A.&Frye, C. A. (2010). Raloxifene and/or estradiol decrease anxiety-like and depressive-like behavior, whereas only estradiol increases carcinogen-induced tumorigenesis and uterine proliferation among ovariectomized rats. *Behav Pharmacol* 21, 231-240. URL:http://www.ncbi.nlm.nih.gov/entrez/query.fcgi?cmd=Retrieve&db=PubMed&dopt=Citation&list_uids=20480545

Walf, A. A., Rhodes, M. E.&Frye, C. A. (2004). Antidepressant effects of ERbeta-selective estrogen receptor modulators in the forced swim test. *Pharmacol Biochem Behav* 78, 523-529. URL:http://www.ncbi.nlm.nih.gov/entrez/query.fcgi?cmd=Retrieve&db=PubMed&dopt=Citation&list_uids=15251261

Weiser, M. J., Foradori, C. D.&Handa, R. J. (2008). Estrogen receptor beta in the brain: from form to function. *Brain Res Rev* 57, 309-320. URL:http://www.ncbi.nlm.nih.gov/entrez/query.fcgi?cmd=Retrieve&db=PubMed&dopt=Citation&list_uids=17662459

Wilkinson, M.&Herdon, H. J. (1982). Diethylstilbestrol regulates the number of alpha- and beta-adrenergic binding sites in incubated hypothalamus and amygdala. *Brain Res* 248, 79-85. URL:http://www.ncbi.nlm.nih.gov/entrez/query.fcgi?cmd=Retrieve&db=PubMed&dopt=Citation&list_uids=6289996

4

Antidepressants and Morphological Plasticity of Monoamine Neurons

Shoji Nakamura
Department of Neuroscience,
Yamaguchi University Graduate School of Medicine, Ube, Yamaguchi,
Japan

1. Introduction

In the 1950s, the monoamines 5-hydroxytryptamine (5-HT) (Woolley & Shaw, 1954), noradrenaline (NA) (Vogt, 1954), and dopamine (DA) (Carlsson, 1958) were identified in the brain. After this discovery, it was identified that the tricyclic compound imipramine and the antituberculosis drug iproniazid were effective in the treatment of clinical depression, and that these drugs can increase the extracellular concentration of monoamines by inhibiting the re-uptake of 5-HT and NA and by blocking monoamine oxidase (MAO) respectively. These findings have led to the catecholamine hypothesis of depression (Schildkraut, 1965), followed by the monoamine hypothesis (Coppen, 1967), which propose that depression is caused by deficiencies within the central catecholaminergic or monoaminergic systems respectively. At present, it is understood that all antidepressants increase monoamine levels in the brain. Other evidence supporting the monoamine hypothesis has also been put forward: reserpine, which depletes monoamines in the synaptic cleft, caused depressive symptoms in some patients taking it for the treatment of hypertension. 5-HIAA, the primary metabolite of 5-HT, was seen as reduced in the cerebrospinal fluid of clinically depressed patients. All these findings suggest that monoamine concentrations in the brain are reduced in depressive patients.

Despite compelling evidence supporting the monoamine hypothesis, there is an enigma which must be resolved. Although antidepressants raise monoamine concentrations immediately after their administration, it takes several weeks or more for their clinical efficacy to become apparent. The delayed onset of action of antidepressants suggests that they induce slowly occurring changes in the monoaminergic systems, rather than simply increasing the monoamine concentrations. It has been reported that chronic (but not acute) treatments with antidepressants cause the down-regulation of postsynaptic β-adrenergic receptors (Banerjee et al., 1977; Vetulani & Sulser, 1975). This finding presumably explained the delayed onset of antidepressant action. However, the down-regulation of β-adrenergic receptors appeared to contradict the monoamine hypothesis of depression, which proposes hypofunction in the monoaminergic systems during depression. The decreased β-adrenergic receptor sensitivity observed following treatments suggests that antidepressants exert clinical effects by attenuating *hyper*function of the noradrenergic system.

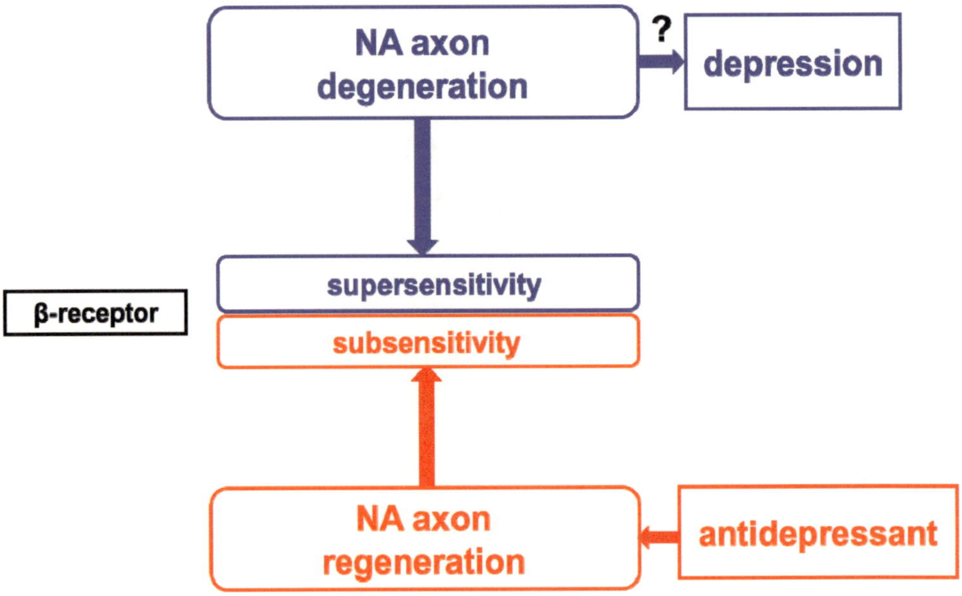

Fig. 1. A link between postsynaptic receptors (β-receptors) and presynaptic axons (NA axons). The degeneration of presynaptic NA axons induced by an NA-specific neurotoxin causes supersensitivity of postsynaptic β-receptors, while repeated administration of noradrenergic antidepressants causes subsensitivity. Based on these findings, the antidepressants have been shown to have the ability to induce NA axon regeneration (Nakamura, 1990,1991). This has led to the view that the degeneration of NA axons is involved in the pathophysiology of depression.

This discrepancy is resolved by considering an association of the receptor sensitivity with morphological changes (Fig. 1). Denervated skeletal muscle becomes supersensitive to acetylcholine due to an increase in the number of acetylcholine receptors on the muscle membrane (denervation supersensitivity). Denervation supersensitivity similar to this occurs in the central noradrenergic system: denervation of cortical NA axons with 6-hydroxydopamine (6-OHDA), a neurotoxin to catecholaminergic neurons, causes supersensitivity (up-regulation) in cortical β-adrenergic receptors (Sporn et al., 1976). As up-regulation of β-adrenergic receptors is associated with denervation of NA axons, it is possible that the converse is also true: down-regulation of β-adrenergic receptors results from an increase in the density of NA axons, i.e., regeneration or sprouting of NA axons. This idea has led to the monoamine axon hypothesis of depression, which proposes the involvement of degeneration or retraction of monoaminergic axons in the pathophysiology of depression (Nakamura, 1990: Harley, 2003). According to the monoamine axon hypothesis, antidepressant drugs exert their effects by inducing regeneration or sprouting of monoaminergic axons.

This review focuses on the effects of antidepressants on the morphological plasticity of monoaminergic axons (mainly 5-HT- and NA-axons) in the adult and developing brain. There is no report showing a link between morphological plasticity and antidepressants in DA axons, although DA neurons have been reported as having the ability to induce axonal sprouting (Hansen et al., 1995; Blanchard et al., 1996; Finkelstein et al., 2000; Stanic et al.,

2003). Therefore, this review is limited to links between antidepressants and the morphological plasticity of 5-HT and NA neurons. In addition, other factors including stress, retinoic acid, and interferon-α that affect morphological plasticity of monoamine neurons are described in relation to clinical depression. This review also discusses slow-acting (monoamininergic) and fast-acting (glutamatergic) antidepressants in relation to a possible link between the monoaminergic and glutamatergic systems.

2. Effects of antidepressants on the density of monoaminergic axons

There is evidence to support the monoamine axon hypothesis of depression. It has been shown that antidepressants that increase extracellular NA concentrations also enhance the regeneration of damaged NA axons (Nakamura, 1990, 1991), and that antidepressants that modulate 5-HT release from 5-HT axon terminals also induce axonal sprouting of 5-HT neurons (Zhou et al., 2006). Focusing on the noradrenergic system, we developed a rat model by which we can assess the ability of antidepressant drugs to induce the regeneration of NA axons (Nakamura, 1990, 1991, 1994). First, to denervate NA axons locally, 6-OHDA (2 μg/0.5 μℓ) was injected bilaterally in the frontal cortex. 6-OHDA was delivered from the tip of a 30-gauge metallic cannula, which was connected to an infusion pump with polyethylene tubing. Two weeks after the toxin infusion, one hemisphere was infused with an antidepressant at the same cortical site, and the other was infused with saline. These drugs were delivered continuously from the tip of an infusion cannula connected to osmotic minipumps (Alzet, model 2002) for more than two weeks (Kasamatsu et al., 1979). To visualize NA axons, we used either fluorescence histochemistry or immunohistochemistry. The size of NA (and DA) axon denervation was then compared between the antidepressant- and saline-infused hemispheres. We showed that antidepressants that increase the extracellular concentration of NA, such as desipramine, maprotiline, and mianserin, have the ability to induce regeneration of NA axons, but fluoxetine, a potent reuptake inhibitor of 5-HT, does not (Nakamura, 1990, 1991). Desipramine and maprotiline are potent reuptake inhibitors of NA, while mianserin has little or no effect on NA reuptake inhibition but enhances NA release by blocking presynaptic α_2-adrenergic receptors. Zhou et al. (2006) have demonstrated the ability of antidepressants to induce axonal sprouting of 5-HT neurons by systemic injections of antidepressants in rats without damaging the 5-HT axons. In this study, they tested three types of antidepressants: the 5-HT reuptake inhibitor fluoxetine, the 5-HT reuptake enhancer tianeptine, and the NA reuptake inhibitor desipramine. These antidepressant drugs were administered intraperitoneally for four weeks. The density of 5-HT axons was examined by visualizing 5-HT axons using antibody immunohistochemistry on 5-HT or 5-HT transporters. They found that fluoxetine and tianeptine, but not desipramine, increased the density of 5-HT axons in the cerebral cortex and some limbic forebrain areas. Using an anterograde labeling technique, they also showed that branching increased in terminal axons from the dorsal raphe. These findings all strongly indicate that antidepressants that modulate 5-HT reuptake also induce axonal sprouting of 5-HT neurons.

These findings appear to suggest that an increased extracellular NA concentration in the synaptic cleft is required to induce axonal regeneration in NA neurons. Regarding 5-HT neurons, however, it is unlikely that an increase in extracellular 5-HT concentration causes axonal sprouting of 5-HT neurons, because the antidepressant-induced sprouting of 5-HT axons occurs after treatments with both 5-HT reuptake inhibitors and facilitators (Zhou et al., 2006). It is worth noting that axonal regeneration in NA neurons is induced by NA antidepressants but not by 5-HT antidepressants (fluoxetine), while 5-HT but not NA antidepressants are able to induce axonal sprouting in 5-HT neurons. This finding suggests the possibility that terminal axons of the monoamine neurons form, at least in part, in relation to changes in the release of their own neurotransmitter.

3. Effects of stress on the morphology of monoaminergic axons

Many studies have demonstrated that 5-HT and NA axons have a great capacity to regenerate in response to brain damage (Nygren et al., 1971; Bjorklund et al., 1973; Nygren et al., 1974; Bjorklund & Lindvall, 1979; Wiklund & Bjorklund, 1980; Fritschy & Grzanna, 1992; Liu et al., 2003). It has been noted that the regeneration of 5-HT axons occurred as early as 28 days after damage from 5-HT neurotoxin injection, while the regeneration of NA axons was not evident 60 days after NA neurotoxin injection (Liu et al., 2003). Furthermore, repeated stress, which is a major cause of depression, has been shown to cause degeneration (or retraction) or regeneration (or sprouting) of monoaminergic axons (Nakamura et al., 1989; Sakaguchi & Nakamura, 1990; Kitayama et al., 1994, 1997; Liu et al., 2004, 2006; Kuramochi et al., 2009). Of interest is that the effects of repeated stress on the morphology of 5-HT and NA axons are not the same. For example, in cortices partially denervated by either 5-HT or NA neurotoxin, repeated stress causes 5-HT axon sprouting and NA axon retraction in cortical regions outside the denervation site (Liu et al., 2004). Moreover, the expression of brain-derived neurotrophic factor (BDNF), reportedly a neurotrophic factor for 5-HT axons (Eaton et al., 1995; Mamounas et al., 1995, 2000), was found to increase in cortical regions where 5-HT axon sprouting had occurred in response to stress. These findings suggest that the molecular mechanism of axonal regeneration or sprouting is different between 5-HT and NA axons. As mentioned earlier, this possibility is also supported by the finding that sprouting of 5-HT and regeneration of NA axons are induced by 5-HT and NA antidepressants, respectively.

4. Link between morphology of monoaminergic axons and depressive behavior

There are reports showing a link between morphological changes in monoaminergic axons and depressive symptoms in animal models of depression. Kitayama et al. (1994, 1997) have demonstrated that an animal model of depression resulted in the degeneration of cortical NA axon terminals. Model animals were subjected to long-term walking stress for two weeks, and showed depressive behaviors including prolonged inactivity, seclusion, aggression, motor retardation, lack of coupling behavior, fitful sleep, weight loss, and hypersensitivity to light and sound (Hatotani et al., 1977, 1979; Kitayama et al., 1994, 1997). In this model, the density of NA axons in the frontal cortex projecting from the locus coeruleus (LC) was examined using retrograde labeling of LC neurons with horseradish peroxidase injected into the cortex and immunohistochemical staining of cortical axons with dopamine-β-hydroxylase antibody. The NA axon density was significantly reduced in the depressed rats, and when subjects were allowed to engage in spontaneous running activity, their recovery rates were positively correlated with the density of NA axons (Kitayama et al., 1997). The density of cortical NA axons in depressed rats was restored by chronic treatment with imipramine (Kitayama et al., 1994, 1997) producing a reversal of depressive behaviors (Kitayama et al., 1987). These findings all support the possibility that degeneration of NA axons is involved in the pathophysiology of depression, and that antidepressants exert their clinical efficacy by inducing the regeneration of NA axons. It is notable that some of the animals subjected to long-term forced walking stress did not demonstrate persistent inactivity but gradually recovered to control levels after the end of the stress treatments (spontaneous recovery rats). The spontaneous recovery rats showed an increase, rather than a decrease, in the density of NA axons as compared to unstressed control rats (Kitayama et al., 1997). This finding suggests that adaptation to stress produces regeneration or sprouting of NA axons. This is consistent with the observation that sprouting of NA axons occurs following chronic mild stress (Nakamura et al., 1989; Sakaguchi & Nakamura, 1990; Nakamura, 1991). It remains to be determined whether morphological plasticity of 5-HT axons is involved in the depression model of long-term forced walking stress.

A recent study has presented a possible link between the density of 5-HT axons and depressive behavior in rats (Kuramochi & Nakamura, 2009). This study examined the effects of postweaning social isolation stress on the density of 5-HT and NA axons and the presence of depressive behavior as assessed by immobility in the forced swim test. Social isolation rearing, which started at postnatal day (PD) 28 and continued until eight to nine weeks later, reduced the density of 5-HT but not NA axons in the central nucleus and basolateral nucleus of the amygdala and CA3 of the hippocampus. Moreover, increased immobility was observed in the forced swim test, suggesting that postweaning social isolation is a possible model of depression containing 5-HT axon deficits. In addition to postweaning social isolation rearing, this study examined the effects of postnatal treatment with the antidepressant clomipramine on the density of 5-HT and NA axons and the presence of depressive behavior. Paradoxically, it has been reported that neonatal treatment with clomipramine induced a rat model of depression as measured by increased immobility in the forced swim test (Velazquez-Moctezuma & Diaz Ruiz, 1992; Bonilla-Jaime et al., 2003). Furthermore, Vijayakumar and Meti (1999) have reported that neonatal treatment with clomipramine caused a decrease in levels of 5-HT and NA in several brain regions, including the frontal cortex and hippocampus. However, following the same treatment protocols, Kuramochi and Nakamura failed to find any changes in either the density of 5-HT and NA axons or the immobility observed in the forced swim test following neonatal treatment with clomipramine. This result is consistent with the finding that neonatal clomipramine treatment had little effect on tryptophan hydroxylase in the dorsal raphe or 5-HT transporter expression in the cerebral cortex (Maciag et al., 2006), and no effect on forced swim immobility (Yoo et al., 2000). The contradictory results may be due to differences in rat strains used for each experiment. The experiments in which neonatal clomipramine induced depression used Wistar rats, whereas the experiments that failed to induce depression used Sprague-Dawley rats or Long-Evans rats. Therefore, it is possible that the Wistar strain is more susceptible to neonatal treatment with clomipramine than other strains (Kuramochi & Nakamura, 2009).

Gonzalez and Aston-Jones (2006, 2008) have reported that light deprivation or long-term exposure to constant darkness in rats (DD) increased apoptosis in LC neurons and decreased the number of NA boutons in the cerebral cortex. The DD rats also demonstrated increased immobility in the forced swim test. The results suggest that the DD rats displaying depressive behaviors could be an appropriate model for seasonal affective disorders (SAD) associated with limited light exposure, and that the pathophysiology of SAD may also involve degeneration or retraction of NA axons. Regarding the molecular mechanism of DD-induced depressive behaviors, Monje et al. (2011) have reported that activation of the proinflammatory cytokine interleukin-6 (IL-6) through the NF-κB signaling pathway plays a pivotal role in causing such behaviors, although it remains unclear whether elevated IL-6 levels are associated with the DD-induced degeneration or retraction of NA axons.

It remains to be determined that the major symptoms of depression, i.e., depressed mood and anhedonia, are induced by changes in the morphology of 5-HT and/or NA axons. It is likely that the degeneration of 5-HT and/or NA axons causes depressed mood rather than anhedonia, because anhedonia is thought to be associated with dysfunction of the dopaminergic reward system.

5. Effects of chemical factors on morphology of monoaminergic axons

To understand the molecular mechanisms of the morphological alterations of monoaminergic axons observed in depression models or induced by antidepressants, it is important to identify the endogenous chemical factors that affect these observed changes. The following are chemicals which have been reported to induce morphological changes of monoaminergic neurons (or axons) in relation to depressive behaviors (Interferon-α, retinoic acids) or effects of antidepressants (phospholipase A2). However, it remains unclear what roles these chemicals play in the molecular mechanisms of stress-related depression.

5.1 Interferon-α

Interferon-α (IFN-α), a proinflammatory cytokine widely used for the treatment of cancers and viral illnesses, is well-known to induce depressive symptoms in 30-50% of patients (Schiepers et al., 2005; Raison et al., 2006). Based on this fact, Ishikawa et al. (2007) have shown that chronic treatments with IFN-α in rats caused significant decreases in the densities of NA axons in the dorsal medial prefrontal cortex, ventral medial prefrontal cortex, and dentate gyrus of the hippocampus and of 5-HT axons in the ventral medial prefrontal cortex and amygdala. The changes in the density of NA axons became apparent after treatments with IFN-α after nine weeks, but not at four weeks. It is not clear why such a long-term administration of IFN-α was necessary to cause the degeneration of the monoaminergic axons. One possibility is that since IFN-α has little ability to cross the blood-brain barrier (BBB) (Collins et al., 1985; Wiranowska et al., 1989), long-term administration of IFN-α may disrupt the BBB so that IFN-α becomes able to enter the brain. Moreover, it is possible that the changes in the densities of the monoaminergic axons induced by chronic administration of IFN-α are not due to IFN-α directly. As IFN-α increases other cytokines such as IL-6 and IL-8, which are also associated with depression (Bonaccorso et al., 2001), the cytokines induced by IFN-α might be responsible for the observed changes in densities (Ishikawa et al., 2007). Taken together with a possible involvement of IL-6 in DD-induced depressive behavior (Monje et al., 2011), proinflammatory cytokines may play a critical role in the pathophysiology of depression because of their association with the degeneration or retraction of monoaminergic axons.

5.2 Phospholipase A2

As mentioned in the Introduction, down-regulation of β-adrenergic receptors induced by chronic administration of antidepressants may be associated with the antidepressant-induced regeneration of NA axons. It has been reported that down-regulation of β-adrenergic receptors following repeated application of β-adrenergic agonists or chronic stress treatment is blocked by phospholipase A2 (PLA2) inhibitors, while this down-regulation can be induced by the activation of PLA2 (Limbird & Lefkowitz, 1976; Mallorga et al., 1980; Hirata & Axelrod, 1980; Torda et al., 1981; Cohen et al., 1985). Manji et al. (1991) demonstrated that PLA2 activation is involved in the down-regulation of β-adrenergic receptors induced by chronic desipramine treatment. Moreover, they suggested that in addition to elevated intrasynaptic levels of NA, desipramine acts directly on the postsynaptic membrane to contribute to the down-regulation. A possible link between down-regulation of β-adrenergic receptors and the regeneration of NA axons raised the possibility that PLA2 is involved in the molecular mechanisms of the antidepressant-induced regeneration of NA axons. Nakamura (1993, 1994) demonstrated that mepacrine or 4-bromphenacyl bromide, which are PLA2 inhibitors, attenuates the regeneration of NA axons induced by desipramine, while the PLA2 activator mellitin induces NA axon regeneration. These findings support the notion that the antidepressant-induced regeneration of NA axons is mediated, at least in part, through PLA2.

PLA2 is an enzyme that generates free fatty acids, such as arachidonic acid (AA), eicosapentenoic acid (EPA) and docosahexaenoic acid (DHA), by acting on membrane phospholipids. AA produces a variety of bioactive substances, such as prostaglandins and leukotrienes, via cycloxygenase or lipoxygenase. Since aspirin, a cycloxygenase inhibitor, had no apparent effect on the desipramine-induced regeneration of NA axons (unpublished data, Nakamura), it seems unlikely that the cycloxygenase system would play a critical role in the desipramine-induced regeneration of NA axons. Many reports have shown lower levels of EPA and/or DHA being associated with clinical depression (Peet et al., 1998; De Vriese et al., 2003; Frasure-Smith et al., 2004; McNamara et al., 2007; Lin et al., 2010; Su et al., 2010). Animal studies demonstrated that administration of EPA and DHA had an antidepressant-like effect, reducing immobility in the forced swim test (Carlezon et al., 2005; Huang et al., 2008). Moreover, a recent study reported that the action of maprotiline, an NA reuptake inhibitor with the same effect, is mediated by EPA or DHA released by activation of calcium-independent PLA2 in the prefrontal cortex (Lee et al., 2011), although it remains unclear whether the EPA or DHA releases are associated with regeneration or sprouting of NA axons. Notably, there is one report which has shown the association between PLA2 genes and the risk of IFN-α-induced depression (Su et al., 2010). All these findings suggest that the PLA2-AA/EPA/DHA signaling pathway plays a crucial role in the occurrence of depressive symptoms, possibly by affecting the morphology of monoaminergic axons.

5.3 Retinoic acids

It has been reported that the acne drug Accutane (isotretinoin), the active component of which is 13-cis-retinoic acid (13-cis-RA), occasionally induces severe depression with suicidal ideation (Wysowski et al., 2001; Hull & D'Arcy, 2003; O'Donnell, 2003). There are conflicting studies to this effect: O'Reilly et al. (2006) demonstrated that chronic administration of 13-cis-RA increased depression-related behavior in adult mice, although

Ferguson et al. (2005) reported that 13-cis-RA or all-trans-RA had no such effect in rats. Based on findings that 13-cis-RA reduced neurogenesis and cell survival in the hippocampi of adult mice (Crandall et al., 2004 Sakai et al., 2004), McCaffery and coworkers have suggested that hippocampal cell loss is a major contributor to the pathophysiology of depression associated with 13-cis-RA use. Regarding the relationship between 13-cis-RA and the morphology of monoamine neurons, Ishikawa et al. (2008) demonstrated that the negative effects on the dendritic morphology of slice-cultured 5-HT neurons created by high doses of 13-cis-RA is mediated via retinoic acid receptor (RAR) and retinoid X receptor (RXR), which are nuclear receptors acting as ligand-inducible transcription factors (Chambon, 1996). It remains unclear whether 13-cis-RA induces the degeneration/retraction of monoaminergic axons through RAR and/or through RXR in the adult animal brain. It is notable that RA stimulates PLA2 activation via RA receptors, suggesting that the morphological effects of RAs such as 13-cis-RA are mediated along the PLA2 signaling pathway (Farooqui et al., 2004).

5.4 1-Bromopropane

1-Bromopropane (1-BP), a commonly used solvent in the dry cleaning industry (CDC, 2008; Blando et al., 2010), is used as an alternative to ozone layer depleting solvents as a cleaning agent for metal parts in electronics factories (Ichihara, 2005). Exposure to 1-BP has been reported to cause various neurological and neurobehavioral symptoms in humans, including numbness in the legs, ataxic gait and memory disturbances (Ichihara, 2005). In addition, workers exposed to 1-BP often display depressive symptoms (Ichihara et al., 2002; Majersik et al., 2007). To see if exposure to 1-BP causes degeneration of monoaminergic axons, Mohideen et al. (2011) examined the effects of repeated exposure to 1-BP on the density of 5-HT and NA axons in the rat brain. Exposure to 1-BP induced dose-dependent reductions in the density of NA axons in the prefrontal cortex and the basolateral nucleus of the amygdala, but no apparent change in the density of 5-HT axons. The results suggest that depressive symptoms in workers exposed to 1-BP may be associated with degeneration of NA axons in the brain, although the link between 1-BP and endogenous chemical factors involved in the degeneration of NA axons is unclear. The findings also suggest that there are exogenous chemical agents, as well as exogenous stressors, which can induce depressive symptoms, possibly by negatively affecting the morphology of monoaminergic axons.

6. Slow-acting and fast-acting antidepressants

In contrast to the delayed onset of the clinical efficacy of classical antidepressants, recent studies have reported that ketamine, an NMDA antagonist, exerts rapid antidepressant effects in humans (Berman et al., 2000; Zarate et al., 2006; Price et al., 2009). In animals, other NMDA antagonists such as MK-801 and CPP as well as ketamine have been reported to cause rapid antidepressant action in animals, though the effects are short-lasting compared to ketamine (Maeng et al., 2008; Autry et al., 2011). Many studies have corroborated the fact that the antidepressant effects of a single injection of ketamine persist up to 1-2 weeks in humans (Berman et al., 2000; Zarate et al., 2006; Price et al., 2009; Phelps et al., 2009; aan het Rot et al., 2010) and animals (Maeng et a., 2008; Li et al., 2010; Autry et al., 2011), while other studies failed to confirm the persistent effects of such an injection in rodents (Popik et al., 2008; Lindholm et al., 2011). Since the fast-acting, sustained antidepressant effects of

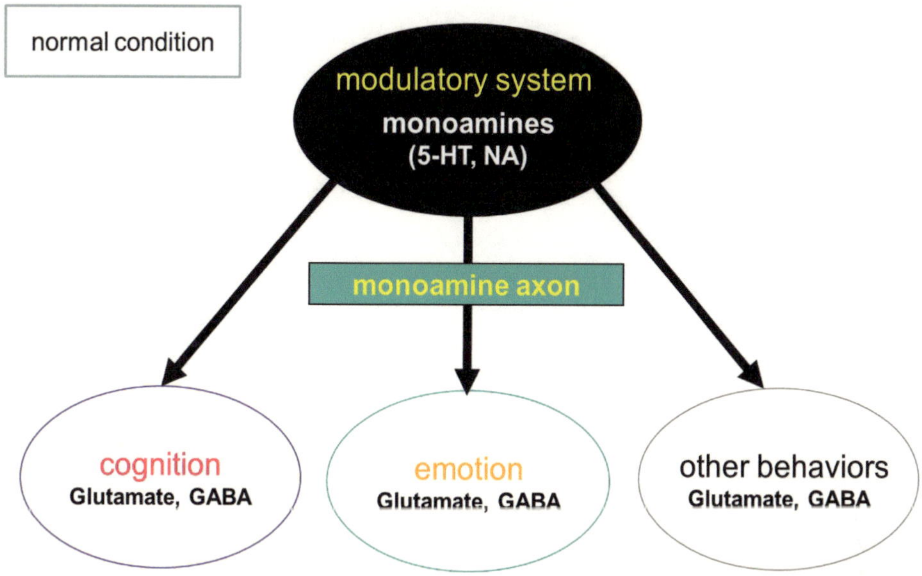

Fig. 2A. All behaviors, including cognition and emotion, are processed by neural circuits mediated by the neurotransmitters glutamate and GABA. The operations of these functional neural circuits are modified by the modulatory systems, which exert their effects by releasing monoamines.

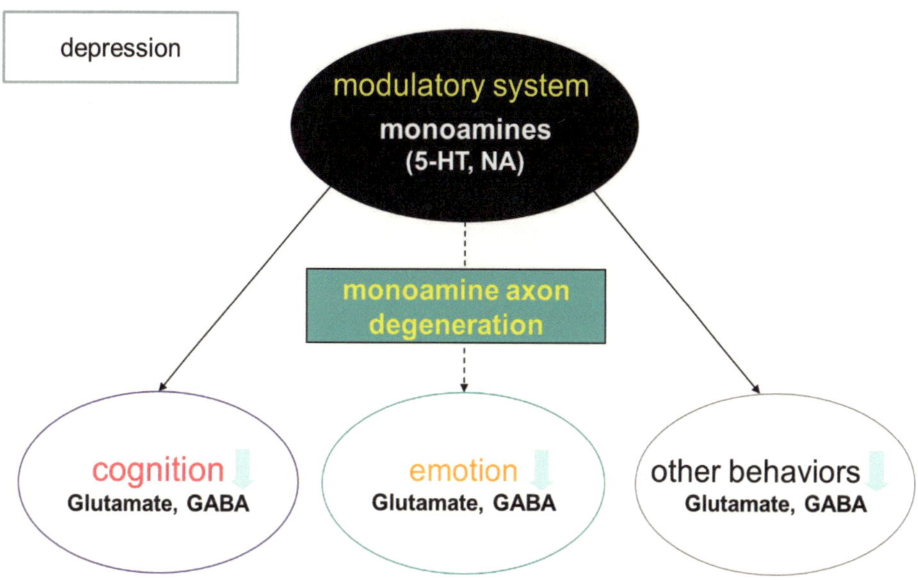

Fig. 2B. In depression, the degeneration of monoaminergic axons containing 5-HT and/or NA may occur, resulting in the disorder of neural circuits that process behaviors such as emotion.

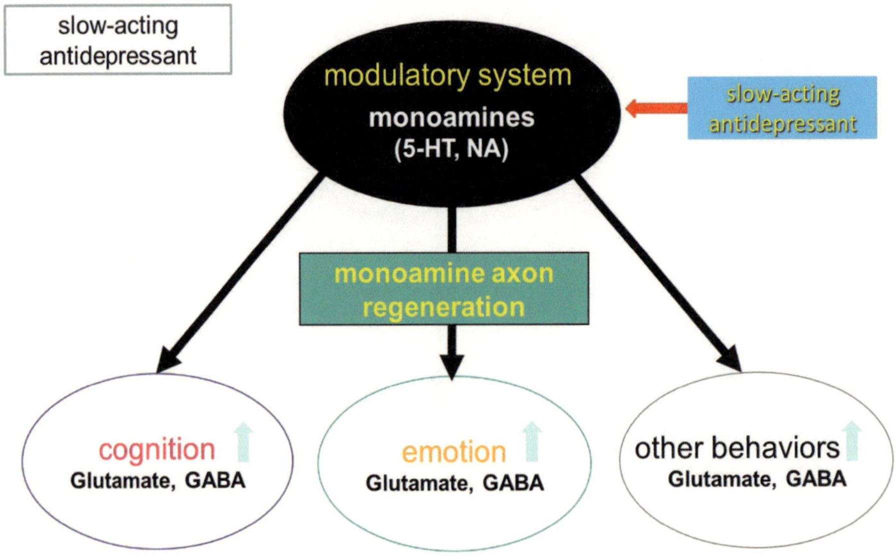

Fig. 2C. Slow-acting antidepressants affecting monoamine activity may exert their effects by inducing the regeneration of monoaminergic axons containing 5-HT and/or NA, thereby taking a few weeks or more to restore the normal conditions and operations of functional neural circuits.

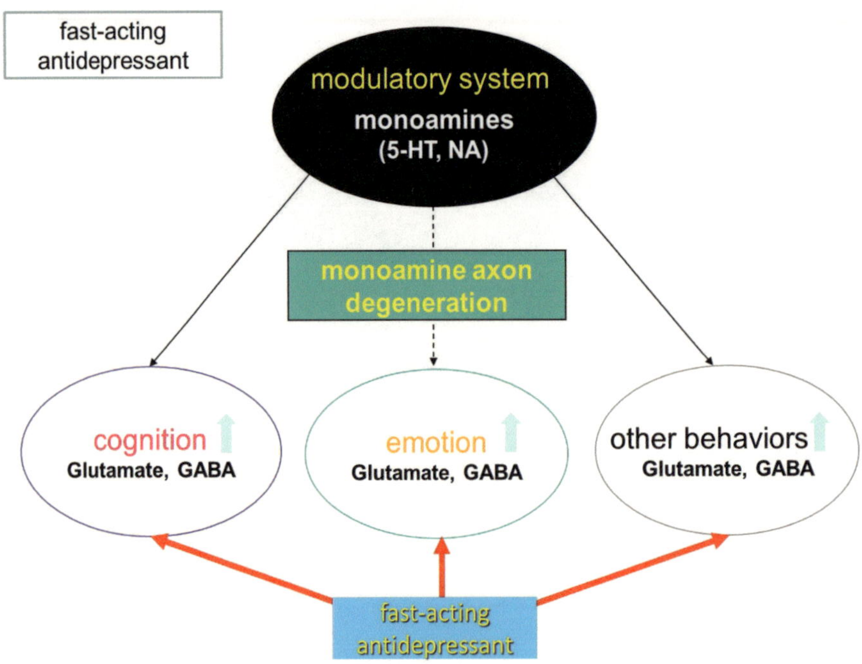

Fig. 2D. Fast-acting antidepressants may restore the normal conditions of functional neural circuits by directly affecting the glutamatergic system. However, the dysregulation of the monoamine system may continue.

ketamine are blocked by AMPA receptor antagonists, activation of AMPA receptors is presumably involved in the cellular mechanism of ketamine's action (Maeng et al., 2008; Autry et al., 2011; Koike et al., 2011). These findings indicate that the rapid antidepressant response of ketamine is associated with the glutamatergic systems, including NMDA and AMPA receptors.

Glutamate and GABA are the major excitatory and inhibitory neurotransmitters in the brain, respectively. The information processing of functional neural circuits is mediated by glutamate and GABA. All behaviors, including cognition and emotion, are performed by the glutamatergic/GABAergic neural circuits. The neurotransmitters of monoaminergic systems influence the activity of glutamate and GABA in these functional neural circuits (Fig. 2A). Thus, glutamate and GABA play a direct role in the expression of behaviors, while the monoaminergic systems, although not directly responsible, play a role in attenuating or strengthening it by modulating the activity of glutamatergic/GABAergic neural circuits. In depression, the degeneration of monoaminergic axons containing 5-HT and/or NA may occur, causing the influence of the monoaminergic systems on the functional neural circuits to continuously decline. Consequently, this may blunt the activity of functional neural circuits that process behaviors, including emotion (Fig. 2B), leading to depression and depressive states. Antidepressants affecting the activity of 5-HT and/or NA neurons induce the regeneration of previously degenerated monoaminergic axons and restore the normal conditions of functional neural circuits (Fig. 2C). The antidepressant effects of these antidepressants occur slowly due to the time required for morphological changes to take

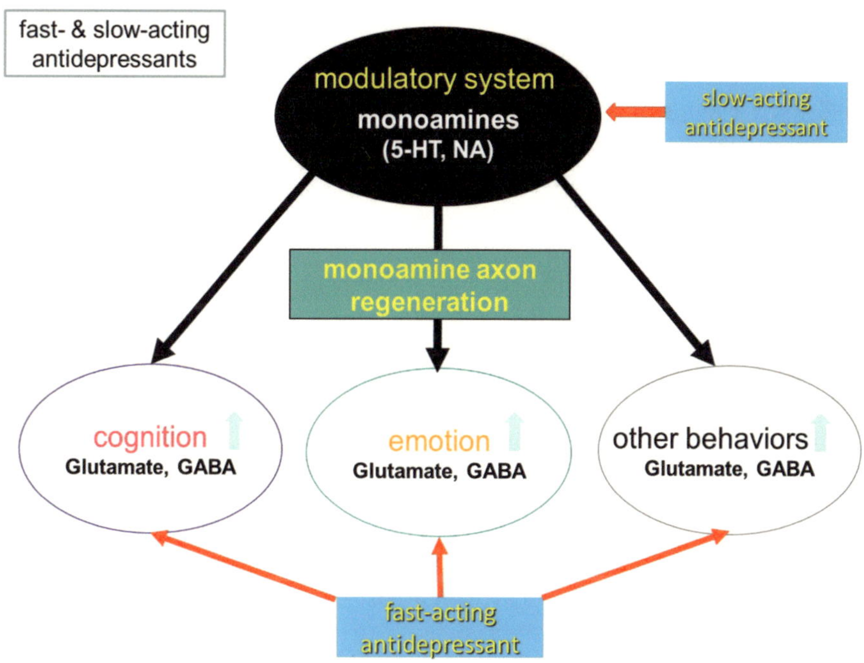

Fig. 2E. Administration of both fast- and slow-acting antidepressants may restore the normal conditions and operations of functional neural circuits within both the glutamatergic and monoaminergic systems.

place, and become manifest over several weeks. In contrast, fast-acting antidepressants such as ketamine, which affect the activity of the glutamatergic system, act directly on functional neural circuits to restore the normal healthy condition, while the monoamine systems remain dysregulated (Fig. 2D). To completely restore functionality of neural circuits, both the glutamatergic and monoaminergic systems must be restored to full capacity through administration of both fast- and slow-acting antidepressants (Fig. 2E).

7. Concluding remarks

The delayed onset of clinical efficacy of classical antidepressants may be explained, at least in part, by the fact that degeneration of 5-HT and/or NA axons is heavily involved in the pathophysiology of depression, and that such antidepressants exert their clinical efficacy by inducing a relatively slow regeneration of these monoaminergic axons. Although newer antidepressants that directly affect the glutamatergic system produce a rapid and sustained antidepressant response, the monoaminergic systems may remain suboptimal and in need of restoration. New antidepressant development should focus on maintaining these immediate effects of action on the glutamatergic system, but also restoring the modulatory activity of the monoaminergic systems in the long-term, possibly by inducing the regeneration of monoaminergic axons.

8. Acknowledgements

The author thanks Mr. Takashi Kudoh for his excellent secretarial assistant.

9. References

Aan het Rot, M., Collins, K.A., Murrough, J.W., Perez, A.M., Reich, D.L., Charney, D.S. & Mathew, S.J. (2010) Safety and efficacy of repeated-dose intravenous ketamine for treatment-resistant depression. Biol Psychiatry, 67, 139-145.

Autry, A.E., Adachi, M., Nosyreva, E., Na, E.S., Los, M.F., Cheng, P., Kavalali, E.T. & Monteggia1, L.M. (2011) NMDA receptor blockade at rest triggers rapid behavioural antidepressant responses. Nature, 475, 91-95.

Banerjee, S.P., Kung, L.S., Riggi, S.J. & Chanda, S.K. (1977) Development of β-adrenergic receptor subsensitivity by antidepressants. Nature, 268, 455-456.

Berman, R.M., Cappiello, A., Anand, A., Oren, D.A., Heninger, G.R., Charney, D.S. & Krystal, J.H. (2000) Antidepressant effects of ketamine in depressed patients. Biol Psychiatry, 47, 351–354.

Bjorklund, A. & Lindvall, O. (1979) Regeneration of normal terminal innervation patterns by central noradrenergic neurons after 5,7-dihydroxytryptamine-induced axotomy in the adult rat. Brain Res, 171, 271—293.

Bjorklund, A., Nobin, U. & Stenevi, U. (1973) Regeneration of central 5-HT neurons after axonal degeneration induced by 5,6-dihydroxytryptamine. Brain Res, 50, 214-220.

Blanchard, V., Anglade, P., Dziewczapolski, G., Savasta, M., Agid, Y. & Raisman-Vozari, R. (1996) Dopaminergic sprouting in the rat striatum after partial lesion of the substantia nigra. Brain Res, 709, 319-325.

Blando, J.D., Schill, D.P., De La Cruz, M.P., Zhang, L. & Zhang, J. (2010) Preliminary study of propyl bromide exposure among New Jersey dry cleaners as a result of a pending ban on perchloroethylene. J Air Waste Manage Assoc, 60, 1049–1056.

Bonaccorso, S., Puzella, A., Marino, V., Pasquini, M., Biondi, M., Artini, M. Almerighi, C., Levrero, M., Egyed, B., Bosmans, E., Meltzer, H.Y. & Maes, M. (2001) Immunotherapy with interferon-alpha in patients affected by chronic hepatitis C induces an intercorrelated stimulation of the cytokine network and an increase in depressive and anxiety symptoms. Psychiatry Res, 105, 45-55.

Bonilla-Jaime, H., Retana-Marquez, S., Vazquez-Palacios, G. & Moctezuma, J. (2003) Corticosterone and testosterone levels after chronic stress in an animal model of depression. Neuropsychobiology, 48, 55-58.

Carlezon, W.A.Jr., Mague, S.D., Parow, A.M., Stoll, A.L., Cohen, B.M. & Renshaw, P.F. (2005) Antidepressant-like effects of uridine and omega-3 fatty acids are potentiated by combined treatment in rats. Biol Psychiatry, 57, 343–350.

Carlsson, A. (1958) A fluorimetric method for the determination of dopamine (3-hydroxytyramine). Acta Physiol Scand, 44, 293-298.

CDC. (2008) Neurologic illness associated with occupational exposure to the solvent 1-bromopropane—New Jersey and Pennsylvania, 2007–2008.

Chambon, P. (1996) A decade of molecular biology of retinoic acid receptors. FASEB J, 10, 940–954.

Cohen, R.M., McLellan, C., Dauphin, M. & Hirata, F. (1985) Glutaraldehyde pretreatment blocks phosphlipase A2 modulation of adrenergic receptors. Life Sci, 36, 25-32.

Collins, J.M., Riccardi, R., Trown, P., O'Neil, D. & Poplack, D.G.. (1985) Plasma and cerebrospinal fluid pharmacokinetics of recombinant interferon alpha A in monkeys: comparison of intravenous, intramuscular, and intraventricular delivery. Cancer Drug Deliv, 2, 247–253.

Coppen, A. (1967) The biochemistry of affective disorders. Brit J Psychiat, 113, 1237-1264.

Crandall, J., Sakai, Y., Zhang, J., Koul, O., Mineur, Y., Crusio, W. E. & McCaffery, P. (2004) 13-cis-Retinoic acid suppresses hippocampal cell division and hippocampal-dependent learning in mice. Proc Natl Acad Sci USA. 101, 5111–5116.

De Vriese, S.R., Christophe, A.B. & Maes, M. (2003) Lowered serum n-3 polyunsaturated fatty acid (PUFA) levels predict the occurrence of postpartum depression: Further evidence that lowered n-PUFAs are related to major depression. Life Sci, 73, 3181–3187.

Eaton, M.J., Staley, J.K., Globus, M.Y. & Whittemore, S.R. (1995) Developmental regulation of early serotonergic neuronal differentiation: the role of brain-derived neurotrophic factor and membrane depolarization. Dev Biol, 170, 169-182.

Ferguson, S., Cisneros, F., Gough, B., Hanig, J. & Berry, K. (2005) Chronic oral treatment with 13-cis-retinoic acid (isotretinoin) or all-trans-retinoic acid does not alter depression-like behaviors in rats. Toxicol. Sci, 87, 451–459.

Finkelstein, D.I., Stanic, D., Parish, C.L., Thomas, D., Dickson, K. & Horne, M.K. (2000) Axonal sprouting following lesions of the rat substantia nigra. Neuroscience, 97, 99-112.

Frasure-Smith, N., Lesperance, F. & Julien, P. (2004) Major depression is associated with lower omega-3 fatty acid levels in patients with recent acute coronary syndromes. Biol Psychiatry, 55, 891- 896.

Fritschy, J.M. & Grzanna, R. (1992) Restoration of ascending noradrenergic projections by residual locus coeruleus neurons: compensatory response to neurotoxin-induced cell death in the adult rat brain. J Comp Neurol, 321, 421-441.

González, M.M. & Aston-Jones, G. (2006) Circadian regulation of arousal: role of the noradrenergic locus coeruleus system and light exposure. Sleep, 29, 1327-1336.

González, M.M. & Aston-Jones, G. (2008) Light deprivation damages monoamine neurons and produces a depressive behavioral phenotype in rats. Proc Natl Acad Sci USA. 105, 4898–4903.

Hansen, J.T., Sakai, K., Greenamyre, J.T. & Moran, S. (1995) Sprouting of dopaminergic fibers from spared mesencephalic dopamine in neurons in the unilateral partial lesioned rat. Brain Res, 670, 197-204.

Harley, C.W. (2003) Norepinephrine and serotonin axonal dynamics and clinical depression: A commentary on the interaction between serotonergic and noradrenergic axons during axonal regeneration. Exp Neurol, 184, 24-26.

Hatotani, N., Nomura, J., Inoue, K. & Kitayama, I. (1979) Psychoendocrine model of depression. Psychoneuroendocrinology, 4, 155-172.

Hatotani, N., Nomura, J., Yamaguchi, T. & Kitayama, I. (1977) Clinical and experimental studies on the pathogenesis of depression. Psychoneuroendocrinology, 2, 115–130.

Hirata, F. & Axelrod, J. (1980) Phospholipid methylation and biological signal transmission. Science, 209, 1082-1090.

Huang, S.Y., Yang, H.T., Chiu, C.C., Pariante, C.M. & Su, K.P. (2008) Omega-3 fatty acids on the forced-swimming test. J Psychiatr Res, 42, 58–63.

Hull, P.R. & D'Arcy, C. (2003) Isotretinoin use and subsequent depression and suicide: presenting the evidence. Am J Clin Dermatol, 4, 493–505.

Ichihara, G., Miller, J., Ziolkowska, A., Itohara, S. & Takeuchi, Y. (2002) Neurological disorders in three workers exposed to 1-bromopropane. J Occup Health, 44, 1–7.

Ichihara, G. (2005) Neuro-reproductive toxicities of 1-bromopropane and 2-bromopropane. Int Arch Occup Environ Health, 78, 79–96.

Ishikawa, J., Ishikawa, A. & Nakamura, S. (2007) Interferon-α reduces the density of monoaminergic axons in the rat brain. NeuroReport, 18, 137-140.

Ishikawa, J., Sutoh, C., Ishikawa, A., Kagechika, H., Hirano, H. & Nakamura, S. (2008) 13-cis-retinoic acid alters the cellular morphology of slice-cultured serotonergic neurons in the rat. Eur J Neurosci, 27, 2363–2372.

Kasamatsu, T., Pettigrew, J.D. & Ary, M. (1979) Restoration of visual cortical plasticity by local microperfusion of norepinephrine. J Comp Neurol, 185, 163-181.

Kitayama, I., Murase, S., Koishizawa, M., Kawaguchi, S. & Nomura, J. (1987) Effect of antidepressant on behavior and central catecholamine of depression-model rats. Jpn J Pshchopharmacol, 7, 433-436.

Kitayama, I., Nakamura, S., Yaga, T., Murase, S., Nomura, J., Kayahara, T. & Nakano, K. (1994) Degeneration of locus coeruleus axons in stress-induced depression model. Brain Res Bull, 35, 573-580.

Kitayama I., Yaga, T., Kayahara, T., Nakano, K., Murase, S., Otani, M. & Nomura, J. (1997) Long-term stress degenerates, but imipramine regenerates, noradrenergic axons in the rat cerebral cortex. Biol Psychiatry, 42, 687-696.

Koike, H., Iijima, M. & Chaki, S. (2011) Involvement of AMPA receptor in both the rapid and sustained antidepressant-like effects of ketamine in animal models of depression. Behav Brain Res, 224, 107-111.

Kuramochi, M. & Nakamura, S. (2009) Effects of postanatal isolation rearing and antidepressant treatment on the density of serotonergic and naoradrenergic axons and depressive behavior in rats. Neuroscience, 163, 448-455.

Lee, L.H., Tan, C.H., Shui, G.., Wenk, M.R. & Ong, W.Y. (2011) Role of prefrontal cortical calcium independent phospholipase A2 in antidepressant-like effect of maprotiline. Int J Neuropsychopharmacol, 11, 1-12.

Li, N., Lee, B., Liu, R., Banasr, M., Dwyer, J.M., Iwata, M., Li, X., Aghajanian, G. & Duman, R.S. (2010) mTOR-dependent synapse formation underlies the rapid antidepressant effects of NMDA antagonists. Science, 329, 959–964.

Limbird, L.E. & Lefkowitz, R.J. (1976) Adenylate cyclase-coupled beta adrenergic receptors: Effect of membrane lipid-perturbing agents on receptor binding and enzyme stimulation by catecholamines. Mol Pharmacol, 12, 559-567.

Lin, P.Y., Huang, S.Y. & Su, K.P. (2010) A meta-analytic review of polyunsaturated fatty acid compositions in patients with depression. Biol Psychiatry, 68, 140-147.

Lindholm, J.S., Autio, H., Vesa, L., Antila, H., Lindemann, L., Hoener, M.C., Skolnick, P., Rantamäki, T. & Castrén, E. (2012) The antidepressant-like effects of glutamatergic drugs ketamine and AMPA receptor potentiator LY 451646 are preserved in bdnf(+/-) heterozygous null mice. Neuropharmacology, 62, 391-397.

Liu, Y., Ishida, Y., Shinoda, K., Furukawa, S. & Nakamura, S. (2004) Opposite morphological responses of partially denervated cortical serotonergic and noradrenergic axons to repeated stress in adult rats. Brain Res Bull, 64, 67-74.

Liu, Y., Ishida, Y., Shinoda, K. & Nakamura, S. (2003) Interaction between serotonergic and noradrenergic axons during axonal regeneration. Exp Neurol, 184, 169-178.

Liu, Y. & Nakamura, S. (2006) Stress-induced plasticity of monoamine axons. Front Biosci, 11, 1794-1801.

Maciag, D., Simpson, K.L., Coppinger, D., Lu, Y., Wang, Y., Lin, R.C. & Paul, I.A. (2006) Neonatal antidepressant exposure has lasting effects on behavior and serotonin circuitry. Neuropsychopharmacology, 31, 47-57.

Maeng, S., Zarate, C.A. Jr., Du, J., Schloesser, R.J., McCammon, J., Chen, G. & Manji, H.K. (2008) Cellular mechanisms underlying the antidepressant effects of ketamine: role of alpha-amino-3-hydroxy-5-methylisoxazole-4-propionic acid receptors. Biol Psychiatry, 63, 349-52.

Majersik, J.J., Caravati, E.M. & Steffens, J.D. (2007) Severe neurotoxicity associated with exposure to the solvent 1-bromopropane (n-propyl bromide). Clin Toxicol (Phila), 45, 270–276.

Mallorga, P., Tallman, J.F., Henneberry, R.C., Hirata, F., Strittmatter, W.T., Axelrod, J. (1980) Mepacrine blocks beta-adrenergic agonist-induced desensitization in astrocytoma cells. Proc Natl Acad Sci USA. 77, 1341-1345.

Mamounas, L.A., Altar, C.A., Blue, M.E., Kaplan, D.R., Tessarollo, L. & Lyons, W.E. (2000) BDNF promotes the regenerative sprouting, but not survival, of injured serotonergic axons in the adult rat brain. J Neurosci, 20, 771-782.

Mamounas, L.A., Blue, M.E., Siuciak, J.A. & Altar, C.A. (1995) Brain-derived neurotrophic factor promotes the survival and sprouting of serotonergic axons in rat bran. J Neurosci, 15, 7929-7939.

Manji, H.K., Chen, G.A., Bitran, J.A. & Potter, W.Z. (1991) Down-regulation of beta receptors by desipramine in vitro involves PKC/phospholipase A2. Psychopharmacol Bull, 27, 247-253.

McNamara, R.K., Hahn, C.G., Jandacek, R., Rider, T., Tso, P., Stanford, K.E. & Richtand N.M. (2007) Selective deficits in the omega-3 fatty acid docosahexaenoic acid in the postmortem orbitofrontal cortex of patients with major depressive disorder. Biol Psychiatry, 62, 17–24.

Mitsumoto, Y., Watanabe, A., Mori, A. & Koga, N. (1988) Spontaneous regeneration of nigrostriatal dopaminergic neurons in MPTP-treated C57BL/6 mice. Biochem Biophy Res Commun, 248, 660-663.

Mohideen, S.S., Ichihara, G.., Ichihara, S. & Nakamura, S. (2011) Exposure to 1-bromopropane causes degeneration of noradrenergic axons in the rat brain. Toxicology, 285, 67-71.

Monje, F.J., Cabatic, M., Divisch, I., Kim, E., Herkner, K.R., Binder, B.R. & Daniela D. Pollak, D.D. (2011) Constant Darkness induces IL-6-dependent depression-like behavior through the NF-κB signaling pathway. J Neurosci, 31, 9075–9083.

Nakamura, S., Sakaguchi, T. & Aoki, F. (1989) Electrophysiological evidence for terminal sprouting of locus coeruleus neurons following repeated mild stress. Neurosci Lett, 100, 147-152.

Nakamura, S. (1990) Antidepressants induce regeneration of catecholaminergic axon terminals in the rat cerebral cortex. Neurosci Lett, 111, 64-68.

Nakamura, S. (1991) Axonal sprouting of noradrenergic locus coeruleus neurons following repeated stress and antidepressant treatment. Prog Brain Res, 88, 587-598.

Nakamura, S. (1991) Effects of mianserin and fluoxetine on axonal regeneration of brain catecholamine neurons. NeuroReport, 2, 525-528.

Nakamura, S. (1993) Involvement of phospholipase A2 in axonal regeneration of brain noradrenergic neurones. NeuroReport, 4, 371-374.

Nakamura, S. (1994) Effects of phospholipase A2 inhibitors on the antidepressant-induced axonal regeneration of noradrenergic locus coeruleus neurons. Microsc Res Tech. 29, 204-210.

Nygren, L.G., Olson, L. & Seiger, A. (1971) Regeneration of monoamine-containing axons in the developing and adult spinal cord of the rat following intraspinal 6-OH-dopamine injections or transactions. Histochemie, 28, 1-15.

Nygren, L.G., Fuxe, K., Jonsson, G. & Olson, L. (1974) Functional regeneration of 5-hydroxytryptamine nerve terminals in the rat spinal cord following 5,6-dihydroxytryptamine induced degeneration. Brain Res, 78, 377-394.

O'Donnell, J. (2003) Overview of existing research and information linking isotretinoin (accutane), depression, psychosis, and suicide. Am J Ther, 10, 148–159.

O'Reilly, K.C., Shumake, J., Gonzalez-Lima, F., Lane, M.A. & Bailey, S.J. (2006) Chronic administration of 13-cis-retinoic acid increases depression-related behavior in mice. Neuropsychopharmacology, 31, 1919–1927.

Peet, M., Murphy, B., Shay, J. & Horrobin, D. (1998) Depletion of omega-3 fatty acid levels in red blood cell membranes of depressive patients. Biol Psychiatry, 43, 315–319.

Phelps, L.E., Brutsche, N., Moral, J.R., Luckenbaugh, D.A., Manji, H. & Zarate Jr., C.A. (2009) Family history of alcohol dependence and initial antidepressant response to an N-methyl-D-aspartate antagonist. Biol Psychiatry, 65, 181-184.

Popik, P., Kos, T., Sowa-Kucma, M. & Nowak, G. (2008) Lack of persistent effects of ketamine in rodent models of depression. Psychopharmacology 198, 421-430.

Price, R.B., Nock, M.K., Charney, D.S. & Mathew, S.J. (2009) Effects of intravenous ketamine on explicit and implicit measures of suicidality in treatment-resistant depression. Biol Psychiatry, 66, 522–526.

Raison, C.L., Capuron, L. & Miller, A.H. (2006) Cytokines sing the blues: inflammation and the pathogenesis of depression. Trends Immunol, 27, 24-31.

Sakaguchi, T. & Nakamura, S. (1990) Duration-dependent effects of repeated restraint stress on cortical projections of locus coeruleus neurons. Neurosci Lett, 118, 193—196.

Sakai, Y., Crandall, J.E., Brodsky, J. & McCaffery, P. (2004) 13-cis Retinoic acid (accutane) suppresses hippocampal cell survival in mice. Ann NY Acad Sci., 1021, 436–440.

Schiepers, O.J., Wichers, M.C. & Maes, M. (2005) Cytokines and major depression. Prog Neuropsychopharmacol Biol Psychiatry, 29, 201-217.

Schildkraut, J. J. (1965) The catecholamine hypothesis of affective disorders: a review of supporting evidence. Am J Psychiat, 122, 509-522.

Sporn, J.R., Harden, T.K., Wolfe, B.B. & Molinoff, P.B. (1976) β-Adrenergic receptor involvement in 6-hydroxydopamine-induced supersensitivity in rat cerebral cortex. Science, 194, 624-626.

Stanic, D., Finkelstein, D.I., Bourke, D.W., Drago, J. & Horne, M.K. (2003) Timecourse of striatal re-innervation following lesions of dopaminergic SNpc neurons of the rat. Eur J Neurosci, 18, 1175-1188.

Su, K., Huang, S., Peng, C., Lai, H., Huang, C., Chen, Y., Aitchison, K.J. & Pariante, C.M. (2010) Phospholipase A2 and cyclooxygenase 2 genes influence the risk of interferon-α–induced depression by regulating polyunsaturated fatty acids levels. Biol Psychiatry, 67, 550–557.

Torda, T., Yamaguchi, I., Hirata, F., Kopin, I.J. & Axelrod, J. (1981) Quinacrine-blocked desensitization of adrenoceptors after immobilization stress or repeated injection of isoproterenol in rats. J Pharmacol Exp Ther, 216, 334-338.

Velazquez-Moctezuma, J. & Diaz Ruiz, O. (1992) Neonatal treatment with clomipramine increased immobility in the forced swim test: an attribute of animal models of depression. Pharmacol Biochem Behav, 42, 737-739.

Vetulani, J. & Sulser, F. (1975) Action of various antidepressant treatment reduced reactivity of noradrenergic cyclic AMP-generating system in limbic forebrain. Nature, 257, 495-496.

Vijayakumar, M. & Meti, B. L. (1999) Alterations in the levels of monoamines in descrete brain regions of clomipramine-induced animal model of endogenous depresson. Neurochem Res, 24, 345-349.

Vogt, M. (1954) Norepinephrine and epinephrine in the central nervous system. Pharmacol Rev, 6, 31-32.

Wiklund, L. & Bjorklund, A. (1980) Mechanisms of regrowth in the bulbospinal 5-HT system following 5,6-dihydroxytryptamine induced axotomy. II. Fluorescence histochemical observations. Brain Res, 191, 109-127.

Wiranowska, M., Wilson, T.C., Thompson, K. & Prockkop, L.D. (1989) Cerebral interferon entry in mice after osmotic alteration of blood–brain barrier. J Interferon Res, 9, 353–362.

Woolley, D.W. & Shaw, E. (1954) A Biochemical and pharmacological suggestion about certain mental disorders. Science, 119, 587-588.

Wysowski, D.K., Pitts, M. & Beitz, J. (2001) An analysis of reports of depression and suicide in patients treated with isotretinoin. J Am Acad Dermatol, 45, 515–519.

Yoo, H.S., Bunnell, B.N., Crabe, J.B., Kalish, L.R. & Dishman, R.K. (2000) Failure of neonatal clomipramine treatment to alter forced swim immobility: chronic treadmill or activity-wheel running and imipramine. Physiol Behav, 70, 407-411.

Zarate, C.A., Jr, Singh, J.B., Carlson, P.J., Brutsche, N.E., Ameli, R., Luckenbaugh, D.A., Charney, D.S. & Manji, H.K. (2006) A randomized trial of an N-methyl-D-aspartate antagonist in treatment-resistant major depression. Arch Gen Psychiatry, 63, 856–864.

Zhou, L., Huang, K.X., Kecojevic, A., Welsh, A.M. & Koliatsos, V.E. (2006) Evidence that serotonin reuptake madulators increase the density of serotonin innervation in the forebrain. J Neurochem, 96, 396-406.

5

Serotonin Noradrenaline Reuptake Inhibitors (SNRIs)

Ipek Komsuoglu Celikyurt,
Oguz Mutlu and Guner Ulak
*Kocaeli University, Medical Faculty, Pharmacology Department,
Psychopharmacology Laboratory, Umuttepe, Kocaeli,
Turkiye*

1. Introduction

Antidepressants that block the reuptake of serotonin (5-HT) and noradrenaline (NA) are called 5-HT and NA reuptake inhibitors (SNRIs). SNRIs are agents that show "dual action" on 5-HT and NA. These drugs bind the 5-HT transporters (SERT) and NA transporters (NAT) similar to tricyclic antidepressants (TCAs). However, SNRIs differ from TCAs in that SNRIs do not exert much affinity for other receptors. Altough SNRIs are called "dual action" 5-HT - NA agents they increase dopamine levels in the prefrontal cortex via NAT inhibition. In this way, they have a third action on neurotransmitters in the prefrontal cortex.

The main use of SNRIs is in the treatment of major depression. Other applications include treatment of pain disorders (including neuropathies and fibromyalgia), generalized anxiety, vasomotor symptoms of menopause and stress urinary incontinence (Susman N, 2003). The class of SNRIs now comprises five medications: venlafaxine (Effexor XR, Efexot XR), its metabolite desvenlafaxine (Pristique), milnacipran (Ixel, Toledomin), duloxetine (Cymbalta, Xeristar) and mirtazapine (Remeron).

1. Venlafaxine XR (Effexor)
   25, 37.5,50, 75,100 mg tablets; 37.5,75,150 mg extended release capsules
2. Desvenlafaxine (Pristique)
   50, 100 mg capsules
3. Milnacipran (Ixel, Toledomin)
   100 mg/day (given as 50 mg 2 times daily,
   with a starting period of 4 days on 25 mg/day).
4. Duloxetine (Cymbalta)
   20, 30, 50 mg capsules
5. Mirtazapine (Remeron)
   15 mg to 45 mg/day

Table 1. Serotonin norepinephrine reuptake inhibitors (SNRIs)

2. Pharmacology

2.1 Pharmacodynamics

SNRIs bind to 5-HT and NA transporters to selectively inhibit the reuptake of these neurotransmitters from the synaptic clefts. They have a "dual mode of action". SNRIs block the reuptake of both 5-HT and NA with differing selectivity. Whereas milnacipran blocks 5-HT and NA reuptake with equal affinity, duloxetine has a 10-fold greater selectivity for 5-HT, and venlafaxine has a 30-fold greater selectivity for 5-HT (Stahl et al., 2005).

Venlafaxine was the first SNRI to be introduced. Venlafaxine inhibits neuronal uptake of 5-HT (most potent, present at low doses), NA (moderate potency, present at high doses) and dopamine (DA) in order of decreasing potency. Venlafaxine has no affinity for α2- or β-adrenoceptors, benzodiazepine or opiate receptors. It has a much greater affinity for the 5-HT transporter than for the norepinephrine (NE) transporter. At low doses, it inhibits the 5-HT transporter almost exclusively, acting like a selective serotonin reuptake inhibitor (SSRI), with significant NE reuptake inhibition only occurring at higher doses (Saletu et al., 1992).

Desvenlafaxine is a synthetic form of the isolated major active metabolite of venlafaxine. The neurotransmitters affected by the drug are 5-HT and NE. It is approximately 10 times more potent at inhibiting 5-HT uptake than NE uptake. It has low affinity for other brain neurotransmitter targets, including muscarinic, cholinergic, histamine (H1) and α-adrenergic receptors (Whyte & Dawson, 2003; Septien-Velez et al., 2007).

Previous studies demonstrated that duloxetine potently inhibits neuronal 5-HT and NE re-uptake. It has been demonstrated that this inhibition is balanced throughout the dosing range compared to venlafaxine, which demonstrates low inhibition of NA at low doses and rises as the dose escalates. Duloxetine is also considered a less potent inhibitor of dopamine re-uptake. Duloxetine has no significant affinity for adrenergic, cholinergic, histaminergic, opioid, glutamate, or GABA receptors. It binds selectively with high affinity to both NA and 5-HT transporters and lacks affinity for monoamine receptors within the central nervous system. Additionally, duloxetine is a more potent 5-HT reuptake inhibitor compared to fluoxetine (SSRI) (Westanmo & Gayken, 2005; Bymaster et al., 2001).

Milnacipran is the most balanced SNRI, and some studies have even found it to be slightly more effective for the NE transporter compared with the 5-HT transporter. Milnacipran inhibits the re-uptake of 5-HT and NA in an approximate 1:3 ratio; in practical use, this means a relatively balanced action upon both neurotransmitters. Milnacipran shows antidepressive activity due to suppression of 5-HT re-uptake and NA in postsynaptic receptors. Milnacipran exerts no significant actions on H1, α1, DA1, DA2, and mACh receptors or on benzodiazepine and opioid binding sites. The biochemical profile of milnacipran and its lack of interaction with other neurotransmitters indicate that the drug may be maximally effective in the treatment of depression while being free of the side-effects associated with other antidepressants. Simultaneous inhibition of both 5-HT and NA works synergistically to treat both fibromyalgia and depression (Vaishnavi & Nemeroff, 2004).

Mirtazapine is a tetracyclic compound with antidepressant activity. It has a unique mechanism of action that is different from classical tricyclic antidepressants, the SSRIs and monoamine oxidase inhibitors. Therefore, it could be described as a noradrenergic and specific serotonergic antidepressant. Mirtazapine's pharmacological profile is characterized by a potent presynaptic alpha-2-adrenergic antagonist activity, 5-HT1 agonist activity, and potent 5-HT2 and 5-HT3 antagonist activities as well as by a potent H1 antagonistic activity. The blockade of presynaptic alpha-2-adrenergic receptors is considered as a possible mechanism for the antidepressant activity of mirtazapine. It is also a strong H1 receptor antagonist, therefore, it causes sedative side effects (Dekeyne & Millan, 2008; Millan et al., 2000).

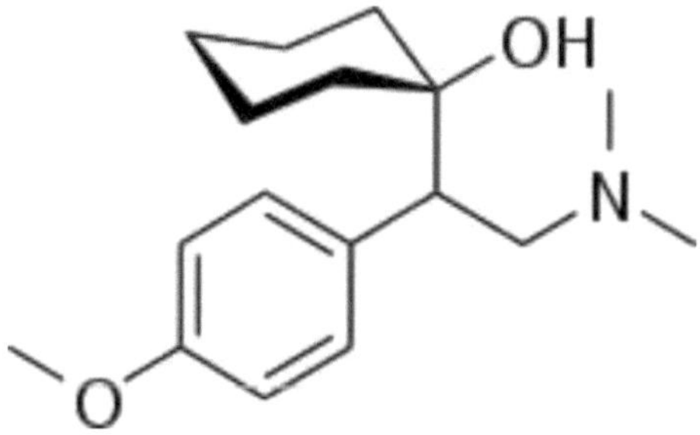

Venlafaxine

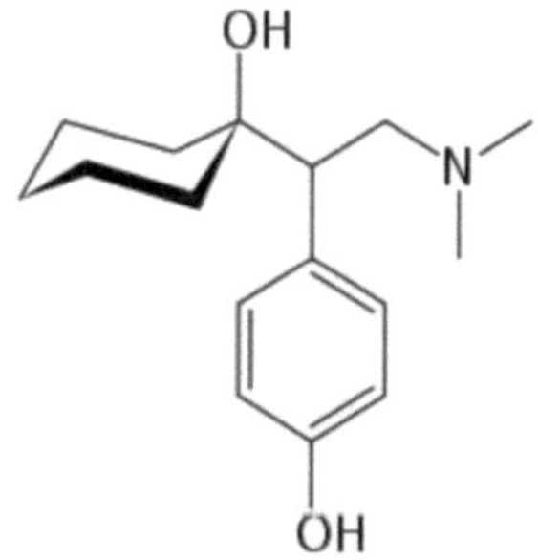

Desvenlafaxine

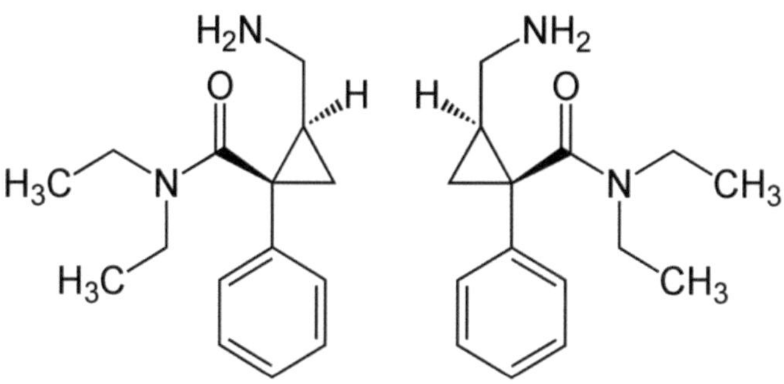

Milnacipran

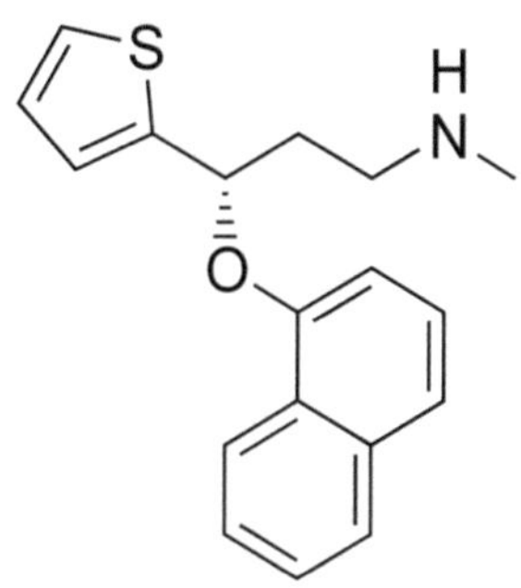

Duloxetine

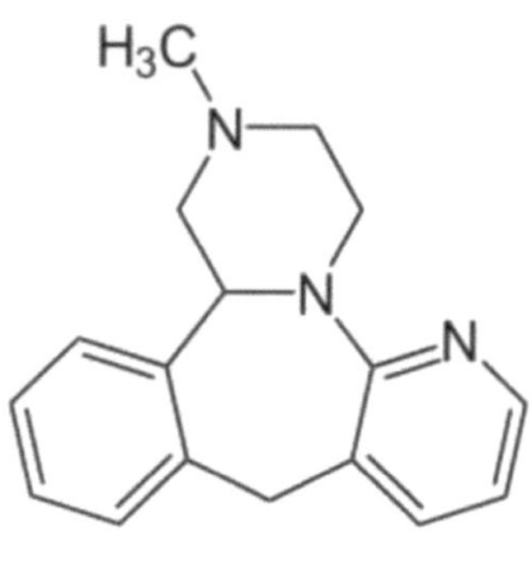

Mirtazapine

Fig. 1. Structure of SNRI-class antidepressants

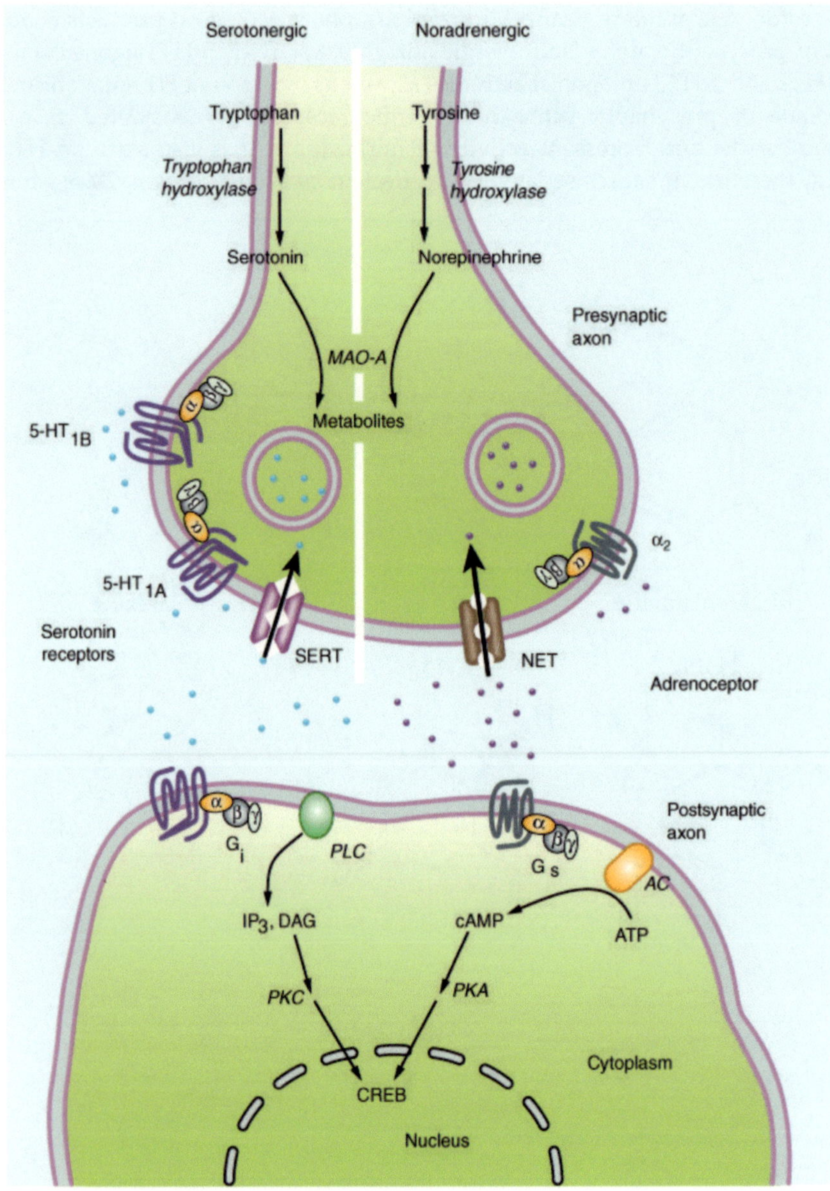

Source: Katzung BG, Masters SB, Trevor AJ: *Basic & Clinical Pharmacology, 11th Edition*: http://www.accessmedicine.com

Fig. 2. The amin hypothesis of major depression. Depression appears to be associated with changes in serotonin and norepinephrine signaling in brain (or both) with significant downstream effects. Most antidepressants cause changes in amine signaling. AC, adenyly cyclase; 5-HT, serotonin; CREB, c AMP response element binding (protein); DAG, diacyl glycerol; IP3, inositol trisphosphate; MAO (monoamine oxidase), NET (norepinephrine transporter), PKC: protein kinase C; PLC, phospholipase C; SERT, serotonin transporter (From: Katzung, B.G.; Masters, S.B.; Trevor, A.J. 11 th edition. Basic and clinical pharmacology. International edition).

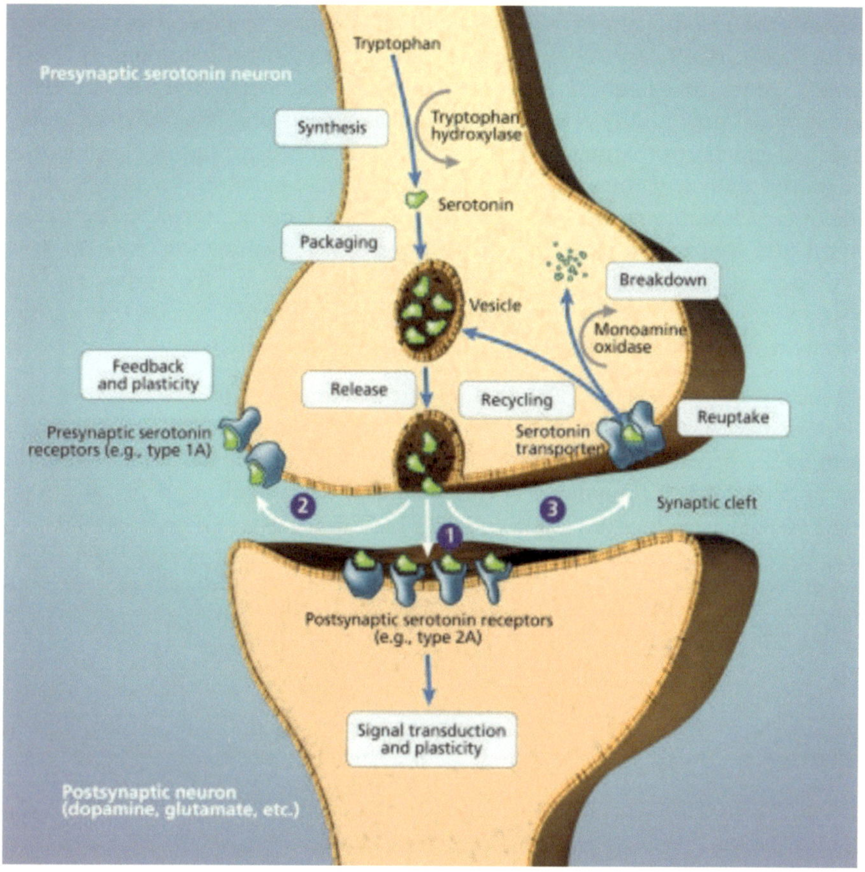

Fig. 3. The serotonin synapse. Serotonin is synthesized from tryptophan by the enzyme tryptophan hydroxylase. Serotonin is then packaged into vesicles for release into the synaptic cleft, which occurs when there is sufficient stimulation of the neuron. Serotonin released from the serotonin neuron into the synaptic cleft has multiple actions. (1) Serotonin binds to its receptors on other neurons. Activation of postsynaptic receptors results in transduction of the signal that initially stimulated the serotonin neuron. (2) Serotonin also binds to presynaptic serotonin receptors on the neuron from which it was released, which provides feedback and regulates plasticity of the neuron. (3) Serotonin is taken up back into the presynaptic serotonin neuron by the serotonin transporter. Serotonin is then recycled for future release or broken down by monoamine oxidase and excreted in urine (From: aan het Rot, M., Mathew, S.J.; Charney, D.S. (2009). Neurobiological mechanisms in major depressive disorder. CMAJ. 3;180(3):305-13).

2.2 Pharmacokinetics

Venlafaxine is a bicyclic phenyetilamine derivative. The mean half-life of venlafaxine is approximately 4 h and is relatively short. Venlafaxine is well-absorbed from the gastrointestinal tract and is a substrate for CYP450. It is extensively metabolized in the liver via the CYP2D6 isoenzyme to desvenlafaxine (O-desmethylvenlafaxine), which is just as potent a 5-HT-NA reuptake inhibitor as the parent compound. This means that the differences in the metabolism between extensive and poor metabolizers are not clinically important in terms of efficacy. Therapeutic effects are usually achieved within 3 to 4 weeks. The primary route of excretion of venlafaxine and its metabolites is via the kidneys (Wellington and Perry, 2001). Desvenlafaxine has linear pharmacokinetics, low protein binding, a half-life of approximately 10 h and is metabolized primarily via glucuronidation and to a minor extent, through CYP3A4. The desvenlafaxine succinate has a good oral bioavailability. Clearance rates are reduced in the elderly, those with severe renal dysfunction and those with moderate to severe hepatic dysfunction, each of which may require dosage adjustments. Desvenlafaxine is excreted in the urine, is minimally metabolized via the CYP450 pathway and is a weak inhibitor of CYP2D6 (De Martinis et al., 2007; Liebowitz & Yeung, 2007; Septien- Velez et al., 2007).

Duloxetine shows linear kinetics. The therapeutic dose range is 60-120 mg/day. Duloxetine has an elimination half-life of approximately 12.5 hours (range of 8 to 17 hours), and its pharmacokinetics are dose proportional over the therapeutic range. Steady-state is usually achieved after 3 days. Elimination of duloxetine is mainly through hepatic metabolism involving two P450 isozymes, CYP2D6 and CYP1A2 (Papakostas GI et al., 2007).

Properties of SNRIs	Venlafaxine	Desvenlafaxine	Duloxetine	Milnacipran	Mirtazapine
Therapeutic dose range	75-375 mg/day	50 mg/day	60-120 mg/day	25-200 mg/day	15-45 mg/day
Biotransformation	CYP2D6	CYP3A4	CYP2D6, CYP1A2	CYP2D6, CYP2C9	CYP2D6,CYP3 A4,CYP1A2
Half -life	4 h	9-10 h	12.5 h	12 h	20-40 h
Elimination route	renal	renal	renal, urine (72%), faeces (19%)	renal	Renal urine (75%), faeces (15 %)
NE/5HT affinity ratio	15:7	13:8	9:3	2:1	-
5HT/NE selectivity	30	3 x higher (NE binding)	10	1	300
Efficacy	SNRI action is dose dependent	Beter efficacy at low doses	May require higher than the approved doses	Beter efficacy at higher doses	Dose dependent
Hepatic side effects	Elevated liver enzymes	-	Complicated by alcohol consumption	Elevated liver enzymes	Hepatic insufficiency
Cardiac side effects	+	QTc interval prolongation	-	-	-
Sexual dysfunction	Loss of libido, anorgasmia	Delayed ejaculation	Loss of libido, anorgasmia	Decrease in sexual desire and ability	Not cause significant sexual dysfunction

Table 1. Quote from: Dell'Osso B, Buoli M, Baldwin DS, Altamura AC. Serotonin norepinephrine reuptake inhibitors (SNRIs) in anxiety disorders: a comprehensive review of their clinical efficacy. Hum Psychopharmacol. 2010 Jan;25(1):17-29.

Milnacipran shows linear pharmacokinetics over a dose range of 25-200 mg/day. Milnacipran is rapidly and extensively absorbed and has a high bioavailability. Peak plasma concentrations are reached 2 hours after oral dosing. The elimination half-life is relatively short (12 hours) and is increased by significant renal disease. Milnacipran is conjugated to an inactive glucuronide and excreted in the urine as an unchanged drug and conjugate. Enzymes of the CYP class do not play a role in the metabolism of this antidepressant drug so the risk of interactions with drugs metabolized by CYP enzymes is minimal (Puozzo & Panconi, 2002).

Mirtazapine has an elimination half-life of 20-40 hours. Like most other antidepressants with a therapeutic-latency mirtazapine may require as long as 2–4 weeks for the therapeutic benefits of the drug to become evident. It is metabolized in the liver by the enzymes CYP2D6, CYP3A4 and CYP1A2. It does not have an active metabolite (Timmer & Ad Sitsen, 2000).

3. Medical uses

3.1 Efficacy and tolerability

Depression is characterized by the presence of depressed mood and anhedonia (decreased pleasure or interest). It is also accompanied by a plethora of other signs and symptoms such as changes in appetite and sleeping, fatigue and loss of energy, psychomotor agitation or retardation, feelings of worthlessness or inappropriate guilt and diminished ability to think or concentrate (Bauer & Bschor, 2007). In general, antidepressants that are used today are effective in treating depression regardless of whether they primarly affect serotonergic or noradrenergic neurotransmission or both. It has been suggested that there may be differences in efficacy of antidepressants among certain patients. Evidence has demonstrated significantly greater remission rates with the SNRI venlafaxine compared with SSRIs (Bauer et al., 2009).

Evidence demonstrates that 5-HT and NA are involved in both the pathogenesis and recovery from depression. Preliminary results showed that dual acting antidepressants may have an advantage over single acting agents in terms of treating patients to remission. Dual acting agents may also be preferable for the treatment of chronic painful conditions and somatic symptoms (Sussman, 2003).

Venlafaxine is used primarily for the treatment of depression, general anxiety disorder, social phobia, panic disorder, and vasomotor symptoms. Venlafaxine inhibits the reuptake of both 5-HT and NA, thus combining two therapeutic mechanisms in one agent. The anticholinergic and cardiotoxic side effects are not as common compared with tricyclic antidepressants. Venlafaxine's serotonergic actions are present at low doses, while its noradrenergic actions are progressively enhanced as the dose increases. Venlafaxine treatment stimulated expression of brain derived neurotrophic factor protein in the frontal cortex and inhibited long-term potentiation in the hippocampus (Cooke et al., 2009).

Desvenlafaxine is a recently introduced antagonist of the human NE and 5HT transporters (hNET and hSERT) that is currently in clinical development for use in the treatment of major depressive disorder and vasomotor symptoms associated with menopause. Desvenlafaxine succinate is the succinate salt of the isolated major active metabolite of venlafaxine. Desvenlafaxine is being tested for the treatment of fibromyalgia with promising results (Wood, 2007).

Duloxetine is a newly developed tiophenpropanamin derivative. It is a SNRI indicated for the treatment of depression and for anxiety disorders but also approved for stress urinary incontinence, diabetic neuropathy and fibromyalgia. Duloxetine is approved for the treatment of major depressive disorder and diabetic peripheral neuropathic pain (Ormseth & Scholz, 2011).

Milnacipran has a balanced activity on NA and 5-HT reuptake inhibition. Its efficacy in mild, moderate, and severe depression and suitable overall tolerability are combined with a low risk of causing pharmacokinetic drug-drug interactions, sexual dysfunction, changes in body weight in normal-weight patients, and toxicity due to overdose. This particular profile qualifies milnacipran as a first-line antidepressant for many depressed patients. Patients who have been withdrawn from SSRIs or other antidepressants due to lack of efficacy or intolerance may find milnacipran to be an effective therapeutic option. Also, milnacipran is an effective treatment option for patients with fibromyalgia. Current studies do not yet provide convincing evidence supporting the efficacy of mirtazapine, reboxetine, milnacipran and duloxetine for the treatment of panic disorder patients (Kasper et al., 2010; Serretti et al., 2010).

Mirtazapine is a piridin analogue of mianserine. Mirtazapine is a newer antidepressant that exhibits both noradrenergic and serotonergic activity. It is a tetracyclic antidepressant used primarily in the treatment of major depressive disorder. It is unlike other agents used for depression both in its mechanism of action as well as its side effects. It is at least as effective as the older antidepressants for treating mild to severe depression. Mirtazapine is relatively safe in overdose. Many clinicians consider mirtazapine a second-line or even third-line antidepressant to be used when older antidepressants are not tolerated or are ineffective. Physicians who are concerned about the risks of elevated lipid levels and agranulocytosis may choose to reserve mirtazapine as a third-line choice. It is particularly useful in patients who experience sexual side effects from other antidepressants. Mirtazapine is also a good choice in depressed patients with significant anxiety or insomnia. (Hartmann, 1999). It has been found to be useful in the treatment of generalized anxiety disorder, social anxiety disorder, obsessive-compulsive disorder, panic disorder and post-traumatic stress disorder (Benjamin & Doraiswamy, 2011).

4. Studies with SNRIs in animal models

Newer dual-acting antidepressants appear to possess analgesic effects similar to that of the TCAs but have a more favorable safety and tolerability profile. These drugs also may have an advantage over SSRIs in treating the painful physical symptoms of depression and in achieving remission of all symptoms of depression. Some animal models have been used to characterize the pathological conditions and the effects of drugs on these conditions. Researchers have compared the performance of SNRIs using novel animal models to evaluate the effects on depression, obsessive compulsive disorder, pain and learning and memory functions.

4.1 Research via SNRIs and depression in animal models

Antidepressants inhibiting the reuptake of both 5-HT and NA may exhibit efficacy superior to that of SSRIs.

Ulak et al. (2008) showed that the neuronal NOS inhibitor, 1-(2-trifluoromethylphenyl)-imidazole, augments the effects of antidepressants acting via the serotonergic system in a forced swimming test (FST) in rats.

The effects of subchronic treatment (24 days) with antidepressants displaying differential effects on NA and 5-HT reuptake on behavior, neurochemistry, and hypothalamic-pituitary-adrenal (HPA) axis activity following FST exposure in the rat were studied. Desipramine significantly decreased immobility in the FST, while paroxetine and venlafaxine were without effect. Nonetheless, treatment with all three antidepressants significantly attenuated stress-related increases in amygdaloid and cortical serotonin turnover. Desipramine attenuated the stress-associated elevation in serum corticosterone. Connor and collegues (2000) concluded that although FST-induced increases in serotonin turnover in the frontal cortex and amygdala were attenuated following treatment with all three antidepressants, FST-induced behavioral changes and increased HPA axis activity were normalized only following desipramine treatment.

The rat forced swimming test distinguishes between selective 5-HT and selective NA reuptake inhibitors, which increase swimming and climbing behaviors, respectively. Since adaptative neurochemical processes occur in the treatment of depression, the influence of long-term antidepressant treatment on these interactions was examined. Fluoxetine, desipramine, milnacipran and mirtazapine were administered subacutely and chronically. A subacute fluoxetine-desipramine combination was administered in rats that were pre-treated with chronic-desipramine. NA system-mediated interactions were further examined by combining clonidine with fluoxetine. Results of this study showed that long-term treatment with either fluoxetine or desipramine did not modify the behavioral response produced by subacute administration. In contrast, whereas subacute-milnacipran increased climbing solely, chronic-milnacipran produced greater anti-immobility effects and increased both climbing and swimming behaviors. Similarly, the fluoxetine-desipramine combination produced climbing solely but increased both climbing and swimming behaviors in animals pre-treated with chronic desipramine. Chronic, but not subacute, mirtazapine increased swimming behavior. Clonidine dose-dependently antagonized fluoxetine-induced anti-immobility effects and swimming behavior. It was concluded that chronic enhancement of NA transmission alters NA system-mediated inhibition of 5-HT-induced behavior in the FST, which may involve alpha (2)-receptors (Rénéric & Bouvard, 2002).

Mochizuki D, et al. (2002) aimed to characterize, both neurochemically and behaviorally, the SNRI milnacipran in the prefrontal cortex in comparison with tricyclic antidepressants and selective serotonin reuptake inhibitors. It was concluded that milnacipran acts as an SNRI in vitro and in vivo and may be useful for the treatment of anxiety as well as depression (Mochizuki et al., 2002).

Researchers aimed to investigate whether estrogen level changes in oviariectomized rats may lead to depression and memory disorders and whether the effects of such changes may be reversible following administration of venlafaxine using the Porsolt forced swimming test and Morris water maze test. It was reported that the regulatory role of estrogen and venlafaxine in antidepressant activity and memory function could be related to the interactions between noradrenergic and serotonergic systems (Nowakowska & Kus, 2005).

In another study, the relationship between the antidepressant effect of venlafaxine and its ability to protect animals against stress-induced oxidative lipid peroxidation and DNA damage was investigated. It was reported that long-term venlafaxine treatment using effective antidepressant doses can protect against stress-induced oxidative cellular and DNA damage. It was concluded that this action may occur by antagonizing oxidative stress and enhancing antioxidant defense mechanisms (Abdel-Wahab & Salama, 2011).

In animal models detecting antidepressant activity, distinct NO synthase inhibitors displayed antidepressant-like action. Previous studies found that pretreatment with L-arginine counteracted the antidepressant-like effect of imipramine and venlafaxine but not the effects of bupropion or fluoxetine. Increasing the dose of L-Arg to 1000 mg/kg attenuated the antidepressant-like effects of bupropion but did not modify the action of fluoxetine. L-Arginine was devoid of any locomotor effects on the animals. In that study, the idea that some antidepressants are able to inhibit nitric oxide synthesis in the brain, an effect that could be mechanistically related to the ability of L-arginine to counteract the antidepressant-like effects, was supported (Krass et al., 2011).

Milnacipran was active in various animal models of depression, such as the forced swimming test in the mouse, learned helplessness in the rat and the olfactory bulbectomized rat model. Milnacipran represents an interesting new therapeutic option for depression being that it is as well tolerated as SSRIs but offers clinical efficacy similar to TCAs (Boyer & Briley, 1998).

Effects of co-treatment with mirtazapine and low doses of risperidone on immobility time in the forced swimming test in mice were evaluated. It was found that MIR (2.5, 5 and 10 mg/kg) and FLU (5 and 10 mg/kg) or risperidone in low doses (0.05 and 0.1 mg/kg) given alone did not change the immobility time of mice in the forced swimming test. Joint administration of MIR (5 and 10 mg/kg) or FLU (10 mg/kg) and risperidone (0.1 mg/kg) produced antidepressant-like activity in the forced swimming test (Rogóż et al., 2010).

The effect of venlafaxine, a dual reuptake inhibitor of 5-HT and NA, was evaluated in a murine model of chronic fatigue. It was concluded that daily treatment with venlafaxine for 15 days produced a significant reduction in the immobility period and reversed various behavioral, biochemical and neurotransmitter alterations induced by chronic fatigue. Therefore, venlafaxine could be of therapeutic potential in the treatment of chronic fatigue (Dhir & Kulkarni, 2008).

4.2 Research via SNRIs and anxiety and obsessive compulsive disorder in animal models

The effects of milnacipran, a 5-HT and NA reuptake inhibitor (SNRI), on the obsessive compulsive disorder (OCD) model and marble burying behavior were investigated in mice. At doses above 10 mg/kg milnacipran inhibited marble burying behavior significantly in mice similar to fluvoxamine. Milnacipran doses inhibiting marble burying behavior did not affect locomotor activity. These results suggest that the inhibition of marble burying behavior may indicate that milnacipran may be useful for OCD therapy (Sugimoto et al., 2007).

Milnacipran has not yet been systematically studied preclinically or clinically for the treatment of anxiety disorders. In the four-plate test (FPT) which is known to predict anxiolytic-like activity in mice, milnacipran demonstrated strong anti-punishment effects following acute administration. It was concluded that the activation of 5-HT2A receptors is critically involved in the anxiolytic activity of milnacipran (Bourin et al., 2005).

Methods for detection of anxiolytic-like behavioral effects of serotonin uptake inhibitors are limited. Venlafaxine dose-dependently suppressed nestlet shredding and marble burying at doses that were generally without effect on rotorod performance. The amine-based antidepressant agents, imipramine and desipramine, as well as the selective NA transport inhibitor, nisoxetine, produced similar qualitative effects on these behaviors (Li & Morrow, 2006).

The effect of chronic treatment with venlafaxine on beta1 and 5-HT2 receptor populations was examined in the frontal cortex of olfactory bulbectomised (OB) and sham operated (SO) animals. The effect of these drugs on the behaviour of the animals on the elevated plus maze and the open field was also assessed. Removal of the bulbs resulted in a characteristic increase in locomotor activity in the OB animals in the open field which was reversed by chronic venlafaxine treatment. Venlafaxine produced a slight reduction in the number of open arm entries made by the OB animals although this failed to reach significance. A decrease in the affinity of beta1-adrenoceptors was found following olfactory bulbectomy and this was normalised by treatment with venlafaxine. Olfactory bulbectomy did not produce any changes in 5-HT2 receptor populations but venlafaxine administration significantly reduced the density of these receptors in both SO and OB animals. It was concluded that the usefulness of the OB as an animal model, for the detection of antidepressants from a wide variety of classes. (McGrath & Norman, 1998). The effect of acute treatment with seven antidepressants covering the classes selective serotonin reuptake inhibitors, serotonin–noradrenaline reuptake inhibitors, noradrenaline reuptake inhibitors and tricyclic antidepressants were compared with the benzodiazepine, chlordiazepoxide, on the mouse zero maze, an unconditioned model of anxiety. Duloxetine was anxiolytic after chronic but not acute treatment, reflecting clinical experience with antidepressants in general (Troelsen, 2005).

Mirtazapine is an antidepressant with a unique mechanism of action and has been categorized as a noradrenergic and specific serotonergic antidepressant. Although numerous clinical trials suggested the usefulness of mirtazapine for not only major depressive disorders but also a variety of anxiety disorders, efficacy studies in animal anxiety models have been rarely reported. A potential anxiolytic-like profile of mirtazapine in rat conditioned fear stress model was investigated. It was reported that the anxiolytic-like action of mirtazapine involves activation of 5-HT1A receptor and alpha1 adrenoceptor to different extents, and are compatible with one aspect of mirtazapine's pharmacological profile (Kakui et al., 2009).

4.3 Research via SNRIs and learning-memory in animal models :

Extensive evidence indicates that noradrenaline and serotonin modulate memory formation. In the literature there are a few works evaluating the effects of SNRIs on cognitive parameters such as learning, memory and habituation to novel environments.

Duloxetine, a potent inhibitor of 5-HT and noradrenaline reuptake with weak effects on dopamine reuptake, is used in the treatment of major depression. It has been recognized that some antidepressants can affect memory in humans, but there are no studies that report duloxetine effects on memory using the inhibitory avoidance method. A recent report investigated the effect of duloxetine on short- and long-term memory (STM and LTM) in the inhibitory avoidance task in mice. Duloxetine did not produce any effect on memory after acute and subacute administration, suggesting that this antidepressant does not affect either memory acquisition or consolidation (Pereira et al., 2009).

The effects of milnacipran in animal models of anxiety and memory were evaluated via Vania K.M. Moojen and collegues, 2006; it was concluded that milnacipran can be useful in the treatment of anxiety disorders. The pharmacological characteristics of milnacipran, in modulation of the synaptic plasticity were investigated. It was found that Milnacipran, suppresses long-term potentiation in the rat hippocampal CA1 field via 5-HT1A receptors and a1-adrenoceptors (Tachibana et al., 2004). It was reported that chronic treatment with milnacipran reverses the impairment of synaptic plasticity induced by conditioned fear stress. And it is concluded that anxiolytic mechanism(s) of chronic treatment with milnacipran may be explained by reversal effects on the psychological stress-induced impairment of synaptic plasticity (Matsumoto et al., 2004).

Effect of venlafaxine on cognitive function and hippocampal brain-derived neurotrophic factor expression in rats with post-stroke depression were evaluated and it was reported that venlafaxine can improve post-stroke depression-induced learning and memory dysfunction, possibly through the enhancement of the BDNF level in the CA3 area of hippocampus. (Dai & Li , 2011).

Ulak et al. (2006) reported that chronic administration of fluoxetine or venlafaxine induces memory deterioration in an inhibitory avoidance task in rats. In this study, the comparison of training latencies versus test latencies showed inhibition of passive avoidance learning in fluoxetine- or venlafaxine-treated rats (e.g., no significant difference between training and test latencies) in a step-through test. There was no significant difference between fluoxetine- and venlafaxine-induced reduction of latency in rats in this test.

4.4 Research via SNRIs and pain in animal models

5-HT and NA are implicated in modulating descending inhibitory pain pathways in the central nervous system. Duloxetine is a selective and potent dual 5-HT and NA reuptake inhibitor (SNRI). Iyengar et al. (2004) reported that inhibition of both 5-HT and NA uptake may account for attenuation of persistent pain mechanisms. Thus, duloxetine may be useful in the treatment of human persistent and neuropathic pain states.

Data from numerous animal and clinical studies suggest that dual acting antidepressants are more active in alleviating pain than specific NA reuptake inhibitors, which themselves are more potent than the SSRI (Fishbain, 2000 & Fishbain, 2000).

Milnacipran, duloxetine and pregabalin (an $\alpha 2$-$\delta 1$ Ca^{2+} channel blocker) are efficacious against fibromyalgia, a condition characterized by diffuse chronic pain and associated with stress. These compounds were compared in the study of Bardin et al. (2010) using rat models of acute/inflammatory pain and stress-induced ultrasonic vocalization. In the formalin test, milnacipran dose-dependently attenuated paw elevation and licking. Duloxetine was slightly more potent. Pregabalin also reduced paw licking/late phase. Milnacipran dose-dependently reduced USV; duloxetine was less potent. Milnacipran, duloxetine and pregabalin possess analgesic activity in the formalin test on paw licking/late phase (corresponding to inflammatory pain with a central sensitization component). In the stress-induced USV model, milnacipran was the most potent and efficacious compound. To summarize, the reduction of formalin-induced paw licking/late phase might constitute a useful indicator of the potential activity against inflammatory/centrally sensitized pain, as might be expressed in fibromyalgia (Bardin et al., 2010).

Milnacipran has shown efficacy against several chronic pain conditions including fibromyalgia. A previous report evaluated its anti-allodynic effects following acute or sub-chronic treatment in a rat model of neuropathic pain (chronic constriction injury (CCI) of the sciatic nerve). It is reported that milnacipran is as efficacious as the reference compound amitriptyline in a pre-clinical model of injury-induced neuropathy and demonstrates, for the first time, that it is active acutely and sub-chronically against cold allodynia. It is also suggested that milnacipran has the potential to alleviate allodynia associated with nerve compression-induced neuropathic pain in the clinic (for example, following discal hernia, avulsion or cancer-induced tissue damage) (Berrocoso et al., 2011).

5. Side effects

Sexual dysfunction is often a side effect of drugs that inhibit 5-HT reuptake in general. Specifically, common side effects with venlafaxine include difficulty becoming aroused, lack of interest in sex, and anorgasmia. Genital anesthesia, loss of or decreased response to sexual stimuli, and ejaculatory anhedonia are also possible. Other side effects include nausea, somnolence, dry mouth, dizziness, insomnia, constipation and yawn. With desvenlafaxine nausea was consistently the most common complaint and the most common reason for discontinuation. Less common mild side effects, but more serious, adverse effects reported includes hypertension, QTc interval prolongation, exacerbation of ischemic cardiac disease, elevated lipids and elevated liver enzymes (Sproule BA and Hazra M, 2008). Nausea, somnolence, insomnia, and dizziness were the main side effects reported by approximately 10% to 20% of patients using duloxetine. In a trial for mild major depressive disorder (MDD), the most commonly reported treatment-emergent adverse events among duloxetine-treated patients were nausea (34.7%), dry mouth (22.7%), headache (20.0%) and dizziness (18.7%), and except for headache, these were reported significantly more often than the placebo group. Duloxetine and SSRIs have been shown to cause sexual side effects in some patients, including both males and females. (Bitter & Filipovits, 2011).

Common side effects of mirtazapine included dizziness, blurred vision, sedation, somnolence, malaise/lassitude, increased appetite and subsequent weight gain, dry mouth, constipation, vivid, bizarre, lucid dreams or nightmares, joint pain (arthralgia), muscle pain (myalgia) and back pain. Less common side effects included agitation/restlessness, irritability, aggression, apathy and/or anhedonia (i.e., inability to experience pleasurable emotions), loss of interest in previously enjoyed activities, excessive mellowness or calmness, difficulty swallowing, shallow breathing, decreased body temperature, miosis, nocturnal emissions, spontaneous orgasm, loss of balance, and restless legs syndrome. Mirtazapine has a lower risk of many of the side effects encountered with other antidepressants, such as decreased appetite, insomnia, nausea and vomiting, diarrhea, urinary retention, increased body temperature, increased perspiration/sweating, mydriasis, and sexual dysfunction (consisting of loss of libido and anorgasmia). Sedation is the most common side effect of mirtazapine. Although agranulocytosis is the most serious side effect, it is rare (approximately one in 1,000) and usually reversible when the medication is stopped. In general, some antidepressants may have the capacity to exacerbate some patients' depression or anxiety or cause suicidal ideation, particularly early in the treatment. It has been proven that mirtazapine has a faster onset of antidepressant action compared to SSRIs (Hartmann, 1999).

With milnacipran the most frequently occurring adverse reactions were nausea, headache, constipation, dizziness, insomnia, hot flush, hyperhidrosis, vomiting, palpitations, heart rate increase, dry mouth, and hypertension. Milnacipran can have a significant impact on sexual function, including both a decrease in sexual desire and ability. Milnacipran can cause pain and swelling of the testicles in men as well as blood in the urine and stools. The incidence of cardiovascular and anticholinergic side effects was significantly lower compared with TCAs in a controlled study with over 3,300 patients. Elevation of liver enzymes without signs of symptomatic liver disease has been infrequent. Mood swing to mania has also been observed and dictates termination of treatment. In psychotic patients, emergence of delirium has been noticed. Milnacipran has a low incidence of sedation but improves sleep (both duration and quality) in depressed patients. In agitated patients or those with suicidal thoughts, additive sedative/anxiolytic treatment is usually indicated (Nakagowa et al., 2009; Montgomery et al., 1996).

6. Conclusion

In this chapter of antidepressants including the SNRIs, pharmacology, medical uses, tolerability, experimental studies and side effects of SNRIs are overviewed. They include venlafaxine, desvenlafaxine, duloxetine, milnacipran and mirtazapine. Pharmacology of SNRIs is characterized by the inhibition of both serotonin and noradrenaline at the presynaptic membrane and by weak affinity with receptors at the postsynaptic membrane, which expects well efficacy on major depressive disorder with less adverse effects in clinical use. SNRIs are well tolerated in general. SNRIs can be considered to be the first-line antidepressant drugs.

7. References

Susman, N. (2003). SNRIs Versus SSRIs: Mechanisms of Action in Treating Depression and Painful Physical Symptoms. *Primary Care Companion J Clin Psychiatry,* 2003;5 [suppl 7]:19–26.

Stahl, S.M.; Grady, MM.; Moret, C. & Briley, M. (2005). SNRIs: their pharmacology, clinical efficacy, and tolerability in comparison with other classes of antidepressants. *CNS Spectr,* 10(9):732-47.

Saletu, B.; Grunberger J.; Anderer P.; Lınzmayer L.; Semlıtsch H. V. & Magnı G. (1992). Pharmacodynamics of venlafaxine evaluated by EEG brain mapping, psychometry and psychophysiology. *Br. J. clin. Pharmac,* 33, 589-601.

Whyte, I.; Dawson, A. & Buckley, N. (2003). "Relative toxicity of venlafaxine and selective serotonin reuptake inhibitors in overdose compared to tricyclic antidepressants". *QJM,* 96 (5): 369–74.

Septien-Velez, L; Pitrosky, B; Padmanabhan, SK; Germain, JM; & Tourian, KA (2007). "A randomized, double-blind, placebo-controlled trial of desvenlafaxine succinate in the treatment of major depressive disorder". *Int Clin Psychopharmacol,* 22 (6): 338–47.

Westanmo, A.D.; Gayken, J. & Haight, R. (2005). Duloxetine: a balanced and selective norepinephrine- and serotonin-reuptake inhibitor. *Am J Health Syst Pharm,* 1;62 (23):2481-90.

Bymaster, F.P.; Dreshfield-Ahmad, L.J.; Threlkeld, P.G.; Shaw, J.L., Thompson, L.; Nelson, D.L.; Hemrick-Luecke, S.K. & Wong, D.T. (2001). Comparative affinity of duloxetine and venlafaxine for serotonin and norepinephrine transporters in vitro and in vivo, human serotonin receptor subtypes, and other neuronal receptors". *Neuropsychopharmacology,* 25(6):871-80

Vaishnavi, S.N.; Nemeroff, C.B.; Plott, S.J.; Rao, S.G.; Kranzler, J. & Owens, M.J. (2004). Milnacipran: A comparative analysis of human monoamine uptake and transporter binding affinity. *Biol Psychiatry,* 55(3):320–322

Dekeyne, A.; Millan, M.J. (2008). Discriminative stimulus properties of the 'atypical' antidepressant, mirtazapine, in rats: A pharmacological characterization. *Psychopharmacology,* 203 (2): 329–41.

Millan, M.J.; Gobert, A.; Rivet, J.M.; Adhumeau-Auclair, A.; Cussac, D.; Newman-Tancredi, A.; Dekeyne, A. & Nicolas, J.P. et al. (2000). Mirtazapine enhances frontocortical dopaminergic and corticolimbic adrenergic, but not serotonergic, transmission by blockade of α2-adrenergic and serotonin2C receptors: a comparison with citalopram. *European Journal of Neuroscience,* 12 (3): 1079–95.

Wellington, K & Perry, C. (2001). Venlafaxine extended-release: a review of its use in the management of major depression. *CNS Drugs,* 15 (8): 643–69.

Shams, M.E. et al. (2006). CYP2D6 polymorphism and clinical effect of the antidepressant venlafaxine. J Clin Pharm Ther, 31 (5): 493–502.

DeMartinis, N.A.; Yeung, P.P.; Entsuah, R. & Manley, A.L. (2007). A double-blind, placebo-controlled study of the efficacy and safety of desvenlafaxine succinate in the treatment of major depressive disorder. *J Clin Psychiatry,* 68 (5): 677–88.

Liebowitz, M.R.; Yeung, P.P. & Entsuah, R. (2007). A randomized, double-blind, placebo-controlled trial of desvenlafaxine succinate in adult outpatients with major depressive disorder. *J Clin Psychiatry,* 68 (11): 1663–72.

Septien-Velez, L.; Pitrosky, B.; Padmanabhan, S.K.; Germain, J.M. & Tourian, K.A. (2007). A randomized, double-blind, placebo-controlled trial of desvenlafaxine succinate in the treatment of major depressive disorder. *Int Clin Psychopharmacol,* 22 (6): 338–47.

Papakostas, G.I.; Thase, M.E.; Fava, M.; Nelson, J.C. & Shelton, R.C. (2007). Are antidepressant drugs that combine serotonergic and noradrenergic mechanisms of action more effective than the selective serotonin reuptake inhibitors in treating major depressive disorder? A meta-analysis of studies of newer agents. *Biol. Psychiatry,* 62 (11): 1217–27.

Puozzo, C.; Panconi, E. & Deprez, D. (2002). Pharmacology and pharmacokinetics of milnacipran. *International clinical psychopharmacology,* 17 Suppl 1: S25–35.

Timmer, Cees J.; Ad Sitsen, J.M.; Delbressine, Leon P. (2000). Clinical Pharmacokinetics of Mirtazapine. Clinical Pharmacokinetics, 38 (6): 461–74.

Bauer, M.; Bschor, T.; Pfennig, A. & et al. (2007). World Federation of Societies of Biological Psychiatry (WFSBP) Guidelines for Biological Treatment Of Unipolar Depressive Disorders in Primary Care. *World J Biol Psychiatry*, 8(2):67–104.

Bauer, M; Tharmanathan, P; Volz, H.P; Moeller, H.J. & Freemantle, N. (2009). The effect of venlafaxine compared with other antidepressants and placebo in the treatment of major depression: a meta-analysis. *Eur Arch Psychiatry Clin Neurosci*, 259(3):172-85.

Cooke, J.D.; Grover, L.M. & Spangler, P.R. (2009). Venlafaxine treatment stimulates expression of brain-derived neurotrophic factor protein in frontal cortex and inhibits long-term potentiation in hippocampus. *Neuroscience*, 15;162(4):1411-9.

Wood, P.B.; Holman, A.J. & Jones, K.D. (2007). Novel pharmacotherapy for fibromyalgia. *Expert Opinion on Investigational Drugs*, 16, 6, 829-841.

Ormseth, M.J.; Scholz, B.A. & Boomershine, C.S. (2011). Duloxetine in the management of diabetic peripheral neuropathic pain. *Patient Prefer Adherence*, 5:343-56.

Kasper, S.F.; Pail, G. (2010). Milnacipran: a unique antidepressant. Neurops(Kyle JA, Dugan BD, Testerman KK. Milnacipran for treatment of fibromyalgia. *Ann Pharmacother*, 44(9):1422-9.

Serretti, A.; Chiesa, A.; Calati, R.; Perna, G.; Bellodi, L. & De Ronchi, D. (2011). Novel antidepressants and panic disorder: evidence beyond current guidelines. *Neuropsychobiology*, 263(1):1-7.

Hartmann, P.M. (1999). Mirtazapine: a newer antidepressant. *Am Fam Physician*, 1;59(1):159-61.

Benjamin, S.; Doraiswamy, P.M. (2011). Review of the use of mirtazapine in the treatment of depression. *Expert Opin Pharmacother*, 12(10):1623-32.

Ulak, G.; Mutlu, O; Akar, F.Y.; Komsuoglu, F.I.; Tanyeri, P & Erden, B.F. (2008). Neuronal NOS inhibitor 1-(2-trifluoromethylphenyl)-imidazole augment the effects of antidepressants acting via serotonergic system in the forced swimming test in rats. *Pharmacol Biochem Behav*, 90(4):563-8.

Rogóż, Z. (2010). Effects of co-treatment with mirtazapine and low doses of risperidone on immobility time in the forced swimming test in mice. *Pharmacol Rep*, 62(6):1191-6.

Dhir, A.; Kulkarni, S.K. (2008). Venlafaxine reverses chronic fatigue-induced behavioral, biochemical and neurochemical alterations in mice. *Pharmacol Biochem Behav*, 89(4):563-71.

Connor, T.J.; Kelliher, P.; Shen, Y.; Harkin, A.; Kelly, J.P. & Leonard, B.E. (2000). Effect of subchronic antidepressant treatments on behavioral, neurochemical, and endocrine changes in the forced-swim test. *Pharmacol Biochem Behav*, 65(4):591-7.

Rénéric, J.P.; Bouvard, M. & Stinus, L. (2002). In the rat forced swimming test, chronic but not subacute administration of dual 5-HT/NA antidepressant treatments may produce greater effects than selective drugs. *Behav Brain Res*, 15;136(2):521-32.

Mochizuki, D., Tsujita, R., Yamada, S., Kawasaki, K., Otsuka, Y., Hashimoto, S., Hattori, T., Kitamura, Y.

& Miki, N. (2002). Neurochemical and behavioural characterization of milnacipran, a serotonin and noradrenaline reuptake inhibitor in rats. *Psychopharmacology (Berl)*, 162(3):323-32.

Nowakowska, E., Kus, K. (2005). Antidepressant and memory affecting influence of estrogen and venlafaxine in ovariectomized rats. *Arzneimittelforschung,* 55(3):153-9.

Abdel-Wahab, B.A.; Salama, R.H. (2011). Venlafaxine protects against stress-induced oxidative DNA damage in hippocampus during antidepressant testing in mice. *Pharmacol Biochem Behav,* 100(1):59-65.

Krass, M.; Wegener, G.; Vasar, E. & Volke, V. (2011). The antidepressant action of imipramine and venlafaxine involves suppression of nitric oxide synthesis. *Behav Brain Res,* 17;218(1):57-63.

Boyer, P.; Briley, M. (1998). Milnacipran, a new specific serotonin and noradrenaline reuptake inhibitor. *Drugs Today (Barc),* 34(8):709-20.

Dhir, A.; Kulkarni, S.K. (2008). Venlafaxine reverses chronic fatigue-induced behavioral, biochemical and neurochemical alterations in mice. *Pharmacol Biochem Behav,* 89(4):563-71.

Sugimoto, Y.; Tagawa, N.; Kobayashi, Y.; Hotta, Y. & Yamada, J. (2007). Effects of the serotonin and noradrenaline reuptake inhibitor (SNRI) milnacipran on marble burying behavior in mice. *Biol Pharm Bull,* 30(12):2399-401.

Bourin, M.; Masse, F.; Dailly, E.; Hascoët, M. (2005). Anxiolytic-like effect of milnacipran in the four-plate test in mice: mechanism of action. *Pharmacol Biochem Behav.* 81(3):645-56.

Li, X.; Morrow, D.; Witkin, J.M. (2006). Decreases in nestlet shredding of mice by serotonin uptake inhibitors: comparison with marble burying. *Life Sci,* 20;78(17):1933-9.

McGrath, C.; Norman, T.R. (1998). The effect of venlafaxine treatment on the behavioural and neurochemical changes in the olfactory bulbectomised rat. *Psychopharmacology (Berl).* 136(4):394-401.

Troelsen, K.B.; Nielsen, E.Ø.; Mirza, N.R. (2005). Chronic treatment with duloxetine is necessary for an anxiolytic-like response in the mouse zero maze: the role of the serotonin transporter. *Psychopharmacology (Berl).* 181(4):741-50.

Kakui, N.; Yokoyama, F.; Yamauchi, M.; Kitamura, K.; Imanishi, T.; Inoue, T.; Koyama T. (2009). Anxiolytic-like profile of mirtazapine in rat conditioned fear stress model: Functional significance of 5-hydroxytryptamine 1A receptor and alpha1-adrenergic receptor. *Pharmacol Biochem Behav.* 92(3):393-8.

Pereira, P.; Gianesini, J.; da Silva Barbosa, C.; Cassol, G.F.; Von Borowski, R.G.; Kahl, V.F.; Cappelari, S.E. & Picada, J.N. (2009). Neurobehavioral and genotoxic parameters of duloxetine in mice using the inhibitory avoidance task and comet assay as experimental models. *Pharmacol Res,* 59(1):57-61.

Moojen, V.K.; Martins, M.R.; Reinke, A.; Feier, G.; Agostinho, F.R.; Cechin, E.M. & Quevedo, J. (2006). Effects of milnacipran in animal models of anxiety and memory. *Neurochem Res.* 31(4):571-7.

Tachibana, K.; Matsumoto, M.; Togashi, H.; Kojima, T.; Morimoto, Y.; Kemmotsu, O. & Yoshioka, M. (2004). Milnacipran, a serotonin and noradrenaline reuptake inhibitor, suppresses long-term potentiation in the rat hippocampal CA1 field via 5-HT1A receptors and alpha 1-adrenoceptors. *Neurosci Lett,* 4; 357(2):91-4.

Matsumoto, M.; Tachibana, K.; Togashi, H.; Tahara, K.; Kojima, T.; Yamaguchi, T. & Yoshioka, M. (2005). Chronic treatment with milnacipran reverses the impairment of synaptic plasticity induced by conditioned fear stress. *Psychopharmacology (Berl),* 179(3):606-12.

Dai, M.H.; Li, D.Q. & Han, Y. (2011). *Zhejiang Da Xue Xue Bao Yi Xue Ban,* 40(5):527-34

Ulak, G., Göçmez, S., Erden, F., Tanyeri, P., Utkan, T., Yildiz, F., Mutlu, O. & Gacar, N. (2006). Chronic administration of fluoxetine or venlafaxine induces memory deterioration in an inhibitory avoidance task in rats. *Drug Development Research,* 67: 456–461.

Iyengar, S.; Webster, A.A.; Hemrick-Luecke, S.K.; Xu, J.Y. & Simmons, R.M. (2004). Efficacy of duloxetine, a potent and balanced serotonin-norepinephrine reuptake inhibitor in persistent pain models in rats. *J Pharmacol Exp Ther.* 311(2):576-84.

Fishbain, D. (2000). Evidence-based data on pain relief with antidepressants. *Ann Med,* 32: 305–316.

Fishbain, D.A.; Cutler, R. & Rosomoff, H.L. (2000). Rosomoff RS. Evidence-based data from animal and human experimental studies on pain relief with antidepressants: a structured). review. *Pain Med,* 1:310–316.

Bardin, L.; Gregoire, S.; Aliaga, M.; Malfetes, N.; Vitton, O.; Ladure, P.; Newman-Tancredi, A. & Depoortère, R. (2010). Comparison of milnacipran, duloxetine and pregabalin in the formalin pain test and in a model of stress-induced ultrasonic vocalizations in rats. *Neurosci Res,* 66(2):135-40.

Berrocoso, E.; Mico, JA.; Vitton, O.; Ladure, P.; Newman-Tancredi, A.; Depoortère, R. & Bardin, L. (2011). Evaluation of milnacipran, in comparison with amitriptyline, on cold and mechanical allodynia in a rat model of neuropathic pain. *Eur J Pharmacol,* 25;655(1-3):46-51.

Sproule, B.A.; Hazra, M. & Pollock, B.G. (2008). Desvenlafaxine succinate for major depressive disorder. *Drugs Today (Barc),* 44(7):475-87.

Bitter, I.; Filipovits, D. & Czobor, P. (2011). Adverse reactions to duloxetine in depression. *Expert Opin Drug Saf,* 10(6):839-50.

Hartmann, P.M. Mirtazapine: a newer antidepressant. (1999). *Am Fam Physician,* 1;59(1):159-61.

Nakagawa, A.; Watanabe, N.; Omori, I.M.; Barbui, C.; Cipriani, A.; McGuire, H.; Churchill, R. & Furukawa, T.A. (2009). Milnacipran versus other antidepressive agents for depression. *Cochrane Database Syst Rev,* 8;(3):CD006529.

Montgomery, S.A.; Prost, J.F.; Solles, A. & Briley, M. (1996). Efficacy and tolerability of milnacipran: an overview. *Int Clin Psychopharmacol,* 11 Suppl 4:47-51.

6

Antidepressants Self-Poisoning in Suicide and Suicide Attempt: Acute Toxicity and Treatment

Sara Santos Bernardes[1], Danielle Ruiz Miyazawa[1],
Rodrigo Felipe Gongora e Silva[1], Danielle Camelo Cardoso[1],
Estefânia Gastaldello Moreira[2] and Conceição Aparecida Turini[1]
[1]Poison Information Centre, University Hospital, State University of Londrina (UEL)
[2]Department of Physiological Sciences, State University of Londrina (UEL)
Brazil

1. Introduction

It is estimated that a quarter of the patients that have been diagnosed with major depression attempt suicide during their lifetime, and 15% of these patients ultimately die from suicide. Antidepressants have been shown to be a highly effective treatment for depression; paradoxically, to achieve compliance, physicians must give patients access to a toxic drug, and a possible suicide method (Gunnell & Frankel, 1994; White, Litovitz & Clancy, 2008; Wong et al., 2010).

Suicide is a serious global public health problem. Nearly 1 million individuals commit suicide every year. The magnitude of the problem is even more significant when the number of attempted but uncompleted suicides - 20 times more common - is included (World Health Organization [WHO], 2010).

Suicide, the act of intentionally killing oneself, ranks among the top 10 causes of death in every country, and is one of the three leading causes of death in 15 to 35-year olds. The number of suicides has increased by 60% between 1955 and 1995, mainly in men (Gunnell & Frankel, 1994; Guo & Harstall, 2004). Risk factors for suicide include psychiatric disorders (depression, personality disorder, alcohol dependence, or schizophrenia), and some physical illnesses.

World Health Organization (WHO) defines suicide attempt or "parasuicide" as an act with a nonfatal outcome, in which an individual deliberately initiates a non-habitual behavior, that without intervention from others will cause self-harm; or deliberately ingests a substance in excess of the prescribed therapeutic dosage, and which is aimed at realizing changes which the subject desired via the actual or expected physical consequences (Guo & Harstall,2004). Young women with a previous episode are at high-risk of another suicide attempt (Kessler,Borges & Walters, 1999; Welch, 2001).

Studies on suicide indicated that suicidal behavior and, in particular, the preferred suicide method varies among countries, gender, and age (Ajdacic-Gross et al., 2008; Towsend et al., 2001). European data showed that suicide by poisoning (mainly poisoning by drugs) is the most common method among women and firearm suicide among men (Ajdacic-Gross et al., 2008). Assuming there is functional equivalence, we are drawn to the conclusion that unplanned or impulsive suicide in European women is mainly achieved by poisoning using drugs. Other suicide methods that are common in Western countries are hanging and jumping from high places. In Asia, there are other commonly used suicide methods, *e.g.*, poisoning by pesticides, or carbon monoxide poisoning through charcoal burning in confined spaces (Gunnell & Eddleston, 2003; WHO, 2010).

Access to suicide methods, especially those of easy access, such as large amounts of drugs and alcohol, facilitates impulsive attempts. This is usually observed in younger adults and women (Baca-Garcia et al. 2005; Gunnell & Frankel, 1994; Wyder & De Leo, 2007).

In general, men with non-affective psychosis have higher risk of suicide, and are more likely to succeed. Conversely, women with an anxiety disorder, poor social contact, and high risk factor exposure are less likely to die by suicide (Beaustrais, 2001). In a recent study, at a tertiary hospital in Korea, Oh and colleagues (2011) observed that women in their twenties, who live without their family, and have a history of psychiatric treatment and antidepressant use, may reattempt suicide by self-poisoning. Most commonly used methods of fatal and non-fatal suicide can be observed in figure 1.

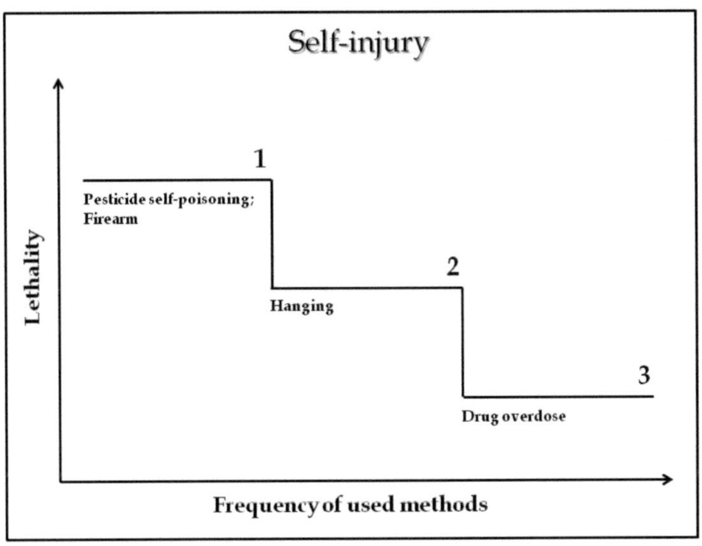

Fig. 1. Most commonly used methods of self-injury worldwide: lethality and frequency of use for suicide attempt. (1) Pesticide self-poisoning and firearm, (2) hanging, and (3) drug overdose. Drug overdose is the most common method of suicide attempt.

Towsend and colleagues (2001) observed that overdose with tranquillizers, sedatives, and antidepressants were more common in older patients and in cases of repeated suicide attempts. These findings are likely to be associated with the accessibility to the drugs. First-timers and younger patients are less likely to have access to prescribed medication, and hence turn to other readily available drugs, whereas repeaters and older patients are more likely to be receiving treatment for psychiatric disorders, and thus have access to psychotropic medication. In addition, the lack of marked variation between suicide intent and overdose of commonly used drugs may reflect the fact that many patients lack knowledge of the relative dangers of overdoses with these substances (Avanci, Pedrão & Costa-Júnior, 2005; WHO, 2010). According to a study conducted by The Poison Information Centre in southern Brazil, suicide attempts were significant among unemployed men, housewives, and retired women. Ingestion of drugs with other substances was responsible for 51.5% of the suicide attempts. Approximately 51.1% of the men mixed the medicine with an alcoholic beverage, and 84.8% of the women used a combination of drugs. The most frequent pharmacological groups were tranquilizers (25.5%), antidepressants (17%), anticonvulsants (15%) and non-steroidal anti-inflammatory drugs (11.9%) (Bernardes, Turini & Matsuo, 2010).

In a systematic review of published follow-up data from observational and experimental studies in Europe, North America and Australasia, Owens, Horrocks & House (2002) found that 16% of the patients repeated the suicide attempt, and only 2% went on to committing fatal suicide in the subsequent year. The risk of suicide following non-fatal deliberate self-harm was greater in men than in women, and the risk increased with age (Hawton, Zahl & Weatherall, 2003). Relative risk of suicide in females who deliberately harm themselves repeatedly is enhanced when compared with those with a single episode of deliberate self-harm. This suggests that repetition status as a risk factor may be particularly relevant when assessing risk in females (Zahl & Hawton, 2004).

Considering patients that commit suicide, about half of them, at some point, had contact with psychiatric services, yet only a quarter had current or recent contact (Andersen et al., 2000; Lee et al., 2008). A study conducted by Gunnell & Frankel (1994) revealed that 20-25% of those committing suicide had contact with a health care professional in the week before death and 40% had such contact one month before death . Bancroft & Marsack (1977) characterized three types of suicide attempters: (a) the chronic, habitual repeater; (b) the individual who repeats several times within a short period, and (c) the "one-off" very occasional repeater.

1.1 Worldwide characteristics of antidepressants self-poisoning

The antidepressants used in deliberate self-poisoning change according to the substances available in each country. In England, the Netherlands, Brazil, and China tricyclic antidepressants (TCAs) are more commonly used, whereas in the United States and Australia, selective serotonin reuptake inhibitors (SSRIs) are more common (Bernardes, Turini & Matsuo, 2010; Bosch et al., 2000; Fernandes et al., 2006; Lam, Lau & Yan, 2010; McKenzie & McFarland, 2007; Neeleman & Wessely, 1997; White, Litovitz & Clancy, 2008; Wong et al., 2010). In these countries, the rates of self-poisoning with SSRIs (particularly citalopram and fluoxetine) and venlafaxine are higher than with tricyclics, especially amongst patients with a history of self-harming and psychiatric treatment (Bergen et al., 2010; Hawton et al., 2010).

Studies carried out in the 90's suggested that some SSRIs antidepressants might selectively increase suicidality (Beasley et al., 1991; Healy, Langmaak & Savage, 1999; Teicher, Glod & Cole, 1990). Khan and colleagues (2003) compared SSRIs with other antidepressants and placebo, and demonstrated that there was no difference in suicide risk among the patients under treatment. This suggests that the prescription of SSRIs does not seem to be associated with higher suicide rates. Nefazodone, mirtazapine, bupropion, venlafaxine, imipramine, amitriptyline, maprotiline, trazodone, mianserin and dothiepin were also evaluated in this study.

Although TCAs have a low therapeutic index, the fact that they are inexpensive and can be prescribed for other pathologies (migraine and polyneuropathy), facilitates their access to suicide attempters (Hawton et al., 2010; Henry, Alexander & Sener, 1995; White, Litovitz & Clancy, 2008). In cases of suicide by drug overdose, TCAs have the highest fatal toxicity, followed by serotonin and noradrenalin reuptake inhibitors (SNRIs), specific serotonergic antidepressants (NaSSA) and SSRIs (Chan, Gunja & Ryan, 2010; Hawton et al., 2010). Therefore, when prescribing antidepressants, the physician should take into consideration the risk of an overdose - especially for patients that have a high risk of suicide attempt - as well as the relative efficacy and acceptability of the drug, possible interactions with other medications and alcohol, and concurrent physical morbidity.

In an analysis of 82.802 cases of suicidal antidepressant overdose registered in the United States between 2000 and 2004, White, Litovitz & Clancy (2008) observed the following:

1. Suicidal overdoses of the newer antidepressants types peaked in younger age groups, especially when compared to antidepressants that had been marketed for decades (SSRIs and SNRIs x TCAs and monoamine oxidase inhibitors);
2. Overdose by lithium peaked in patients in their twenties, TCAs and tetracyclics in their thirties, and MAO inhibitors in their forties;
3. Fatal cases peaked at 40 to 49 years of age. This may be due to the fact that more toxic and older antidepressants are more frequently prescribed in older age groups.

2. Tricyclic and cyclic antidepressants

2.1 History

Tricyclic antidepressants were the first group of drugs used to treat depression to appear in the 60's, being amitriptyline and imipramine the main representatives of this class of drugs (Baldessarini, 2010). In the late 40's Hafliger and Schindler synthesized a series of more than 40 iminodibenzyl derivatives for possible use as an antihistamine, sedative, analgesic and antiparkinson. One of these derivatives was imipramine, a benzazepine with a three-ring chemical structure, very similar to the chemical structure of some drugs that are used to treat schizophrenia, *e.g.*, chlorpromazine (Baldessarini, 2010; Stahl, 2006).

Currently, TCAs are being used not only in the treatment of depression, but also in various other pathologies such as panic disorders, anxiety, obsessive-compulsive disorder, eating disorders, attention deficit hyperactivity disorder, chronic pain, migraine prophylaxis and, enuresis (bed-wetting) (Leke et al., 2004; Cunha-Jr, Barrucand & Verçosa, 2009; Margalho et al., 2007; Liebelt, 2010).

2.2 Acute toxicity and clinical manifestations

The determination of TCAs' toxic dose is a challenging task because in most cases, there is concurrent ingestion of these drugs and alcohol or even other drugs, and interindividual differences in weight and pharmacokinetics. However, the main limitation found is due to the fact that, even therapeutic doses of TCAs, may cause adverse effects and signs of intoxication (Woolf et al., 2007). It is also difficult to determine the toxic dose of TCAs because there is a lack of appropriate studies that specifically investigate the toxic threshold for these drugs, and correlate dose and effect. Data in the literature report that the ingestion of 10-20 mg/kg is considered moderate to severe exposure and cardiovascular symptom may appear (Woolf et al., 2007).

The clinical signs and symptoms that can occur in acute TCAs intoxications are often complex. A short stage of excitement and agitation is common, sometimes with myoclonus, tonic-clonic seizures or dystonia, followed by the rapid development of coma, usually with respiratory depression, hypoxia, depressed reflexes, and hypotension. Some authors report that scores less than 8 for Glasgow Coma Scale may indicate serious complications (Baldessarini, 2010; Bateman, 2005).

The toxicity of TCAs is mainly anticholinergic and cardiovascular (Baldessarini, 2010; Leke et al., 2004; Woolf et al., 2007). The main clinical consequences of anticholinergic effects are dry mouth, sour or metallic taste, epigastric pain, mydriasis, constipation, delayed gastric emptying and slow bowel movements, tachycardia, blurred vision, urinary retention, weakness, and fatigue. Although excessive sweating is a common complaint, the mechanism is still unknown.

The clinical picture reported may be manifested in different degrees of intensity. When the central nervous system (CNS) is affected, the signs and symptoms observed are loss of consciousness, delusions, and hallucinations, increased sensitivity to sounds, dizziness, agitation, and hyperthermia. The hyperthermia that occurs as a consequence of the disturbance in the regulation of body temperature may be due to, among other causes, the central anticholinergic effects of these drugs in overdoses (Baldessarini, 2010; Leke et al., 2004; Bateman, 2005).

In cases of TCA poisoning, patients may present cardiac toxicity and hypotension, and these effects can be especially difficult to control. Arrhythmias, tachycardia, fibrillation, atrioventricular and intraventricular block, and other electrocardiographic changes can also occur. Sinus tachycardia is the most common electrocardiographic abnormality. Other changes such as prolongation of the PR, QRS and QTc intervals may also occur. Prolongation of the QRS is related to clinical manifestations such as seizures and arrhythmias, and when this prolongation is greater than 100 ms it may indicate cardiac toxicity. Therefore, the electrocardiogram (ECG) can be a useful tool as a prognostic indicator in these types of intoxications (Baldessarini, 2010; Kiran et al., 2010; Thanacoody & Thomas, 2005; Liebelt, 2010).

It is considered to be sinus tachycardia when the heart rate exceeds 100 beats per minute and this is mainly due to the inhibition of norepinephrine reuptake, or both. Sinus tachycardia can occur intermittently during the first three days after the intoxication and persist for up to seven days. In more severe cases of poisoning, tachycardia can be caused by myocardial depression, hypovolemia or hypotension (Thanacoody & Thomas, 2005). According to these authors, in the early stages of the intoxication, blood pressure may be elevated, probably as result of the inhibition of norepinephrine reuptake. Posteriorly, blood pressure reduces to very low levels as a consequence of the hypovolemia, reduced peripheral resistance by alpha-adrenergic blockade, cardiac output and impaired myocardial contractility and catecholamine depletion that occur. The hypotension that occurs, which is independent of serum tricyclic levels and prolongation of the QRS interval, is strongly associated with the development of arrhythmias and pulmonary edema.

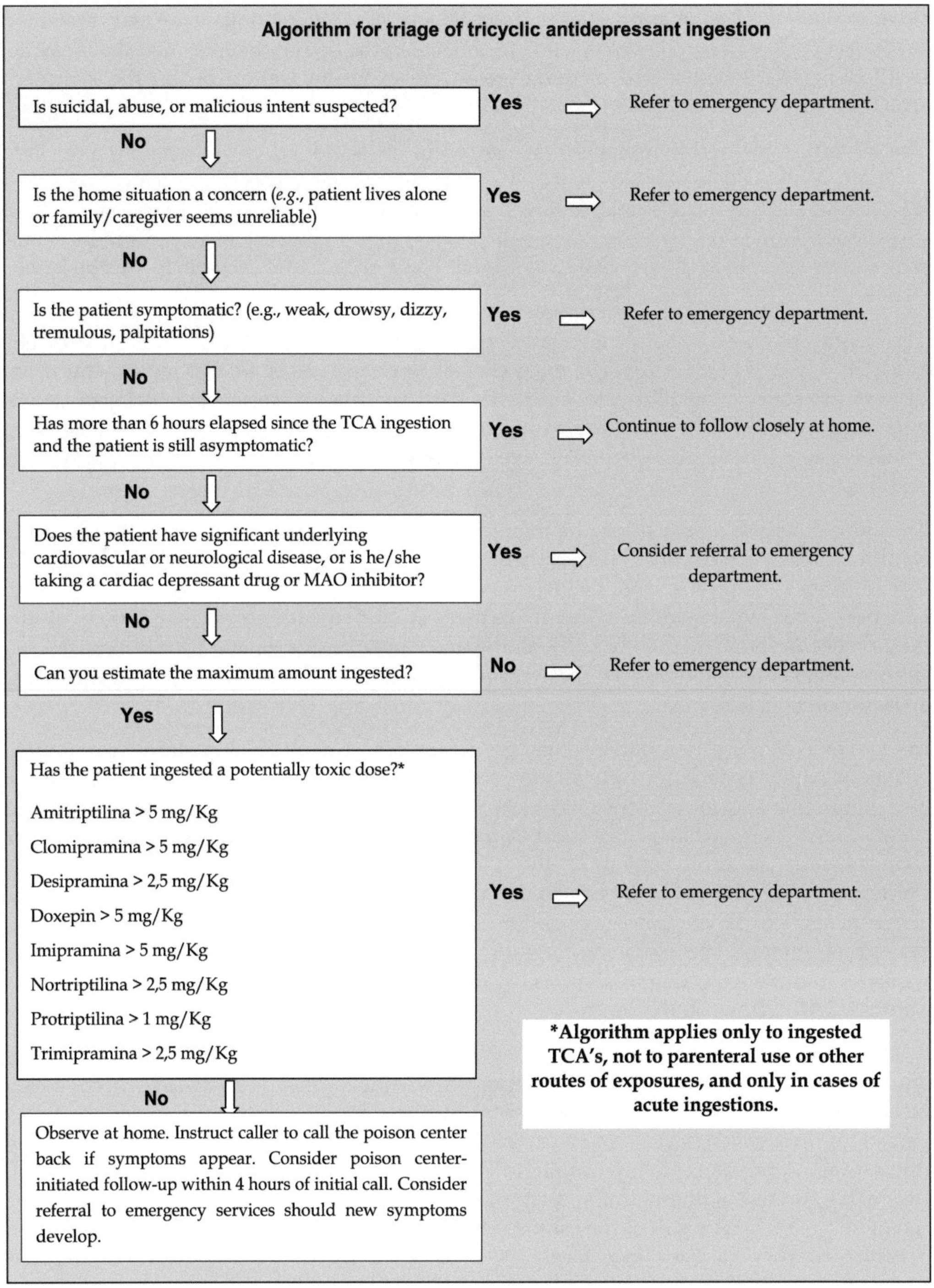

Fig. 2. Algorithm for triage of tricyclic antidepressants poisoning. Adapted from Woolf and colleagues, 2007. With permission from Taylor & Francis INC Publisher (Order License Id: 2813741221934). TCA: Tryciclic antidrepressants.

Thanacoody and Thomas (2005) also reported that cardiac toxicity may be enhanced in patients that develop metabolic acidosis, seizures, and hypotension. Acidosis contributes to the increase in the bioavailability of tricyclics. This provides a higher concentration of free fractions of these drugs, thus potentiating the action of tricyclics, especially on the sodium channels in myocardial cells. These antidepressants can change the conformation of sodium channels and slow cardiac conduction.

Increased risk of tonic-clonic seizures is considered to be one of the most serious toxic effects of tricyclics. The pathophysiology of these seizures is not fully elucidated, however they may occur due to a combination of factors such as the antidopaminergic and anticholinergic properties of TCAs, increased concentration of monoamines (particularly noradrenaline) and inhibition of sodium channels in neurons and interactions with GABA receptors.

Seizures usually occur in 4 out of 100 cases of tricyclic overdose and, as it is an early complication, it is unlikely to occur after 12 hours of the intoxication. If the seizures worsen, hyperthermia and rhabdomyolysis may occur as consequences of muscle hyperactivity and myoclonus. The onset of seizures can lead to brain damage and multiple organ failure. In cases of overdose, the incidence of seizures caused by amoxapine and dothiepin is especially high (Baldessarini, 2010; Stahl, 2006; Citak et al., 2006; Bateman, 2005; Liebelt, 2010).

The duration of signs and symptoms of poisoning vary according to the severity of the case. In prospective case series of 24 adults admitted with TCA overdose, only two patients developed transient supraventricular tachycardia 2 - 4 days after ingestion (Sedal et al, 1972). In retrospective studies, it was observed that only a small number of hospitalized patients developed symptoms such as hypotension and seizures more than 24 hours after ingestion of the drugs. In most of these cases, the clinical manifestations occurred within 24 hours of ingestion (Starkey & Lawson, 1980; Biggs et al., 1977)

The duration of clinical monitoring of asymptomatic patients was also studied. Most authors agree that a six-hour period of observation, after presentation to a healthcare facility, is sufficient to monitor them for the development of major signs of toxicity (Callaham & Kassel, 1985; Fasoli & Glause, 1981).

Studies conducted by The Poison Control Centers in the United States, led to the elaboration of a protocol on the most adequate measures to be taken in cases of poisoning by TCAs. These researchers reached the consensus that decisions about referring patients to emergency services should be based on the patient's clinical status within the first six hours of the ingestion (Woolf et al., 2007). According to this protocol, asymptomatic patients with deliberate TCAs overdose that have not yet sought a health care unit, and after six hours remain asymptomatic, can be easily monitored at home

3. Serotonin reuptake inhibitors

3.1 History

The rate of SSRIs prescription has increased steadily since its introduction in the 80's (Ranchandani et al., 2000). In the U.S., SSRIs are considered first-line treatment of depressive disorders, and are as effective as TCAs and monoamine oxidase inhibitors (MAOIs). The commercial success of the SSRIs is due to their improved side-effect profile and reduced toxicity following overdoses when compared to TCAs. The relative safety in overdose of

SSRIs is supported both by case series and studies of deaths/ number of prescriptions (Isbister et al., 2004; Stork, 2011).

Physicians use SSRIs to treat many other psychiatric disorders, *e.g.*, panic disorder, obsessive compulsive disorder, social anxiety, post-traumatic stress disorder, body dysmorphic disorder, bulimia nervosa, somatoform disorders, pre-menstrual dysphoric disorder, and binge eating. Patients should be informed that the full clinical effect may take more than two weeks to occur (Hirsch & Birnbaum,2011; Stork, 2011).

3.2 Acute Toxicity and clinical manifestations

SSRIs are considered to be less toxic than TCAs and MAOIs because they have an extended therapeutic window. The ingestion of up to 30 times its recommended daily dose produces little or no symptoms. The intake of 50 to 70 times the recommended daily dose can cause vomiting, mild depression of the CNS or tremors. Death rarely occurs, even at very high doses (greater than 150 times) or when SSRIs are ingested with ethanol or benzodiazepines (Hirsch & Binrnaum, 2011).

The symptoms observed following SSRIs overdose are typically mild and manifest primarily as CNS depression. Seizures and cardiac electrophysiological abnormalities (generally QTc interval prolongation) can occur, and they are the most widely reported symptoms following citalopram overdose. Uncommonly, any agent of this class can lead to some clinical effects. These occur as consequences of the development of the serotonin syndrome, which manifests as autonomic instability, altered mental status, seizures, extrapyramidal syndrome including muscle rigidity, hyperthermia, and, rarely, death (Nelson et al., 2007; Stork, 2011).

SSRIs rarely lead to seizures, and are only reported in 1-2% of the cases of SSRI poisoning. These seizures are usually short-lived and self-limited (Hirsch & Birnbaum,2011). SSRIs are safer drugs than tricyclics since they have been related to less expansion of the QT interval and cardiotoxic side effects, (Açikalin et al., 2010).

Severe arrhythmia is unlikely to happen if the patient does not present any of the risk factors and the SSRIs are used at recommended doses. Some of the risk factors are enlargement of the QT, underlying cardiac disease, bradycardia, hypokalemia and hypomagnesemia, use of more than one drug that increases the QT interval, gender , and advanced age (Hirsch & Birnbaum.,2011). The only important exception is citalopram, which can cause QTc prolongation. This provides a biologically plausible basis for the reports of increased morbidity and mortality associated with citalopram overdose (Isbister et al., 2004)

Serotonergic Syndrome

Serotonin syndrome may occur when there is concomitant use of serotonergic drugs or in cases of overdose. It consists of neuromuscular and autonomic changes that result from excessive stimulation of serotonin receptors (5-HT1A and 5-HT2A) in the CNS (Graudins, Sterman & Chan, 1998). Signs of excess serotonin are tremor and diarrhea in mild cases, and delirium, neuromuscular rigidity, and hyperthermia in life-threatening cases (Boyer & Michael, 2005; Poisindex, 2011).

In cases of moderate serotonin syndrome vital sign abnormalities such as tachycardia, hypertension, and hyperthermia may appear. A core temperature as high as 40° C is common in moderate intoxications. Signs and symptoms commonly observed in physical examinations are mydriasis, hyperactive bowel sounds, diaphoresis, and normal skin color. Interestingly, overactive reflexes and clonus in moderate cases may be greater in the lower limbs than in the upper limbs; patellar deep-tendon reflexes often demonstrate clonus for several seconds after a single tap of the tendon, whereas the brachioradialis reflex is only slightly increased. Patients may exhibit horizontal ocular clonus. Changes in mental status include mild agitation or hypervigilance, as well as slightly pressured speech. Patients may easily startle or adopt a peculiar head-turning behavior characterized by repetitive rotation of the head with the neck held in moderate extension (Boyer & Michael, 2005).

In contrast, a patient with a severe case of the serotonin syndrome may present severe hypertension and tachycardia that may abruptly deteriorate into frank shock. These patients may have agitated delirium as well as muscular rigidity and hypertonicity. As motioned above, the increase in muscle tone is considerably greater in the lower limbs. In life-threatening cases, muscle hyperactivity may produce a core temperature of more than 41.1°C. The laboratory abnormalities that are present in severe cases, occur when there is metabolic acidosis, rhabdomyolysis, seizures, and renal failure. Many of these abnormalities arise as a consequence of poorly treated hyperthermia (Boyer & Michael, 2005).

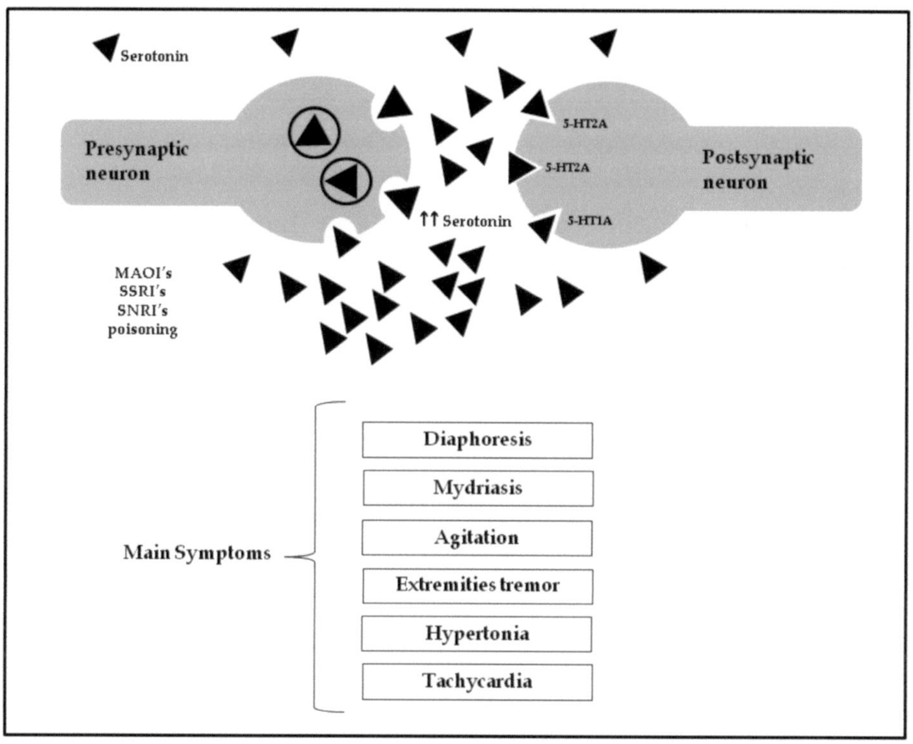

Fig. 3. Findings in moderately severe serotonergic syndrome. The excessive stimulation of serotonin receptors leads to the symptoms listed above. Neuromuscular findings should lead the clinician to consider the diagnosis of the serotonergic syndrome.

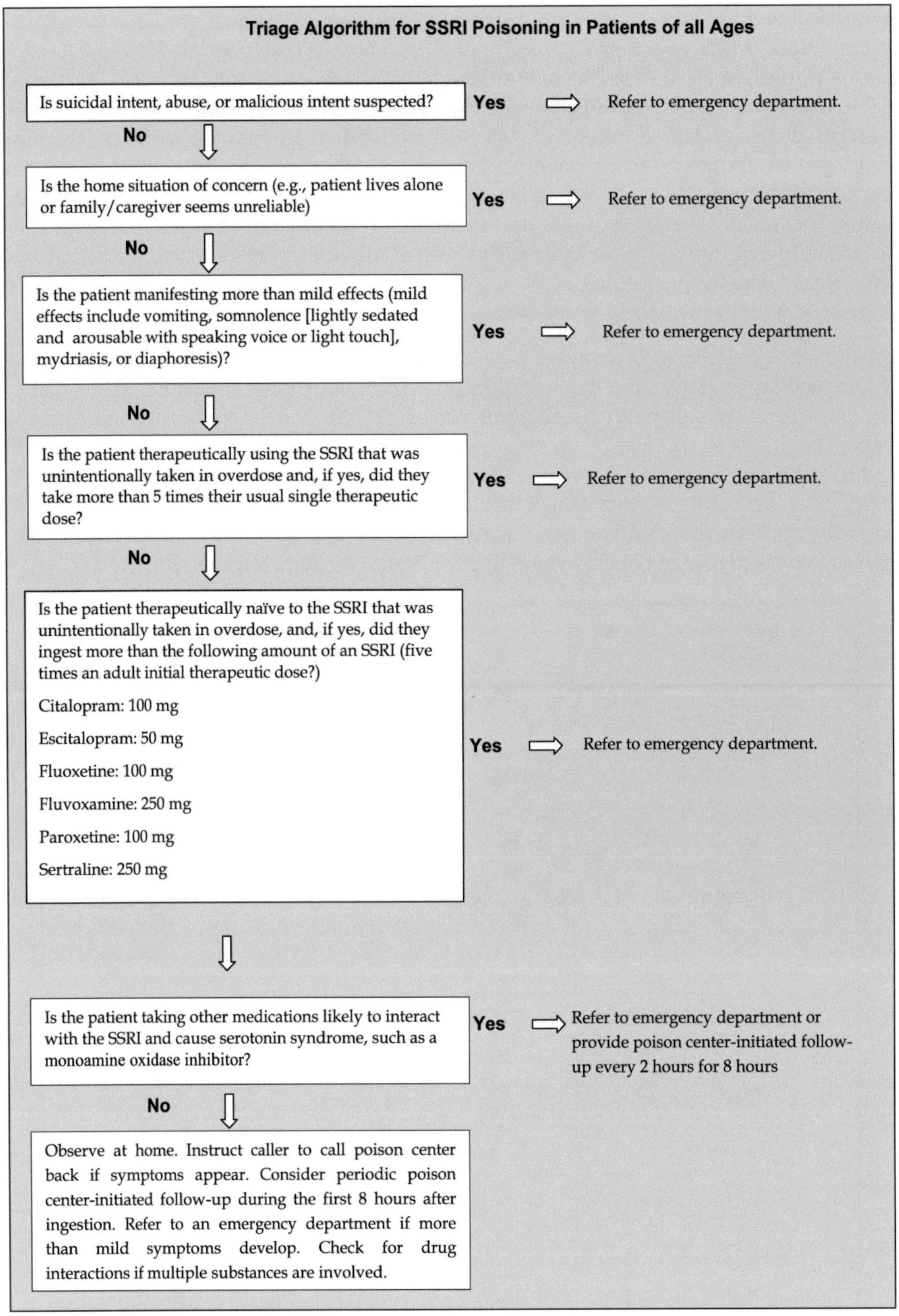

Fig. 4. Triage algorithm for SSRIs poisoning. Adapted from Nelson and colleagues, 2007. With permission from Taylor & Francis INC Publisher (Order License Id: 2813750292586).

According to Boyer (2011), the criteria for diagnosis of serotonin syndrome, known as Hunter criteria are:

- Spontaneous clonus
- Inducible clonus plus agitation or diaphoresis
- Ocular clonus plus agitation or diaphoresis
- Tremor and hyperreflexia
- Hypertonia

Nelson and colleagues (2007) published a triage algorithm for SSRIs poisoning based on an assessment of current scientific and clinical information, to help in clinical judgment (Figure 4).

4. Serotonin and norepinephrine reuptake inhibitor

4.1 History

Venlafaxine is the main antidepressant of the Serotonin and Norepinephrine Reuptake Inhibitor class. Low doses of this bicyclic antidepressant inhibits presynaptic reuptake of serotonin, and medium to high doses inhibits norepinephrine reuptake, therefore the term serotonin norepinephrine reuptake inhibitor (Pacher & Kecskemeti, 2004). Venlafaxine and the structurally unrelated group of SSRIs represent a class of serotoninergic antidepressants developed and marketed, in part, on the basis of a lower risk of toxicity in overdose, when compared to TCAs and MAOIs.

SNRIs became one of the most prescribed antidepressants, especially by psychiatrists. Many symptoms of depression are caused by low dopamine levels. This class of antidepressants treats depression by stimulating dopamine in the pre-frontal cortex (Stahl, 2011). The use of venlafaxine has increased progressively since it was first introduced in 1994, especially in patients who do not respond adequately to SSRIs (Ciuna et al., 2004). In this chapter, we will focus on the most prescribed substances of the SNRI class: venlafaxine, milnacipran, duloxetine, and sibutramine. Sibutramine, however, has been used in the treatment of obesity.

Venlafaxine is a phenethylamine derivative, and was the first SNRI to be used in the U.S. This drug has different levels of serotonin reuptake inhibition when compared to norepinephrine. The inhibition of serotonin reuptake is stronger and occurs even in small doses of the drug. The inhibition of norepinephrine reuptake, on the other hand, is not as strong, so larger doses are required. Venlafaxine does not interact with any other receptor. This drug is metabolized and converted into desvenlafaxine in the liver (CYP450 2D6).

Milnacipran and duloxetine are prescribed to treat not only depression, but also algic disorders. Milnacipran was the first SNRI available in Japan and many European countries. It is more commonly used to treat algic disorders because of its singular characteristic of being a stronger inhibitor of the norepinephrine transporter than the serotonin one (Clauw et al, 2008).

SNRIs can be used to treat different clinical conditions, and may vary according to the drug, dosage, and patient's comorbidities. Some indications were already mentioned in the last section of the chapter. In general, SNRI are useful in cases of psychiatric disorders, such as panic disorder, social anxiety disorder, obsessive compulsive disorder, trichotillomania, attention deficit hyperactivity, and also in cases of chronic pain and fibromyalgia (Ninan, 2000). Since some antidepressants are more important to treat specific clinical conditions, physicians should analyze which antidepressant should be used to treat each case, and then decide on the best drug for the patient.

When comparing poisonings by SNRIs and SSRIs, patients who overdosed with venlafaxine were older (37.4 ±13 *vs.* 28.8 ± 10.1, *P*= 0.001), had higher degree of suicidal intent, and had ingested more pills (Chan, Gunja & Ryan, 2010). However, these observations were explained by studies that suggested that venlafaxine is prescribed to patients with higher risk of suicidal ideation.

4.2 Acute toxicity and clinical manifestations

SNRIs produce rapid down regulation of central beta-adrenergic receptors, and may result in a more rapid onset of toxic effects (Stork, 2011). Sodium and potassium channel blocking promotes membrane-stabilization in the heart (Charniot et al, 2010), which is rarely clinically apparent. However, QRS prolongation, QT prolongation, and ventricular tachycardia have resulted in death (Stahl, 2011). Toxicity is associated with serum concentration of venlafaxine, and chronic side-effects are alopecia, yawning, focal myositis facial flushing, and dose-related increases in blood pressure.

SNRIs are well absorbed orally and suffer no relevant influence of concurrent food ingestion, except in the case of duloxetine. All the drugs of this class are distributed through protein-biding, metabolized in the liver (P450), and excreted in the urine and feces. The elimination half-life of these drugs is 6-10 hours (except for sibutramine: 1,1 hour), and depends on existing comorbidities, such as liver disease or renal insufficiency.

Toxic doses are different among SNRIs. For instance, venlafaxine is considered toxic when doses are greater than 1500 mg (adults) and 5.5 mg/kg (children), milnacipran, on the other hand, is toxic when doses are greater than 2800 mg.

According to Micromedex (2011), a mild to moderate intoxication can cause tremor, hyperreflexia, anxiety, and agitation. Palpitations, hypertension, tachycardia, and exacerbation of congestive heart failure have been reported in cases of ingestion of therapeutic doses and overdose. Somnolence is common in mild toxicity and delirium is more likely to happen as the toxicity increases.

Severe intoxications can lead to serotonergic syndrome (described in subitem 3.2). Cardiovascular toxicity includes PR, QRS, and QT prolongation and can occasionally culminate in ventricular tachycardia, fibrillation, and cardiac arrest. Although interval prolongations are common, ventricular dysrhythmias are rare, and are associated with large drug intake (greater than 8 g). Seizures are common in patients taking over 1 g of the drug.

Venlafaxine can induce direct skeletal muscle toxicity and lead to severe rhabdomyolysis (Pascale et al., 2005). A case of a young adult that developed eosinophilic pneumonia after venlafaxine overdose was reported. Coma and hypotension are rare effects of severe toxicity. Sibutramine can cause thrombocytopenia and ALT, AST, and alkaline phosphatase elevations (Micromedex, 2011). Rajapakse and colleagues (2010) reported rhabdomyolysis and, consequently, renal failure, probably induced by a therapeutic dose of venlafaxine, in a patient with idiopathic Parkinson disease. Since this occurred in the absence of seizures, it lead the researchers to believe that this antidepressant has a certain degree of muscle toxicity. The authors also reported that the ingestion of a therapeutic dose of venlafaxine led to serotonin syndrome, which is unusual at this dose.

A case of cardiogenic shock in a middle-aged man with prior normal cardiac function was reported. Good prognosis occurs when the drug is withdrawn, the patient is treated adequately, and an ECG and echocardiography are conducted (Charniot et al, 2010).

5. General treatment for acute antidepressants poisoning

There is no specific antidote for acute poisoning by antidepressants, but there are ways of reducing the patient's exposure to the toxic agent. This can be done by promoting gastric decontamination and decreasing intestinal absorption. Although these procedures have been performed for many years, there are several controversies regarding their real effectiveness. The clinical manifestations of acute poising by antidepressants are complex, and depend on different factors related to the patient, such as previous diseases, and the conditions of intoxication. Therefore, it is essential that the physician understands the complexity of the situation, and that it is virtually impossible to treat all the symptoms at the same time.

5.1 Support

Benzodiazepines are indicated in cases of agitation, mild serotonergic effects, hyperadrenergic signs, seizures and agitation. The administration of an intravenous dose of benzodiazepine, usually diazepam, as prophylaxis in patients with potential risk for seizures is not scientifically proven. The physicians should keep in mind that the use of benzodiazepines may contribute to respiratory depression and worsen the patient's condition (Bateman, 2005; Woolf et al., 2007). Obtunded patients should be intubated and dysrhythmias, hypoventilation, and hypoperfusion should be treated with the Advanced Cardiac Life Support (ACLS). If hyperthermia persists, even after the administration of an adequate sedative, induced neuromuscular paralysis with continuous EEG monitoring should be considered. In addition, isotonic fluids should be given to replace large losses, facilitate myoglobin clearance, and promote renal clearance of the agent (Micromedex, 2011).

5.2 Decontamination

Gastric lavage is one of the most common gastrointestinal decontamination methods, and has been widely used for over 180 years. Recommended dose is 10 ml of 0.9% saline per kg of body weight. The saline should be heated to 38°C in order to avoid hypothermia. If there is neurological or respiratory depression, the patient's airways should be protected before beginning the procedure. Since TCAs delay gastric emptying, this procedure can be done even after twelve hours of ingestion of the drugs (Liebelt, 2010). Gastric lavage is also recommended in massive overdoses of SNRIs, but it is only effective within 1 hour of ingestion. However, in cases of SSRI overdose, orogastric lavage usually is not recommended because it is rarely fatal (Poisindex, 201; Stork, 2011).

Another method of decontamination often employed is the administration of actived charcoal (AC). AC absorbs toxic substances and, therefore, reduces the availability of the drug for absorption by the digestive system. Teenagers and adults are usually treated orally with 50 grams of AC, but the conventionally accepted optimal ratio is approximately 10:1 (dose of AC/amount of drug ingested by weight) (Olson, 2010). AC may be effective in reducing the absorption of TCAs if administered shortly after the ingestion. In cases of SSRIs and SNRIs poisoning, there is greater effectiveness of AC treatment if it is given within 1-2 hours of the ingestion (Stork, 2011).

Studies analyzing the clinical course of patients receiving AC after several hours of TCAs overdose have shown a lack of efficacy in this procedure (Woolf et al., 2007). The administration of multiple doses of AC is based on the concept that the use of repeated doses may increase gastrointestinal elimination of substances present in toxic levels in the systemic circulation and have a long half life, low volume of distribution, enterogastric secretion, enteroenteric or enterohepatic circulation. Although there is no evidence of the effectiveness of multiple doses of AC, studies suggest it may increase the elimination of amitriptyline (Olson, 2010; Woolf, 2007).

In general, acute intoxications by TCAs are the most serious, for this reason alternative forms of decontamination in severe acute poisonings have been studied. Plasmapheresis is an effective method of decontamination in cases of poisoning by substances that bind to plasma proteins with high affinity, *e.g.*, TCAs (Kolsal et al., 2009; Belen et al., 2009). Kolsal and colleagues (2009) reported a case of a two year old girl with signs and symptoms of severe intoxication by amitriptyline, with plasma concentration of 70 mg / kg. The patient was in a coma and had generalized tonic clonic seizures, ventricular tachycardia and QRS interval prolongation. After conventional life support treatment, gastric lavage and AC, the patient did not have a good clinical response. However, after plasmapheresis the patient progressed well and presented no complications. Belen and colleagues (2009) also reported a case in which plasmapheresis was performed in a fifteen-year-old patient intoxicated with amitriptyline, with plasma concentration of 18 mg / kg. They confirmed a reduction of 59.5% of serum level of the drug and significant improvement of electrocardiographic changes after a single session of plasmapheresis. These authors concluded that the presence of signs and symptoms such as respiratory depression, seizures, arrhythmias with QRS prolongation, or ventricular tachycardia may be considered as a criterion for choosing plasmaphereisis. This technique can be very effective in severe cases of poisoning by these drugs and when life support treatment does not contribute to a good clinical outcome. Nevertheless, it is important to conduct randomized clinical trials to analyze the efficiency of this method and substantiate these results.

5.3 Toxic syndromes

5.3.1 Cardiac

Patients with acute TCAs poisoning should undergo careful cardiac monitoring throughout their hospitalization, because of the high cardiotoxicity of these drugs. Patients with massive SSRIs and SNRIS overdose are at greater risk of cardiotoxicity, so they should have their heart monitored during 24 hours (Stahl, 2011; Stork, 2011). If the overdose was of citalopram or escitalopram, patients should have an ECG at least 6 hours after ingestion. If the ECG changes or shows any arrhythmia, the patient should be admitted until the normalization of the ECG. (Isbister et al., 2004). Tachycardia can be treated with fluids and sedative drugs, like benzodiazepines, and unstable ventricular dysrhythmias should be treated according to ACLS protocols. Lidocaine has been suggested as the antiarrhythmic of choice for ventricular tachycardia or ventricular fibrillation (Stork, 2011).

Sodium bicarbonate has been indicated for the treatment of the cardiovascular effects of intoxication and recommended as a preventive treatment when various clinical indicators are present, including seizures and QRS interval prolongation greater than 100 ms. The use of sodium bicarbonate is important for the treatment of patients with TCAs poisoning. It acts as a sodium channel antagonist and corrects metabolic acidosis. The recommended dose for administration is 1 to 2 mEq / kg IV (Blackman, Brown & Wilkes, 2001; Calkins et al., 2003). The effectiveness of sodium bicarbonate in treating cardiotoxic and neurotoxic effects has been demonstrated in experimental studies in animals and a few studies in humans. (Woolf et al. 2007; Bradberry et al. 2005; Blackman, Brown & Wilkes, 2001, Calkins et al., 2003). According to the literature, prophylactic alkalinization in asymptomatic patients and that are not at risk of cardiovascular events is not recommended (Bradberry et al. 2005; Blackman, Brown & Wilkes, 2001).

5.3.2 Hyperthermia

Benzodiazepines should be used to control agitation. During severe hyperthermia, enhance heat loss using evaporation (keep skin damp and use fans to encourage air circulation), ice water immersion or packing the patient in ice. In severe cases, the patient should be intubated and higher doses of sedatives, such as propofol, should be administrated. Occasionally, paralysis is necessary to eliminate the neuromuscular hyperactivity and rhabdomyolysis and fever (Micromedex, 2011).

5.3.3 Serotonin syndrome

Benzodiazepines should be given to control neuromuscular hyperactivity. Cyproheptadine has been used as a serotonin receptor antagonist, minimizing the serotonergic effects in overdose. It is only available in an oral formulation; it can be crushed and administered via nasogastric tube if the patient is unable to ingest the medication orally (Boyer & Shannon, 2005; Boyer, 2011; Micromedex, 2011).

5.3.4 Monitoring the patient

In severe poisoning, patients with altered mental status, hypotension, cardiac conduction abnormalities or seizures should be monitored in an Intensive Care Unit (ICU) for five days, or longer if necessary. Complementary tests to evaluate the clinical outcome can be requested: exam to detect TCAs in the urine, ionogram (mainly sodium and potassium), complete blood cell count, aspartate aminotransferase (AST), alanine aminotransferase (ALT), creatine phosphokinase (CK), creatine kinase-MB fraction (CK-MB), lactate dehydrogenase (LDH), urea, creatinine and urinalysis (particularly if patient has rhabdomyolysis), blood glucose, arterial blood gases and chest radiograph. Determining the serum levels TCAs is not recommended since there is poor correlation between serum levels and clinical effects (Liebelt, 2010; Micromedex, 2011; Poisindex, 2011; Stork, 2011).

6. Conclusion

In general, antidepressants are one of the most widely used chemical agents in deliberate self-poisonings. When we talk about suicide and suicide attempt with antidepressants overdose, we are referring mainly to women in their twenties - thirties who are suicide repeaters. The antidepressants used in self-poisoning may differ in each country, however TCAs and SSRIs antidepressants are the most common. TCAs have the highest fatality rates in suicide overdose cases, followed by SNRIs and SSRIs.

Physicians treating cases of tricyclic poisoning should monitor the patients' cardiac functions, and in cases SSRIs poisoning, the physician should be aware for the development of serotonin syndrome.

The relative safety of the SSRIs when taken in overdose, when compared with TCAs and MAOIs, make them desirable drugs to be prescribed. Furthermore, SSRIs does not seem to increase suicidality, differently from what was believed two decades ago. The only important exception in toxicity is citalopram, which is associated with QTc prolongation, and this provides a biological basis for the reports of increased morbidity and mortality associated with citalopram overdose.

7. Acknowledgments

The authors are grateful to Miriam de Cássia Tóffolo, Poison Information Centre - University Hospital - for excellent technical assistance, and Secretaria de Estado da Saúde (SESA) for the financial support.

8. References

Açikalin A, Satar S, Avc A, Topal M, Kuvandk G, Sebe A. QTc Intervals in Drug Poisoning Patients with Tricyclic Antidepressants and Selective Serotonin Reuptake Inhibitors. *American Journal of Therapeutics*, Vol.17, No. 1, (Jan-Feb 2010), pp. 30–33.

Ajdacic-Gross V, Weiss MG, Ring M, Hepp V, Bopp M, Gutzwiller F, Rössler W. Methods of suicide: international suicide patterns derived from the WHO mortality database. *Bulletin of the World Health Organization*, Vol. 86, No. 9, (Sep 2008), pp. 726-732.

Andersen UA, Andersen M, Rosholm JU, Gram LF. Contacts to the health care system prior to suicide: a comprehensive analysis using registers for general and psychiatric hospital admissions, contacts to general practitioners and practising specialists and drug prescriptions. *Acta Psychiatrica Scandinavica*, Vol.102, No.2, (Aug 2000), pp.126-134.

Avanci RC, Pedrão J, Costa-Jr ML. Perfil do adolescente que tenta suicídio em uma unidade de emergência. *Revista Brasileira de Enfermagem*, Vol. 58, No. 5, (Sep-Oct 2005), pp. 535-539.

Baca-Garcia E, Diaz-Sastre C, Resa EG, Blasco H, Conesa DB, Oquendo MA, Saiz-Ruiz J, Leon J. Suicide attempts and impulsivity. *European Archives of Psychiatry and Clinical Neuroscience*. Vol. 255, No. 2, (Apr 2005), pp.152-156.

Baldessarini RJ, (Eds. Brunton LL, Lazo JS, Parker KL). (2010). Tratamento Farmacológico da Depressão e dos Transtornos de Ansiedade. *Goodman & Gilman: As Bases Farmacológicas da Terapêutica*. McGraw-Hill, 8577260011, Porto Alegre.

Bancroft J, Marsack P. The Repetitiveness of self-poisoning and self-injury. *British Journal of Psychiatry*, Vol.131, (Oct 1977),:394-9.

Bateman DN. Tricyclic Antidepressant Poisoning: Central Nervous Effects and Management. *Toxicology Reviews*, Vol. 24, No. 3, (2005),p p.181-186.

Beasley CM, Dornseif BE, Bosomworth JC, Sayler ME, Rampey AH, Heiligenstein JH, Thompson VL, Murphy DJ, Masica DN. Fluoxetine and suicide: a meta-analysis of controlled trials of treatment for depression. *British Medical Journal*, Vol. 303, No. 6804, (Sep 1991), pp.685–692

Beautrais AL. Suicides and serious suicide attempts: two populations or one? *Psychological Medicine*, Vol. 31, No. 5, (Jul 2001), pp. 837-845.

Belen B, Akman A, Yüksel N, Dilsiz G, Yenicesu I, Olguntürk R. A Case Report of Amitriptyline Poisoning Successfully Treated With the Application of Plasma Exchange. Therapeutic Apheresis and Dialysis, Vol. 13, No. 2, (Apr 2009), p. 147-149.

Bergen H, Murphy E, Cooper J, Kapur N, Stalker C, Waters K, Hawton K.A comparative study of non-fatal self-poisoning with antidepressants relative to prescribing in three centres in England. *Journal of Affective Disorders*, Vol. 123, No. 1-3, (Jun 2010), pp. 95-101.

Bernardes SS, Turini CA, Matsuo T. Profile of suicide attempts using intentional overdose with medicines, treated by a poison control center in Paraná State, Brazil. *Cadernos de Saúde Pública*, Vol. 26, No. 7, (Jul 2010), pp. 1366-1372.

Biggs JT, Spiker DG, Petit JM, Ziegler VE. Tricyclic antidepressant overdose: incidence of symptoms. *The Journal of the American Medical Association*, Vol. 11. No. 2, (Jul 1977), pp. 135–138.

Blackman K, Brown SG, Wilkes GJ. Plasma alkalinization for tricyclic antidepressant toxicity: A systematic review. *Emergency Medicine*, Vol. 13, No. 2 (Jun 2001), p. 204-210.

Bosch TM, van der Werf TS, Uges DR, Ligtenberg JJ, Fijen JW, Tulleken JE, Zijlstra JG. Antidepressants self-poisoning and ICU admissions in a university hospital in The Netherlands. *Pharmacy World & Science*, Vol. 22, No. 3, (Jun 2000), pp. 92-95.

Boyer EW, Shannon M. Current Concepts: The Serotonin Syndrome. *The New England Journal of Medicine*, Vol. 352, No. 1, (Mar 2005), pp. 1112-1120.

Boyer EW. Serotonin syndrome (2011). *In* Up to date, 2011. Available in: http://www.uptodate.com. Acessed in Oct, 2011.

Bradberry SM, Thanacoody HK, Watt BE, Thomas SH, Vale JA. Management of the Cardiovascular Complications of Tricyclic Antidepressant Poisoning. *Toxicology Reviews*, Vol. 24, No. 3, (2005), p. 195-204.

Callaham M, Kassel D. Epidemiology of fatal tricyclic antidepressant ingestion: implications for management. *Annals of Emmergency Medicine*, (Jan 1985), Vol. 14, pp. 1-9.

Calkins T, Chan T, Clark R, Stepanski B, Vilke G. Review of prehospital sodium bicarbonate use for cyclic antidepressant overdose. *Emergency Medicine Journal*, Vol. 20, No. 5, (Sep 2003), pp. 483-486.

Chan AN, Gunja N, Ryan CJ. A Comparison of Venlafaxine and SSRIs in Deliberate Self-poisoning. *Journal of Medical Toxicology*, Vol. 6, No. 2, (Jun 2010), pp. 116–121.

Charniot JC, Vignat N, Monsuez JJ, Kidouche R, Avramova B, Artigou JY, Albertini JP. Cardiogenic shock associated with reversible dilated cardiomyopathy during therapy with regular doses of venlafaxine. *The American Journal of Emergency Medicine*, Vol. 28, No. 2, (Feb 2010) pp. 256.e1–256.e5.

Citak A, Soysal DD, Uçsel R, Karaböcüoglu M, Uzel N. Seizures associated with poisoning in children: tricyclic antidepressant intoxication. *Pediatrics International*, Vol. 48, No. 6, (Dec 2006), p. 582-585.

Ciuna A, Andretta M, Corbari L, Levi D, Mirandola M, Sorio A, Barbui C. Are we going to increase the use of antidepressants up to that of benzodiazepines? *European Journal of Clinical Pharmacoly*, Vol. 60, No. 9, (Nov 2004), pp. 629- 634.

Clauw DJ, Mease P, Palmer RH, Gendreau RM, Wang Y. Milnacipran for the treatment of fibromyalgia in adults: a 15-week, multicenter, randomized, double-blind, placebo-controlled, multiple-dose clinical trial. Clin Ther. 2008; 30(11):1988-2004.

Cunha-Jr RJ, Barrucand L, Verçosa N. A Study on Electrocardiographic Changes Secondary to the Use of Tricyclic Antidepressants in Patients with Chronic Pain. Revista Brasileira de Anestesiologia, Vol. 59, No.1, (Jan-Feb 2009), p. 46-55.

Fasoli RA, Glauser FL. Cardiac arrhythmias and ECG abnormalities in tricyclic antidepressant overdose. *Clinical Toxicology*, Vol. 18, No. 2, (Feb 1981), pp. 155–163.

Fernandes G, Palvo F, Pinton FA, Dourado DAN, Mendes CAC. Impacto das intoxicações por antidepressivos tricíclicos comparados aos depressores do "sistema nervoso central". Arquivos de Ciências da Saúde, Vol. 13, No.3 (Jul-Set 2006), p. 61-65.

Graudins A, Sterman A, Chan B. Treatment of the Serotonin Syndrome with Cyproheptadine. *The Journal of Emmergengy Medicine*, Vol. 16, No. 4, (Jul-Aug. 1998), pp. 615-619).

Gunnell D, Frankel S. Prevention of suicide: aspirations and evidence. *British Medical Journal*, Vol. 308, No. 6938, (May 1994), pp. 1127-1233.

Gunnell D, Eddleston M. Suicide by intentional ingestion of pesticides: a continuing tragedy in developing countries International. *Journal of Epidemiology*, Vol. 32, No. 6, (Dec 2003), pp. 902-909.

Guo B, Harstall C. *For which strategies of suicide prevention is there evidence of effectiveness?* (2004). Copenhagen, Denmark, WHO Regional Office for Europe (Health Evidence Network report; http://www.euro.who.int/__data/assets/pdf_file/0010/74692/E83583.pdf, accessed 15 July 2011.

Hawton K, Zahl D, Weatherall R. Suicide following deliberate self-harm: long termfollow-upstudy of patients who presented to a general hospital. *British Journal of Psychiatry*, Vol. 182, (Jun 2003), pp. 537-542.

Hawton K, Bergen H, Simkin S, Cooper J, Waters K, Gunnell D, Kapur N. Toxicity of antidepressants: rates of suicide relative to prescribing and non-fatal overdose. *British Journal of Psychiatry*, Vol. 196, No. 5, (May. 2010), pp. 354-358.

Healy D, Langmaak C, Savage M: Suicide in the course of the treatment of depression. *Journal of Psychopharmacoly*, Vol. 13, (Jan 1999), pp. 94–99

Henry JA, Alexander CA, Sener EK. Relative mortality from overdose of antidepressants. *British Medical Journal*, Vol. 310, No. 6974, (Jan 1995), pp. 221-224.

Hirsh M, Birnbaum RJ. Selective serotonin reuptake inhibitors (SSRIs) for treating depressed adults. Available in: http://www.uptodate.com. Acessed in Oct, 2011.

Howell C, Wilson AD, Waring WS. Cardiovascular toxicity due to venlafaxine poisoning in adults: a review of 235 consecutive cases. *British Journal of Clinical Pharmacology*, Vol. 64, No. 2, (Aug 2007), pp. 192–197.

Isbister GK, Bowe SJ, Dawson A, Whyte IM. Relative Toxicity of Selective Serotonin Reuptak Inhibitors (SSRIs) in Overdose. *Clinical Toxicology*, Vol. 42, No. 3, (2004), pp. 277-285.

Kessler RC, Borges G, Walters EE. Prevalence of and risk factors for lifetime suicide attempts in the national comorbidity survey. *Archives of General Psychiatry*, Vol. 56, No. 7, (Jul 1999), pp.617-626.

Khan A, Khan S, Kolts R, Brown WA.Suicide Rates in Clinical Trials of SSRIs, Other Antidepressants, and Placebo: Analysis of FDA Reports. *The American Journal of Psychiatry*, Vol. 160, No. 4, (Apr 2003), pp. 790-792.

Kiran HS, Ravikumar YS, Jayasheelan MR, Prashanth. Brugada Like Pattern in ECG with Drug Overdose. *Journal of the Association of Physicians of India*, Vol. 58, (Feb 2010), p. 114-115.

Kolsal E, Tekin IO, Piskin E, Aydemir C, Akyüz M, Cabuk H, Eldes N, Numanoglu V. Treatment of Severe Amitriptyline Intoxication With Plasmapheresis. *Journal of Clinical Apheresis*,Vol. 24, No. 1, (Jan 2009), p. 21-24.

Lam SM, Lau AC, Yan WW. Over 8 years experience on severe acute poisoning requiring intensive care in Hong Kong, China. *Human & Experimental Toxicology*, Vol. 29, No. 9, (Sep 2010), pp. 757-765.

Lee HC, Lin HC, Liu TC, Lin SY. Contact of mental and nonmental health care providers prior to suicide in Taiwan: a population-based study. *Canadian Journal of Psychiatry*, Vol. 53, No. 6, (Jun 2008), pp. 377-383.

Leke R, Portela LVC, Souza DO, Lara DR, Thiesen FV. Tricycles antidepressants: a review about pharmacological characteristics and therapeutic dry monitoring importance. *Revista Brasileira de Toxicologia,* Vol. 17, No. 2, (Dec 2004), pp. 51-54.

Liebelt EL, (Eds. Nelson LS, Lewin NA, Howland MA *et al*). (2011). Cyclic Antidepressants. *Goldfrank's toxicologic emergencies,* MCGrawHill, 978-0-07-160593-9, New York.

Margalho C, Barroso M, Gallardo E, Monsanto P, Vieira DN. Massive intoxication involving unusual high concentration of amitriptyline. *Human & Experimental Toxicology,* Vol. 26, No. 8, (Aug 2007), p.667-670.

Mastrogianni O, Theodoridis G, Spagou K, Violante D, Henriques T, Pouliopoulos A, Psaroulis K, Tsoukali H, Raikos N. Determination of venlafaxine in post-mortem whole blood by HS-SPME and GC-NPD. *Forensic Science International,* (Jun 2011), Epub Ahed of print.

McKenzie MS, McFarland BH. Trends in antidepressant overdoses. *Pharmacoepidemiology and drug safety,* Vol. 16, No. 5, (May 2007), pp. 513-523.

Micromedex. Venlafaxine, 2011. In Micromedex healthcare series, 2006. Available in: http://www.micromedex.com.br. Acessed in Oct, 2011.

Mines D, Hill D, Yu H, Novelli L. Prevalence of risk factors for suicide in patients prescribed venlafaxine, fluoxetine, and citalopram. *Pharmacoepidemiology and Drug Safety,* Vol. 14, No. 6, (Jun 2005), pp. 367–372.

Neeleman J, Wessely S. Drugs taken in fatal and non-fatal self-poisoning: a study in South London. *Acta Psychiatrica Scandinavica,* Vol. 95, No. 4, (Apr 1997), pp. 283-287.

Nelson LS, Erdman AR, Booze LL, Cobaugh DJ, Chyka PA, Woolf AD, Scharman EJ, Wax PM, Manoguerra AS, Christianson G, Caravati EM, Troutman WG..Selective serotonin reuptake inhibitor poisoning: an evidencebased consensus guideline for out-of-hospital management. *Clinical Toxicology,* Vol. 45, No. 4, (May 2007), pp. 315-332.

Ninan PT. Use of venlafaxine in other psychiatric disorders. *Depression and Anxiety,* Vol. 12, S. 1 (2000), pp. 90-94.

Oh SH, Park NK, Jeong SH, Kim HJ, Lee CC. Deliberate self-poisoning: factors associated with recurrentself-poisoning. *The American Journal of Emergency Medicine.* Vol. 29, No. 8 (Oct 2011), pp. 908-912.

Olson KR. Activated Charcoal for Acute Poisoning: One Toxicologist's Journey. Journal of Medical Toxicology, Vol. 6, No. 2, (Jun 2010), pp. 190-198.

Owens D, Horrocks J, House A. Fatal and non-fatal repetition of self-harm : Systematic review. *British Journal of Psychiatry,* Vol. 181 (Sep 2002), pp. 181-193.

Pacher P, Kecskemeti V. Trends in the development of new antidepressants. Is there a light at the end of the tunnel? Current Medical Chemistry, Vol.11, No. 7, (Apr 2004), pp. 925–943.

Pascale P, Oddo M, Pacher P, Augsburger M, Liaudet L. Severe Rhabdomyolysis Following Venlafaxin Overdose. *Therapeutic drug Monitoring,* Vol. 27, No. 5, (Oct. 2004), pp. 562-565.

Poisindex. Serotonin Syndrome. *In* Micromedex healthcare series, 2006. Available in: http://www.micromedex.com.br. Acessed in Oct, 2011.

Rajapakse S, Abeynaike L, Wickramarathne T. Venlafaxine-Associated Serotonin Syndrome Causing Severe Rhabdomyolysis and Acute Renal Failure in a Patient With Idiopathic Parkinson Disease. *Journal of Clinical Psychopharmacoly*, Vol. 30, No. 5, (Oct 2010), pp. 620-622.

Ramchandani P, Murray B, Hawton K, House A. Deliberate self poisoning with antidepressant drugs: a comparison of the relative hospital costs of cases of overdose of tricyclics with those of selective-serotonin re-uptake inhibitors. *Journal of Affective Disorders*, Vol.60, No.2, (Nov 2000), pp. 97–100.

Sedal L, Korman MG, Williams PO, Mushin G. Overdosage of tricyclic antidepressants. A report of two deaths and a prospective study of 24 patients. *The Medical Journal of Australia*, Vol. 2, No. 2, (Jul 1972), pp. 74-79.

Stahl SM.(2010). *Psicofarmacologia: Bases neurocientíficas e aplicações práticas* (3rd edition). Guanabara Koogan, 978-85-277-1609-3, Rio de Janeiro.

Starkey IR, Lawson AA. Poisoning with tricyclic and related antidepressants-a ten-year review. *The Quartely Journal of Medicine*, Vol. 49, No. 193, (1980), pp. 33-49.

Stork CM, (Eds. Nelson LS, Lewin NA, Howland MA *et al*). (2011). Serotonin reuptake inhibitors and atypical antidrepressants. *Goldfrank's toxicologic emergencies*, MCGrawHill, 978-0-07-160593-9, New York.

Thanacoody HK, Thomas SH. Tricyclic Antidepressant Poisoning: Cardiovascular Toxicity. *Toxicology Reviews*, Vol. 24, No. 3, (2005), p. 205-214.

Teicher MH, Glod C, Cole JO: Emergence of intense suicidal preoccupation during fluoxetine treatment. The *American Journal of Psychiatry*,Vol. 147, No.2, (Feb 1990), pp. 207-210.

Townsend E, Hawton K, Harriss L, Bale E, Bond A. Substances used in deliberate self-poisoning 1985–1997: trends and associations with age, gender, repetition and suicide intent. *Social Psychiatry and Psychiatric Epidemiology*, Vol. 36, No. 5 (May 2001), pp. 228-234.

Welch SS. A review of the literature on the epidemiology of parasuicide in the general population. *Psychiatric Services*, Vol. 52, No. 3, (March 2001), pp. 368-375.

White NC, Litovitz T, Clancy C. Suicidal antidepressant overdoses: A comparative analysis by antidepressant type. *Journal of Medical Toxicology*, Vol. 4. No. 4, (Dec 2008), pp. 238-250.

Wyder M, De Leo D. Behind impulsive suicide attempts: Indications from a community study. *Journal of Affective Disorders*. Vol. 104, No. 1-3, (Dec 2007), pp. 167-173.

Woolf AD, Erdman AR, Nelson LS, Caravati EM, Cobaugh DJ, Booze LL, Wax PM, Manoguerra AS, Scharman EJ, Olson KR, Chyka PA, Christianson G, Troutman WG. Tricyclic antidepressant poisoning: an evidence-based consensus guideline for out-of-hospital management. *Clinical Toxicology*, Vol. 45, No. 3, (Mar 2007), pp. 203-233.

Wong A, Taylor DMD, Ashby K, Robinson J. Changing epidemiology of intentional antidepressant drug overdose in Victoria, Australia. *Australian and New Zealand Journal of Psychiatry*, Vol. 44, No. 8, (Aug 2010), pp. 759-764.

World Health Organization - Western Pacific Region. *Towards evidence-based suicide prevention programmes* (2010). World Health Organization [WHO], ISBN - 9789929061463, Geneva, Switzerland.

Zahl DL, Hawton K. Repetition of deliberate self-harmand subsequent suicide risk: long-termfollow-up study of 11583. *British Journal of Psychiatry*, Vol. 181, (Sep 2002), pp. 181-193.

7

Rational Polypharmacy in the Acute Therapy of Major Depression

Per Bech and Claudio Csillag
Psychiatric Research Unit, Mental Health Centre North Zealand,
University of Copenhagen
Denmark

1. Introduction

Monotherapy is a basic principle in all branches of clinical medicine, including psychiatry. It is a scientific principle where we are making an attempt to clarify one single therapeutic step, its wanted and unwanted effects, in isolation. According to this principle we make sure to start with the least aggressive approach. However, in daily clinical practice polypharmacy might be considered when treating patients who have only a partial response to the first prescribed monotherapeutic trial.

With the introduction of the antidepressive medication in the 1960s we had access to two different classes of antidepressants: the tricyclic antidepressants (TCAs) and the monoamine oxidase inhibitors (MAO-Is). Together these drugs cover serotonin, noradrenaline and dopamine effects in the brain, which we still consider important to stabilize in the acute therapy of major depression. On the other hand, both classes of drugs have many other actions which are often considered as side-effects.

The new generation of antidepressants became available in the late 1980s and most of them are much more selective in their action than the first generation antidepressants. Therefore they have less severe side effects, but must often be combined to obtain the same antidepressive effectiveness as the first generation antidepressants.

In the following text we will introduce the most patient-friendly approach to obtain a rational polypharmacy in the acute therapy of major depression. This is based not only on the traditional classification of drugs by receptor profile and expected mechanism of action in the brain, but also on clinical monitoring by use of valid rating scales for both the wanted and unwanted effects upon the mind.

2. The disease-centre model of antidepressants

The tricyclic antidepressants (TCAs) and the monoamine oxidase inhibitors (MAO-Is) are the first generation of effective antidepressants. These types of drugs showed that major depression could be treated like other medical conditions, by covering the acute short-term treatment of four to eight weeks followed by a medium-term treatment, and the continuation phase of four to eight months (the relapse-prevention phase).

It was from this evidence that a "disease-centred" model emerged, in which antidepressants were seen to help the brain of the depressed patient by restoring the neuropathological states.

Over the fifty years since the TCAs and MAO-Is were first marketed, their biological mechanisms of action in the brain have been extensively studied. All the TCAs are both serotonin and noradrenaline reuptake inhibitors, but also act on many other mechanisms (e.g. histamine blockers). However, they have no action on dopamine. At the receptor level they all stimulate the serotonin 1A receptor and the most potent of them, amitriptyline, is also a serotonin receptor 2A blocker. The MAO-Is, as they inhibit the enzyme monoamine oxidase, act on both serotonin and noradrenaline as well as on dopamine. The MAO-Is probably also act on other processes in the brain, e.g. vitamin B6. We do know, however, that the MAO-Is are not antihistamines.

Taken together the TCAs and the MAO-Is can be considered to be non-selective or multidimensional drugs, comparable to a more or less rational polypharmacy at the receptor level. This is even when used as monotherapy in the acute therapy of major depression.

The new generation of selective antidepressants (the selective serotonin reuptake inhibitors (SSRIs)), or the selective noradrenaline and serotonin reuptake inhibitors (SNRIs) have a selective mechanism of action, thus avoiding polypharmacy. However, the new generation antidepressants such as the SSRIs or SNRIs are less effective than the TCAs. Even within the TCAs, amitriptyline was found to be superior to imipramine both in the acute therapy of depressed patients and in the relapse-prevention phase .

3. Using the Hamilton depression scale (HAM-D_{17}) to direct polypharmacy

When discussing the difference between the first generation and the second generation of antidepressants, Moncrieff and Cohen claimed that the Hamilton Depression Scale (HAM-D) contains many items that are not specific to depression, for example: "… three items on sleep, two on anxiety and one on agitation can score up to 18 points (a total score between 19 - 22 on the Hamilton Rating Scale for Depression indicates severe depression). On these items, any drug with sedative effects would be likely to outperform placebo…"

However, with correct clinical use, the Hamilton Depression Scale covers the three clinical dimensions that have to be taken into account in the acute therapy of major depression in order to institute rational polypharmacy within the "disease-control" model of antidepressants. This correct clinical approach is obtained by use of the tripartite A,B,C HAM-D.

The HAM-D_{17} is a multidimensional depression rating scale, implying that a total summed score of all the 17 items is not always a sufficient statistic, i.e. a profile score is needed.

Recently Santen *et al.* studied all placebo-controlled trials with the SSRI drug paroxetine and demonstrated that the most sensitive items in the HAM-D_{17} to discriminate between paroxetine and placebo were the six items in the HAM-D_6. Actually, when using the HAM-D_{17}, the difference from baseline to endpoint between paroxetine 20 mg daily and placebo did not reach the level of $P < 0.05$, in contrast to HAM-D_6 ($P = 0.03$) . Furthermore, they found that with paroxetine 10 mg daily no difference to placebo was reached at the level of $P < 0.05$ for either HAM-D_{17} or HAM-D_6, indicating a dose response pattern.

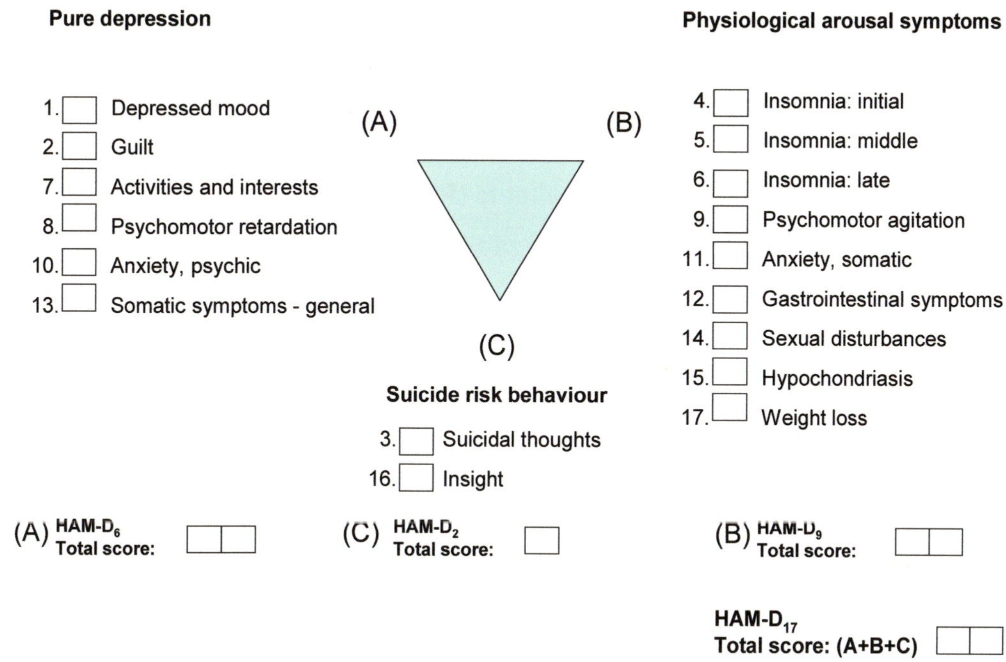

Fig. 1. ABC version of the depression scale (HAM-D)

Fig. 1. Shows the three major components A, B, C in the $HAM\text{-}D_{17}$. Domain A in Figure 1 covers the six pure depression symptoms in the HAM-D as used by experienced psychiatrists when measuring the severity of depressive states. Using item response theory models, the invariant item ordering of the $HAM\text{-}D_6$ items was found by their prevalence at baseline and at the endpoint in clinical trials of antidepressants. In the archetypical trial with the TCA amitriptyline in the setting of general practice, Paykel showed that all items in the $HAM\text{-}D_6$ discriminated between the TCA and placebo in both mild and moderate degrees of depression. Among the other HAM-D items only the sleep symptom showed discrimination, implying that amitriptyline is a sedative antidepressant. When comparing amitriptyline with the most sedative new generation antidepressant mirtazapine in placebo-controlled trials, it was the $HAM\text{-}D_6$ items that significantly differentiated between the active drugs and placebo, thereby prefiguring Moncrieff and Cohen's critical remarks on the use of the $HAM\text{-}D_{17}$ in measured outcome.

Domain B in Figure 1 covers the physiological arousal symptoms, including the "sedative" HAM-D items selected by Moncrieff and Cohen. These nine symptoms ($HAM\text{-}D_9$) in Figure 1 were included by Hamilton in his $HAM\text{-}D_{17}$ because they were found very common and distressing by the depressed patients themselves. As non-sedative antidepressants both the SSRIs and the SNRIs as well as the MAO-Is have to be combined with the antidepressants with antihistaminic action and/or serotonin receptor 2 blockers when the $HAM\text{-}D_9$ profile is in operation in the depressed patients, i.e. when polypharmacy is rationally needed. In therapy-resistant depression it is often the physiological arousal symptoms that have been inadequately reduced.

Domain C in Figure 1 covers the two remaining items in HAM-D_{17} (suicidal thoughts and lack of insight). Due to the obvious clinical relevance of these items, their assessment is crucially important in the acute therapy of patients with major depression. It has even been questioned that SSRIs might induce suicidal thoughts over the first weeks of therapy.

4. Patient related inventory of side effects ($PRISE_{20}$)

Table 1 shows the Patient Rated Inventory of Side Effects (PRISE), modified to monitor domain B selectively with 20 items ($PRISE_{20}$).

The first 17 items listed in Table 1 are derived from the original PRISE and the remaining 3 items at the bottom in Table 1 are derived from the UKU (Udvalg for Kliniske Undersøgelser) subscale for antidepressants. The UKU scale is a clinician-rated scale whereas the PRISE is a patient-reported questionnaire.

Have you had any of these side effects over the past two weeks?			
	No	Yes, but tolerable	Yes – Distressing
1. Dry mouth	☐	☐	☐
2. Nausea	☐	☐	☐
3. Diarrhoea	☐	☐	☐
4. Constipation	☐	☐	☐
5. Dizziness	☐	☐	☐
6. Palpitations	☐	☐	☐
7. Sweating	☐	☐	☐
8. Headache	☐	☐	☐
9. Tremor	☐	☐	☐
10. Difficulty sleeping	☐	☐	☐
11. Sleeping too much	☐	☐	☐
12. Loss of sexual desire	☐	☐	☐
13. Trouble achieving orgasm	☐	☐	☐
14. Trouble with erections	☐	☐	☐
15. Anxiety	☐	☐	☐
16. Restlessness	☐	☐	☐
17. Decreased energy	☐	☐	☐
18. Increased appetite	☐	☐	☐
19. Increased weight	☐	☐	☐
20. Emotional indifference	☐	☐	☐

$PRISE_{20}$ (Patient related Inventory of Side Effects) modified after Wisniewski *et al.*

Table 1.

This patient-administrated questionnaire was included in the STAR-D study (Bech *et al.* 2012) so that the baseline score was used to evaluate before augmentation of citalopram with either bupropion or buspirone to ensure that the side effects to eight weeks treatment with citalopram were tolerable. In rational polypharmacy it is important to accept only tolerable side effects before any augmentation with other drugs.

In a post-hoc analysis of the STAR-D study, decreased energy was significantly reduced when citalopram was combined with bupropion (Bech *et al.* 2012). This symptom seems therefore to be an indication of lack of effect of citalopram rather than a side effect.

In a similar way, many of the items in $PRISE_{20}$ can be considered as physiological arousal symptoms of depression as covered by $HAM\text{-}D_9$, e.g. difficulty sleeping, restlessness, anxiety, gastrointestinal symptoms or sexual symptoms. In the therapy-resistant depressed patients it is important to understand the nature of these symptoms, i.e. part of the depressive illness or drug-induced symptoms.

5. Polypharmacy as a rational treatment with antidepressants monitored by the $HAM\text{-}D_{17}/PRISE_{20}$.

Typically, antidepressants as monotherapy are now approved by the regulators (e.g. FDA) with reference to placebo-controlled clinical trials of patients with major depression. This makes comparative analyses between individual new generation antidepressants difficult. In some trials an active comparator (e.g. a TCA) has been included, which however, is compared with placebo using only the total HAM-D score as an outcome, not the profile score in accordance with the ABC version.

In clinical practice, if a patient with major depression has failed to respond fully to the initial antidepressant, the treating physician can either augment by adding another drug to the initial antidepressant as part of a polypharmacy approach, or switch to another antidepressant with a quite different mechanism of action.

The Sequenced Treatment Alternatives to Relieve Depression, the STAR*D study, is probably the most evidence-based trial to reflect the daily clinical practice. After failure to respond to monotherapy with the SSRI citalopram, patients went on to receive medication augmentation with bupropion-SR (sustained release) or buspirone in a controlled, double-blind trial.

Bupropion is a non-sedative second generation antidepressant with a selective reuptake inhibition of noradrenaline and dopamine (Table 2). It has a profile on the A, B and C $HAM\text{-}D_{17}$ similar to that of the SSRIs or SNRIs. This profile is also similar to the first generation of MAO-Is. Bupropion, like the MAO-Is, has an effect on dopamine in contrast to the TCAs or SSRIs/SNRIs..

Within the antidepressants referred to as first generation, concomitant treatment with a TCA and an "irreversible" MAO-I (e.g. phenelzine or isocarboxazid) has rarely been used. If a patient with major depression fails to respond fully on the $HAM\text{-}D_6$ with a TCA but still had some benefit on $HAM\text{-}D_9$, it is then acceptable to add phenelzine or isocarboxazid. However, it is not considered acceptable to add a TCA in a patient with only partial response to a MAO-I due to the risk of cardiovascular problems (e.g. severely increased blood pressure leading to stroke). On the other hand, if the MAO-I has been stopped for 2 weeks, then combination therapy with a TCA and the reinstated treatment with MAO-I is acceptable. The most frequently used TCA in this situation is amitriptyline.

If initial therapy has been with an SSRI/SNRI, then the combination with a MAO-I, either an irreversible (e.g. isocarboxazid) or a reversible (e.g. moclobemide), might prove fatal. As shown in the post hoc analysis of the STAR*D study data, there is no problem in a combination therapy with citalopram and bupropion SR.

The TCAs were found to be superior to the MAO-Is. Because of their antihistamine action, the TCAs have a very strong and early onset effect on the arousal symptoms compared to citalopram, paroxetine or the MAO-I moclobemid. The most effective antidepressant is still amitriptyline.

In Table 2 the second generation antidepressants mianserin and mirtazapine are also antihistaminergic, but with a less pronounced effect on HAM-D_6. However, mianserin differs from the TCAs by having no anticholinergic effect, which is important when treating elderly depressed patients due to the side effects of anticholinergics on cognitive functioning. However, as shown in Table 2, all antihistamines have weight gain as a serious side effect.

- No clear effect **+** Clear effect, mild to moderate **++** Clear effect, moderate to marked **+++** Clear effect, marked to excellent/severe		**HAM-D**		**Side effects**
		A Pure depression symptoms	B Arousal symptoms	Weight gain
MONOTHERAPY				
First generation antidepressants	TCAs (amitriptyline)	+++	++	++
	MAO-Is (isocarboxazid)	+	-	-
Second generation antidepressants Specific reuptake inhibitors	SSRIs (citalopram/ sertraline)	+	-	-
	SNRIs (venlafaxine/ duloxetine)	++	-	-
	DNRI (bupropion)	+	-	-
	NRI (reboxetine)	+	-	-
Second generation antidepressants Other	Mianserin	+	++	++
	Mirtazapine	+	++	++
	Agomelatine	+	+	-
CONCOMITANT THERAPY				
Specific	SSRI plus NRI	++	-	-
	SSRI plus DNRI	++	-	-
	SNRI plus DNRI plus agomelatine	++	+	-
Non-specific	Mianserin/ mirtazapine plus SSRI/SNRI	+++	++	++
	Mianserin/ mirtazapine plus MAO-I	++	++	++
Monotherapy Mood stabilizers	Lithium	+	-	-
	Olanzapine	+	++	++
Concomitant therapy	Olanzapine plus SSRI	+ +	++	++
	Lithium plus SSRI	+ +	-	-

Rational polypharmacy of antidepressants in the acute therapy of major depression with reference to ABC HAM-D_{17}. Concerning the optimal dose of the included drugs, see Papakostas *et al.*

Table 2.

Concomitant therapy with mianserin and the MAO-I isocarboxazid has been found safe, but with weight gain as a problem. Concomitant therapy with mianserin and the SSRI fluoxetine has been evaluated in placebo-controlled trials by Dam *et al.* In this pilot study 13 patients received fluoxetine plus mianserin, while 17 patients received fluoxetine plus placebo. On the HAM-D_{17} the distance from baseline to endpoint (six weeks) was greatest for fluoxetine plus mianserin. However, even in this study approximately 30% had increased weight gain on the combination of mianserine plus fluoxetine whereas no weight gain was seen in the fluoxetine plus placebo treated group. A re-analysis of the data set has shown that it is on the arousal symptoms (HAM-D_9, domain B, Figure 2) that the effect of the combination therapy is greatest. In a comprehensive study Blier *et al.* have investigated the effect of monotherapy with fluoxetine compared to the combination of mirtazapine with fluoxetine or of mirtazapine with venlafaxine or of mirtazapine with bupropion. The results showed that the rate of remitters (HAM-$D_{17} \leq 7$) increased from 25% with monotherapy to approximately 50% with any of the three mirtazapine combinations. However, in all these combination therapies weight gain was significantly increased compared to monotherapy with fluoxetine. Otherwise the combination therapy was safe.

A HAM-D_6 (depression)

	Flu + Mian	Flu + Pla	P
Baseline	12.6 (2.2)	12.0 (1.4)	
% improvement at endpoint	56.3%	57.5%	0.35

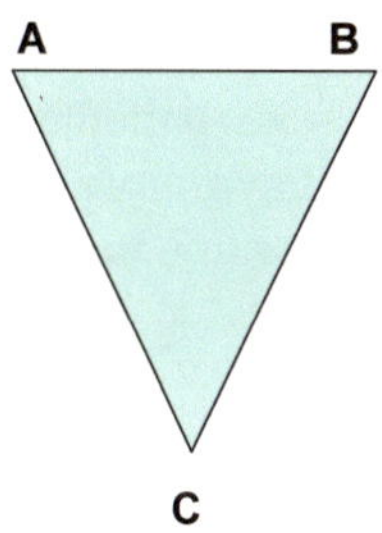

B HAM-D_9 (arousal)

	Flu + Mian	Flu + Pla	P
Baseline	11.2 (3.1)	9.1 (3.7)	
% improvement at endpoint	71.4%	53.8%	0.08

C HAM-D_2 (suicide)

	Flu + Mian	Flu + Pla	P
Baseline	2.0 (1.5)	1.3 (1.3)	
% improvement at endpoint	80.0%	76.9%	0.23

Fig. 2. A re-analysis of the dataset in Dam et al. 1998

In Table 2 the new generation antidepressant agomelatine is included. So far this drug has not been approved by the FDA as an antidepressant, but it is on the market in many European countries. Agomelatine acts by blocking the serotonin receptor 2, as mianserin or mirtazapine, but in contrast to these two drugs, without any antihistaminergic effects and therefore without weight gain as a side effect. However, agomelatine also has a selective effect on melatonin, thereby acting on sleep within the arousal symptoms in the HAM-D_9. We still have no firm data from controlled clinical trials on concomitant therapy with agomelatine and SSRIs/SNRIs, but clinical experience is indicated in Table 2. An anecdotal report of a safe combination of agomelatine and MAO-I is now available.

Table 2 also includes the mood-stabilizing drug lithium. The major indication for lithium therapy is its prophylactic effect in both bipolar and unipolar affective disorder. However, in the acute therapy of major depression, in a low dose (serum concentration of 0.4 - 0.5 mmol/l), lithium is one of the most effective drugs, helping to obtain a response in therapy-resistant depression. Its anti-suicidal effect is especially well-documented. The use of lithium in the acute therapy of major depression is referred to as augmentation, i.e. a non-concomitant initial use, in which the decision to start lithium treatment follows an initial treatment trial with one antidepressant resulting in only partial response.

Whereas concomitant therapy of lithium and an antidepressant seems most obvious in bipolar depression or depressed patients with hidden bipolarity , a concomitant therapy of olanzapine and an antidepressant (fluoxetine) has been shown to be effective not only in bipolar depression , but also in major depression . In the latter study, the HAM-D_{24} version was actually used, in this version specific items for hopelessness, helplessness and worthlessness have been included to strengthen domain A (Figure 1).

The term 'atypical antidepressants' refers to the use of MAO-Is (especially phenelzine) in the treatment of atypical major depression - i.e. patients with pure depression symptoms (A in Figure 1) but with inverse physiological symptoms (hypersomnia and increased appetite). As a non-antihistaminergic drug, agomelantine might be used in combination with MAO-Is in the treatment of atypical depression.

6. Polypharmacy: Pharmacokinetic considerations

According to pharmacokinetic studies the TCAs are mainly metabolized by CYP 450 enzyme system with the 2D6 substrate. Both agomelatine and mirtazapine are metabolized by the 1A2 substrate and therefore have no problems with CYP2D6 genetic polymorphisms. Among SSRIs we have listed citalopram and sertraline in brackets in Table 2 because these two antidepressants have the most acceptable pharmacokinetic profile. Among the SNRIs we have included both duloxetine and venlafaxine although desvenlafaxine might turn out to have the fewest drug-drug interactions in this class of antidepressants. Reboxetine and bupropion are metabolized through CTP3A4 but this seems only to be a problem when combined with the SSRI fluvoxamine. It is, however, recommended to consult specific reviews on pharmacokinetics when starting rational polypharmacy. In this review we have considered practical experience to be a valid guide. Thus, no problems with mirtazapine were found in the Blier *et al.* study. Mianserine was found to be safe both when combined with MAO-Is and with SSRIs (fluoxetine or citalopram). A combination of olanzapine and fluoxetine is also acceptable.

7. Conclusion

The most selective second generation antidepressants have not proved in monotherapy to be more effective on the core symptoms of depression than the first generation TCAs or MAO-Is. It is by their safety profiles, either in overdose or in terms of long term side effects, that the second generation antidepressants have outperformed the first generation.

If we accept that amitriptyline is the most effective antidepressant ever marketed, we need to use rational polypharmacy with the second generation antidepressants in the acute therapy of major depression in order to obtain effectiveness similar to that of amitriptyline, but without problematic side effects such as anticholinergic actions. A combination of mianserine/mirtazapine and SSRI/SNRI (Table 2) is the most rational polypharmacy when compared to amitriptyline. On the other hand, weight gain as a serious side effect is also prevalent here.

If a sedative effect on the HAM-D subscale of arousal symptoms (HAM-D_9) is needed, agomelatine might be used in combination with the specific reuptake inhibitors (Table 2). Reboxetine, for example, is a very weak antidepressant but when combined with an SSRI there is anecdotal evidence that patients respond much more favourably than on the SSRI in monotherapy.

The A,B,C HAM-D combined with $PRISE_{20}$ should be used whenever rational polypharmacy is employed.

8. References

[1] Trivedi MH, Fava M, Wisniewski SR, Thase ME, Quitkin F, Warden D, et al. Medication augmentation after the failure of SSRIs for depression. N Engl J Med. 2006 Mar 23;354(12):1243-52.

[2] Papakostas GI, Bech P, Fava M. Pharmacological treatment of major depressive disorder: A review. In: Herman H, Maj M, Sartorius N, editors. WPA Series Evidence and Experience in Psychiatry. Chichester: Wiley-Blackwell; 2009. p. 47-74.

[3] Barbui C, Hotopf M. Amitriptyline vs. the rest: Still the leading antidepressant after 40 years of randomised controlled trials. Br J Psychiatry. 2001;178:129,129-144.

[4] Larsen JK, Bendsen BB, Bech P. Vitamin B6 treatment of oedema induced by mirtazapine and isocarboxazid. Acta Psychiatr Scand. 2011 Jul;124(1):76,7; discussion 77.

[5] DUAG. Citalopram: Clinical effect profile in comparison with clomipramine. A controlled multicenter study. danish university antidepressant group. Psychopharmacology (Berl). 1986;90(1):131-8.

[6] DUAG. Paroxetine: A selective serotonin reuptake inhibitor showing better tolerance, but weaker antidepressant effect than clomipramine in a controlled multicenter study. Danish University Antidepressant Group. J Affect Disord. 1990 Apr;18(4):289-99.

[7] Hordern A, Burt CG, Holt NF, Cade JF. Depressive states: A pharmacotherapeutic study. Springfield: Charles C Thomas; 1965.

[8] Moncrieff J, Cohen D. Do antidepressants cure or create abnormal brain states? PLoS Med. 2006 Jul;3(7):e240.
[9] Hamilton M. Development of a rating scale for primary depressive illness. Br J Soc Clin Psychol. 1967 Dec;6(4):278-96.
[10] Bech P. The ABC profile of the HAM-D17. Revista Brasileira de Psiquiatria. 2011;33(2):109-10.
[11] Bech P. The threefold Hamilton Depression Scale. Acta Psychiatrica Scandinavica. 2012 In press.
[12] Bech P. Fifty years with the Hamilton scales for anxiety and depression. A tribute to Max Hamilton. Psychother Psychosom. 2009;78(4):202-11.
[13] Bech P, Gram LF, Dein E, Jacobsen O, Vitger J, Bolwig TG. Quantitative rating of depressive states. Acta Psychiatr Scand. 1975 Mar;51(3):161-70.
[14] Bech P, Allerup P, Gram LF, Reisby N, Rosenberg R, Jacobsen O, et al. The Hamilton Depression Scale. evaluation of objectivity using logistic models. Acta Psychiatr Scand. 1981 Mar;63(3):290-9.
[15] Bech P, Allerup P, Reisby N, Gram LF. Assessment of symptom change from improvement curves on the Hamilton Depression Scale in trials with antidepressants. Psychopharmacology (Berl). 1984;84(2):276-81.
[16] Paykel ES. Use of the Hamilton Depression Scale in general practice. In: Bech P, Coppen A, editors. The Hamilton Scales. Berlin: Springer; 1990. p. 40-9.
[17] Bech P. Meta-analysis of placebo-controlled trials with mirtazapine using the core items of the Hamilton Depression Scale as evidence of a pure antidepressive effect in the short-term treatment of major depression. Int J Neuropsychopharmacol. 2001 Dec;4(4):337-45.
[18] Santen G, Gomeni R, Danhof M, Della Pasqua O. Sensitivity of the individual items of the Hamilton Depression Rating Scale to response and its consequences for the assessment of efficacy. J Psychiatr Res. 2008 Oct;42(12):1000-9.
[19] Andreasson K, Liest V, Lunde M, Martiny K, Unden M, Dissing S, et al. Identifying patients with therapy-resistant depression by using factor analysis. Pharmacopsychiatry. 2010 Sep 6;43:252-6.
[20] Healy D. Did regulators fail over selective serotonin reuptake inhibitors? BMJ. 2006 Jul 8;333(7558):92-5.
[21] Rush AJ, Fava M, Wisniewski SR, Lavori PW, Trivedi MH, Sackeim HA, et al. Sequenced treatment alternatives to relieve depression (STAR*D): Rationale and design. Control Clin Trials. 2004 Feb;25(1):119-42.
[22] Wisniewski SR, Rush AJ, Balasubramani GK, Trivedi MH, Nierenberg AA, for the STAR*D Investigators. Self-rated global measure of the frequency, intensity, and burden of side effects. J Psychiatr Pract. 2006 Mar;12(2):71-9.
[23] Bech P. Rating scales for psychopathology, health status and quality of life. A compendium on documentation in accordance with the DSM-III-R and WHO systems. Berlin: Springer; 1993.
[24] Bech P, Gefke M, Lunde M, Lauritzen L, Martiny K. The pharmacopsychometric triangle to illustrate the effectiveness of T-PEMF concomitant with antidepressants in treatment resistant patients: A double-blind, randomised, sham-controlled trial

revisited with focus on the patient-reported outcomes. Depression Research and Treatment. 2011:Article ID 806298, 6 pages doi:10.1155/2011/806298.
[25] Bech P, Fava M, Trivedi MH, Wisniewski SR, Rush AJ. Outcomes on the pharmacopsychometric triangle in bupropion-SR vs. buspirone augmentation of citalopram in the STAR*D trial. Acta Psychiatr Scand. 2011 Nov 12.
[26] Bech P, Boyer P, Germain JM, Padmanabhan K, Haudiquet V, Pitrosky B, et al. HAM-D17 and HAM-D6 sensitivity to change in relation to desvenlafaxine dose and baseline depression severity in major depressive disorder. Pharmacopsychiatry. 2010;43(7):271-6.
[27] White K, Simpson G. Combined MAOI-tricyclic antidepressant treatment: A reevaluation. J Clin Psychopharmacol. 1981 Sep;1(5):264-82.
[28] Stern SL, Mendels J. Drug combinations in the treatment of refractory depression: A review. J Clin Psychiatry. 1981 Oct;42(10):368-73.
[29] Neuvonen P, Pohjola-Sintonen S, Tacke U. Five fatal cases of serotonin syndrome after moclobemide-citalopram or moclobemide-clomipramine overdoses. Lancet. 1993;342:1419.
[30] Medical Research Council. Clinical trial of the treatment of depressive illness. BMJ. 1965;1:881-6.
[31] DUAG. Moclobemide: A reversible MAO-A-inhibitor showing weaker antidepressant effect than clomipramine in a controlled multicenter study. danish university antidepressant group. J.Affect.Disord. 1993;28:105-116.
[32] Riise IS, Holm P. Concomitant isocarboxazid/mianserin treatment of major depressive disorder. J Affect Disord. 1984 Apr;6(2):175-9.
[33] Dam J, Ryde L, Svejso J, Lauge N, Lauritsen B, Bech P. Morning fluoxetine plus evening mianserin versus morning fluoxetine plus evening placebo in the acute treatment of major depression. Pharmacopsychiatry. 1998 Mar;31(2):48-54.
[34] Blier P, Ward HE, Tremblay P, Laberge L, Hebert C, Bergeron R. Combination of antidepressant medications from treatment initiation for major depressive disorder: A double-blind randomized study. Am J Psychiatry. 2010 Mar;167(3):281-8.
[35] Olié J-. Combining agagomelatine in the evening + iproniazide in the morning. 2011.
[36] Bech P. The full story of lithium. A tribute to Mogens Schou (1918-2005). Psychother Psychosom. 2006;75(5):265-9.
[37] Bech P, Christensen EM, Vinberg M, Bech-Andersen G, Kessing LV. From items to syndromes in the Hypomania Checklist (HCL-32): Psychometric validation and clinical validity analysis. J Affect Disord. 2011 Feb 22;132:48-54.
[38] Tohen M, Vieta E, Calabrese J, Ketter TA, Sachs G, Bowden C, et al. Efficacy of olanzapine and olanzapine-fluoxetine combination in the treatment of bipolar I depression. Arch Gen Psychiatry. 2003 Nov;60(11):1079-88.
[39] Rothschild AJ, Williamson DJ, Tohen MF, Schatzberg A, Andersen SW, Van Campen LE, et al. A double-blind, randomized study of olanzapine and olanzapine/fluoxetine combination for major depression with psychotic features. J Clin Psychopharmacol. 2004 Aug;24(4):365-73.

[40] Årsland D, Larsen JP, Lim NG, Wermuth L, Bech P. a_2-adrenoreceptor antagonism and serotonin reuptake inhibition in patients with parkinson disease and depression. Nord J Psychiatry. 2000;54:411-5.
[41] Eyding P, Lelgemann M, Grouven U, Härter M, Kromp M, Kaiser T, et al. Reboxetine for acute treatment of major depression: Systematic review and meta-analysis of published and unpublished placebo and selective serotonin reuptake inhibitor controlled trials. British Medical Journal. 2010;341:4737.

8

Antidepressant Drugs and Pain

Blanca Lorena Cobo-Realpe[1], Cristina Alba-Delgado[1,2], Lidia Bravo[1,2], Juan Antonio Mico[1,2] and Esther Berrocoso[2,3]

[1]Neuropsychopharmacology Research Group, Department of Neuroscience (Pharmacology and Psychiatry), University of Cádiz
[2]Centro de Investigación Biomédica en Red de Salud Mental (CIBERSAM), Instituto de Salud Carlos III, Madrid
[3]Neuropsychopharmacology Research Group, Psychobiology Area, Department of Psychology, University of Cádiz, Spain

1. Introduction

Physical pain is one of the most common somatic symptoms in patients that suffer depression and conversely, patients suffering from chronic pain of diverse origins are often depressed. Indeed, symptoms of physical pain in depressed patients are associated with a more severe prognosis of longer duration, greater functional impairment, a poorer clinical outcome and increased health-care costs. Moreover, the intensity of pain has been correlated with the severity of the symptoms of depression. While these data strongly suggest that depression is linked to altered pain perception, pain management has received little attention to date in the field of psychiatric research (Elman et al., 2011).

The monoaminergic system influences both mood and pain (Delgado, 2004), and since many antidepressants modify properties of monoamines, these compounds may be effective in managing chronic pain of diverse origins in non-depressed patients and to alleviate pain in depressed patients. There are abundant evidences in support of the analgesic properties of tricyclic antidepressants (TCAs), particularly amitriptyline, and another TCA, duloxetine, has been approved as an analgesic for diabetic neuropathic pain. By contrast, there is only limited data regarding the analgesic properties of selective serotonin reuptake inhibitors (SSRIs) (Saarto & Wiffen, 2007). In general, compounds with noradrenergic and serotonergic modes of action are more effective analgesics (Saarto & Wiffen, 2005), although the underlying mechanisms of action remain poorly understood, antidepressants appear to enhance endogenous analgesia and they are thought to increase the activity of the descending inhibitory bulbospinal pathway, which is compromised in chronic pain (Mico et al., 2006a).

While the utility of many antidepressant drugs in pain treatment is well established, it remains unclear whether antidepressants alleviate pain by acting on mood (emotional pain) or nociceptive transmission (sensorial pain). Indeed, in many cases, no correlation exists between the level of pain experienced by the patient and the effect of antidepressants on mood. Thus, in this chapter we will summarize our current knowledge relating to the use of antidepressants in chronic pain conditions and in the treatment of pain as a somatic symptom of depression. We will review the pharmacological mechanisms and the neurobiological substrates underlying the analgesic properties of antidepressants, and discuss the varying analgesic effects of specific types of antidepressants.

2. Depression and pain: Linked diseases

Depression and pain are two reciprocally linked and highly prevalent conditions (Figure 1). Epidemiological studies in pain clinics indicate that major depressive disorder has a prevalence of 52%, ranging from 1.5-100% depending on the chronic pain condition considered, and the prevalence of pain in depressed patients ranges from 15-100% (Bair et al., 2003). Depression is defined as an affective disorder characterized by ill mood, feelings of worthlessness, diminished interest in pleasurable stimuli and impaired decision making abilities. Moreover, depression involves a somatic dimension that is characterized by weight change, fatigue, sleep disturbances, headaches, stomach aches and other painful symptoms (DSM-IVR, 2000), such as back pain, neck-shoulder pain and musculoskeletal pain (Leino & Magni, 1993). Depressed patients may also experience an heightened response to pain or in the associated suffering, and in a primary care setting, they frequently complaining of specific types of pain, including abdominal, joint and chest pain, and headaches (Kroenke et al., 1994; Mathew et al., 1981). Indeed, lower back pain is twice as likely to be reported by depressed versus non-depressed patients (Croft et al., 1995).

According to the IASP (*International Association for Study of Pain*), pain is defined as "an unpleasant sensory and emotional experience associated with actual or potential tissue damage, or described in terms of such damage" (Merskey, 1994). The experience of pain can also be significantly influenced by emotional and psychosocial factors. Accordingly, depression may exacerbate the response to painful stimuli (Berna et al., 2010).

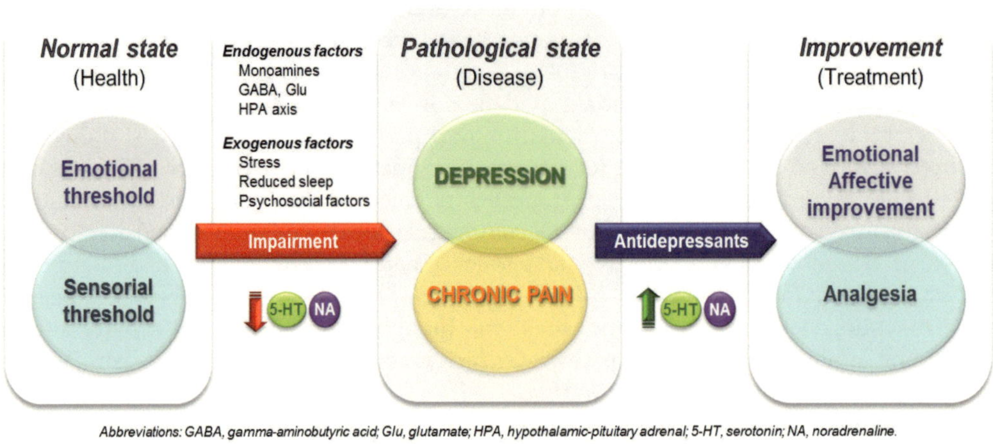

Fig. 1. Pain and depression. Pathological conditions of chronic pain and depression are associated with a decrease in the levels of both noradrenaline and serotonin. Treatment with some antidepressant drugs can improve both conditions.

3. Evidence of the analgesic effects of antidepressants

Currently, drugs that increase monoamine levels by inhibiting neurotransmitter reuptake represent the first line of treatment for depression, constituting a pharmacologically heterogeneous group known generically as "antidepressants". Typical antidepressant drugs are classified according to their mechanism of action (see Table 1) and they include the classical TCAs, SSRIs, noradrenaline reuptake inhibitors (NRIs) and mixed non-TCA antidepressants (SNRIs - serotonin and noradrenaline reuptake inhibitors). This group also includes dopamine and noradrenaline reuptake inhibitors (DNRIs), and reversible monoamine oxidase inhibitors (MAOIs) that inhibit both A and B subtypes of enzyme monoamine oxidase (MAO-A and MAO-B). The effects of atypical antidepressants include or rely exclusively on blocking of the α2-adrenoceptor and/or 5-HT2A receptors.

	Pharmacological action	Observations
Tricyclic antidepressants (TCAs)		
Desipramine Clomipramine Amitriptyline Nortriptyline Imipramine	Inhibitor of serotonin and noradrenaline reuptake Desipramine is essentially noradrenergic Clomipramine is principally serotonergic	Demethylated metabolites are associated with a more noradrenergic action The affinity for cholinergic, histaminergic and α_1-adrenergic receptors limits their use (side effects) Widely used in the treatment of pain
Selective serotonin reuptake inhibitors (SSRIs)		
Citalopram Escitalopram Fluoxetine Fluvoxamine Paroxetine Sertraline	Inhibitor of serotonin reuptake	Highly selective. Most commonly used in the treatment of depression. Not useful for pain treatment.
Noradrenaline reuptake inhibitors (non-tricyclic) *(NRIs)*		
Reboxetine	Inhibitor of noradrenaline reuptake	Low activity at histaminergic, cholinergic and α_1-adrenergic receptors. Some evidence of analgesic activity
Serotonin and noradrenaline reuptake inhibitors (non-tricyclic) *(SNRIs)*		
Venlafaxine Duloxetine Milnacipran	Inhibitor of serotonin and noradrenaline reuptake	No affinity for cholinergic, histaminergic or α_1-adrenergic receptors Widely used in the treatment of pain
Dopamine and noradrenaline reuptake inhibitors (DNRI)		
Bupropion	Inhibitor of dopamine and noradrenaline reuptake Minimal effect on serotonin reuptake	Highly selective. Currently used for smoking cessation treatment. Some studies have demonstrated efficacy in pain treatment
Inhibitors of monoamine oxidase (IMAOs)		
Phenelzine Tranylcyppromine	Irreversible inhibition of MAO-A and MAO-B	First generation drugs. Rarely used nowadays.
Moclobemide	Selective and reversible blockade of MAO-A	Less effective. Not currently used
Others		
Mianserin Mirtazapine	Noradrenergic receptor antagonists	Increase in noradrenergic transmission
Trazodone	Antagonist of postsynaptic 5-HT_2 receptors	Some inhibitory effects on serotonin reuptake
Tianeptine	Increases serotonin reuptake and dopamine release	

Table 1. Classification and general characteristics of antidepressants

3.1 Clinical studies

Several studies have demonstrated the intrinsic analgesic effects of antidepressants (McQuay et al., 1996; Onghena & Van Houdenhove, 1992; Smith et al., 1998). However, it remains unclear whether antidepressants are efficacious for the treatment of all types of pain or only for specific subtypes. Pain is a heterogeneous disorder that may have different origins: 1) nociceptive pain: caused by a lesion or potential tissue damage; 2) inflammatory: occurred as a consequence of an inflammatory process, 3) neuropathic pain: induced by an injury to the nervous system and finally, 4) pain that is not originated by a neurological disorder or peripheral tissue abnormality (irritable bowel syndrome, fibromyalgia and tension headache). The evidence currently available suggests that the antinociceptive effect of antidepressants is particularly relevant for the management of chronic pain, specifically neuropathic pain. Thus, antidepressants constitute the first line of pharmacological treatment of this disease, together with anticonvulsants such as gabapentin and pregabalin (Baidya et al., 2011; Moore et al., 2011). Neuropathic pain is a condition of chronic pain caused by injury to the nervous system. Currently, TCAs (amitriptyline, nortriptiline, imipramine and clomipramine) are the most common antidepressants used in the treatment of neuropathic pain processes associated with diabetes, cancer, viral infections and nerve compression. Among the TCAs, amitriptyline is considered the "gold standard" (Fishbain, 2003), with a demonstrated analgesic effect in several pain conditions, including headaches and fibromyalgia (Arnold et al., 2000; Descombes et al., 2001; Reisner, 2003). Other clinical studies have demonstrated also the efficacy of venlafaxine in several conditions, such as migraine, fibromyalgia and neuropathic pain, as well as cancer pain (Dwight et al., 1998; Tasmuth et al., 1998; Taylor & Rowbotham, 1996). Despite being a SNRI, at lower doses venlafaxine primarily acts on serotonergic transmission and it has no affinity for cholinergic or histaminergic receptors, providing an advantage over TCAs in terms of unwanted side effects. Following recent positive findings in controlled clinical studies, duloxetine has also been proposed as a suitable treatment for diabetic neuropathy (Goldstein et al., 2005; Leo & Barkin, 2003), while another SNRI with analgesic effects, milnacipran, has proved effective in the treatment of fibromyalgia (Leo & Brooks, 2006). SSRIs were successfully introduced in the 1980´s as effective treatments for depression, although in terms of chronic pain, these compounds have proved no more effective than traditional TCAs (McMahon, 2006). Moreover, some authors have proposed that SSRIs may enhance the process underlying acute pain (Dirksen R, 1998). A meta-analysis of antidepressant-induced analgesia by Onghena and colleagues found that selective NRIs were no more efficacious than dual-action antidepressants (Onghena & Van Houdenhove, 1992). However, based on the evidence described here, we can conclude that drugs that inhibit the reuptake of monoamines are likely to be effective in the treatment of chronic pain. In chronic pain it is known that there is a higher rate of action potential firing in nociceptors (Emery et al., 2011) that activate multiple pathophysiological mechanisms that lead to the different cluster of symptoms (spontaneous pain, hyperalgesia, allodynia…) in every pain condition. Evidences up-to-date are limited to the association of pain types with categories of drugs; for example, non-steroidal anti-inflammatory drugs (NSAIDS) with inflammatory pain or antidepressants and anticonvulsants with neuropathic pain. However, the distinction of different types of symptoms remains relevant for mechanism-based pain assessment and management. This makes difficult to identify the correlation of different pain symptoms to differently neurotransmission system (noradrenergic, sertonergic, opioid…).

In addition to their use in the treatment of chronic pain, antidepressants also alleviate physical symptoms (pain) associated with depression. This analgesic effect is typical of antidepressants that augment the levels of noradrenaline and serotonin. In general, TCAs demonstrated analgesic efficacy in a variety of pain conditions (*e.g.*, back pain, fibromyalgia and migraine) in patients with depression (Barbui et al., 2007; Hansen et al., 2005; McDermott et al., 2006; Mico et al., 2006b). In clinical studies, the SNRI venlafaxine was more efficacious in treating the physical symptoms of depression than SSRIs, suggesting that the emotional and physical symptoms of depression are modulated by distinct mechanisms (Nemeroff CN, 2003; Thase et al., 2001). Duloxetine also improves physical symptoms in depression (Detke et al., 2002a; 2002b) and thus, together these findings demonstrate that antidepressants that act on serotonergic and noradrenergic systems are useful to treat the physical symptoms of depression.

Many issues associated with the analgesic properties of antidepressants remain unclear. For example, are the antidepressant and analgesic effects of these compounds exerted at equivalent doses? It has been generally assumed that all antidepressants exert analgesic effects at doses lower than those at which antidepressant activity is induced, as demonstrated for TCAs (Lynch, 2001). However, more recent studies of the antidepressant/analgesic effects of non-TCA SNRIs (venlafaxine and duloxetine) do not support this hypothesis. While venlafaxine is effective in treating depression at doses of 75-225 mg/day (Golden & Nicholas, 2000), higher doses are required to relieve pain for review see (Briley, 2004; Sumpton & Moulin, 2001), although effective pain relief has been obtained with venlafaxine in the upper dose range of 150-225 mg/day (Rowbotham et al., 2004). In humans, venlafaxine inhibits preferentially serotonin uptake at 75 mg/kg, while doses of 150 mg/kg inhibit the uptake of both serotonin and noradrenaline (Roseboom & Kalin, 2000). These data are consistent with preclinical data suggesting that the contribution of both monoamines is required for the analgesic effect of venlafaxine (Berrocoso et al., 2009). By contrast, duloxetine inhibits the reuptake of serotonin and noradrenaline at similar doses, and exerts antidepressant and analgesic effect within the same dose range (Brannan et al., 2005; Goldstein et al., 2005). Thus, TCAs appear to provide effective pain relief at lower doses than those required for their antidepressant effects, while medium to high doses of SNRIs are necessary to produce analgesia (Sansone & Sansone, 2008).

3.2 Animal studies

The mechanisms by which antidepressants produce analgesic effects have been primarily studied in experimental animal models that reproduce the pathophysiological changes that occur in patients suffering pain (Yalcin et al., 2009b). While it is difficult to develop animal models that encompass all the processes associated with chronic pain, a variety of methodological approaches have been developed to model individual aspects of neuropathic pain, including chronic constriction injury of the sciatic nerve (Bennett & Xie, 1988) and induction of diabetic neuropathy through the administration of streptozotocin (Jakobsen & Lundbaek, 1976). These animal models permit the pain thresholds in response to different painful stimuli to be determined (mechanical, thermal, electrical, etc.) and using such approaches, it was demonstrated that diverse antidepressants reduce allodynia in a model of peripheral neuropathy, such as desipramine, venlafaxine, reboxetin and nortriptyline (Yalcin et al., 2009a; 2009b). Moreover, anti-allodynic effects of amitriptyline and nortriptyline (TCAs) have been described in models of chronic but not acute pain (Benbouzid et al., 2008a), and fluoxetine (SSRI) was seen to be ineffective at relatively high doses. Hence, inhibition of serotonin reuptake appears to be insufficient to alleviate allodynia associated to neuropathy, further evidence of the analgesic effects of inhibiting noradrenaline reuptake (Benbouzid et al., 2008a).

Anti-depressant	Treatment (dose)*	Pain model#	Behavioural test	Effect	References
Amitriptyline	Acute (10 mg/kg i.p.)	Neuropathic	Tail flick	Analgesia	(Iyengar et al., 2004)
Imipramine	Acute (5 mg/kg i.p.)	Tonic	Acetic acid	Analgesia	(Aoki et al., 2006)
	Acute (25 mg/kg i.p.)	Tonic (carrageenan)	Paw oedema	Analgesia	(Abdel-Salam et al., 2004)
Fluoxetine	Acute (30 mg/kg i.p.)	Phasic	Tail flick	Analgesia	(Pedersen et al., 2005)
	Acute (30 mg/kg i.p.)	Tonic (formalin)	Second phase	Analgesia	(Pedersen et al., 2005)
	Acute (10 mg/kg i.p.)	Neuropathic	Von Frey	Analgesia	(Pedersen et al., 2005)
	Acute (20 mg/kg i.p.)	Tonic (carrageenan)	Paw oedema	Analgesia	(Abdel-Salam et al., 2004)
	Chronic (20 mg/kg i.p.)	Tonic (carrageenan)	Paw oedema	Analgesia	(Abdel-Salam et al., 2004)
Fluvoxamine	Chronic (10 mg/kg i.p.)	Neuropathic	Paw pressure	No analgesic effect	(Gutierrez et al., 2003)
	Acute (40 mg/kg i.p.)	Tonic	Acetic acid	Analgesia	(Aoki et al., 2006)
	Acute (0.1 M i.t.)	Neuropathic	von Frey	Analgesia	(Ikeda et al., 2009)
Reboxetine	Acute (30 mg/kg i.p.)	Phasic	Tail flick	Analgesia	(Pedersen et al., 2005)
	Acute (10 mg/kg i.p.)	Tonic (formalin)	Second phase	Analgesia	(Pedersen et al., 2005)
Paroxetine	Acute (0.1 M i.t.)	Neuropathic	Von Frey	Analgesia	(Ikeda et al., 2009)
Duloxetine	Acute (10 mg/kg i.p.)	Neuropathic	Place escape/ avoidance	Improvement in the emotional dimension of pain	(Pedersen & Blackburn-Munro, 2006)
	Acute (3 mg/kg i.p.)	Neuropathic	Tail flick	Analgesia	(Iyengar et al., 2004)
	Acute (10 mg/kg p.o.)	Neuropathic	von Frey	Analgesia	(Iyengar et al., 2004)
	Acute (10 mg/kg i.p.)	Phasic	Hot-plate	Analgesia	(Jones et al., 2005)
	Acute (30 mg/kg p.o.)	Tonic	Acetic acid	Analgesia	(Jones et al., 2005)
Venlafaxine	Acute (10 mg/kg i.p.)	Neuropathic	Tail flick	Analgesia	(Iyengar et al., 2004)
	Acute (100 mg/kg p.o.)	Neuropathic	von Frey	Analgesia	(Iyengar et al., 2004)
	Acute (30 mg/kg i.p.)	Tonic (formalin)	Second phase	Analgesia	(Pedersen et al., 2005)
Milnacipran	Acute (10 mg/kg i.p.)	Neuropathic	Tail flick	Analgesia	(Iyengar et al., 2004)
	Acute (200 mg/kg p.o.)	Neuropathic	von Frey	Analgesia	(Iyengar et al., 2004)
	Acute (5 mg/kg i.p.)	Tonic	Acetic acid	Analgesia	(Aoki et al., 2006)
	Acute (60 mg/kg i.p.)	Neuropathic	Paw pressure	Analgesia	(Barbui et al., 2007)
	Acute (0.1 M i.t.)	Neuropathic	von Frey	Analgesia	(Ikeda et al., 2009)

** The dose and route of administration is shown in parentheses (i.p., intraperitoneal; i.t., intrathecal; p.o., oral)*

 # Pain models are categorized as phasic (short-duration pain), tonic (long-duration pain) and neuropathic, according to (Le Bars et al., 2001).

Table 2. Analgesic effects of antidepressant drugs in animal models of pain

The role of the monoaminergic system in antidepressant-induced analgesia has been demonstrated in several studies. Inhibition of noradrenergic, serotonergic or dopaminergic tone significantly attenuates the analgesic effect of antidepressants. For example, the inhibition of tyrosine hydroxylase (an essential enzyme for noradrenaline synthesis) or tryptophan hydroxylase (an essential enzyme for serotonin synthesis) antagonizes the analgesic effect of antidepressants in a wide range of experimental models (Valverde et al., 1994). Monoamines act on multiple receptor subtypes in the nervous system, some of which mediate the analgesic effect of antidepressants, such as α-adrenoceptors (Ghelardini et al., 2000; Yokogawa et al., 2002) and β-adrenoceptors (Mico et al., 2006b), 5-HT_{1A}, 5-HT_2 and 5-HT_3 serotonin receptors (Bonnefont et al., 2005; Yokogawa et al., 2002), and D2 dopamine receptors (Gilbert & Franklin, 2001).

4. Analgesic mechanism of action

Although antidepressants have been used as pain-relieving drugs for over 40 years, the mechanism of action underlying their analgesic effects remains unknown. Although their primary effect on neural circuits is to increase the availability of noradrenaline and/or serotonin, direct and indirect effects of antidepressants on other systems have also been proposed, including opioid neurotransmission. Given the established links between chronic pain and depression, it is plausible that antidepressants may act on substrates common to both conditions.

4.1 The monoaminergic system

Several common biological processes are deregulated in depression and chronic pain, producing hypothalamic-pituitary adrenal axis dysfunction (Blackburn-Munro, 2004), increases in plasma pro-inflammatory cytokines (Omoigui, 2007; Raison et al., 2006), alterations in brain-derived neurotrophic factor (BDNF) expression (Duman & Monteggia, 2006; Geng et al., 2010) and opioid signalling (Gold et al., 1982; Spetea et al., 2002). Nonetheless, the monoaminergic system is the predominant biological substrate linking both conditions, as witnessed by the key role played by serotonin and noradrenaline in pain and depression (Gormsen et al., 2006; Robinson et al., 2009). These observations strongly suggest that pain transmission may be compromised in depression and vice versa.

Serotonin and noradrenaline neurotransmitters are primarily synthesized in the dorsal raphe nuclei and locus coeruleus, respectively. Ascending projections from these two brainstem nuclei (mainly to the hypothalamus, anterior cingulate cortex and amygdala) are involved in the regulation of anxiety, mood and emotion. Moreover, deterioration in mood appears to be associated with impaired transmission along ascending serotonergic and noradrenergic pathways (Figure 1). Descending projections from the raphe nuclei and locus coeruleus project to the spinal cord (descending pain pathway), where they exert inhibitory influences on pain threshold. Furthermore, projections from the nucleus raphe magnus, locus coeruleus and A5 (also a noradrenergic centre) control the release of serotonin and noradrenaline at the level of the spinal cord. As a general rule, when these monoamines augment in synaptic clefts within the spinal cord there is a decrease in the pain threshold (Figure 1). However, it should be noted that serotonin can both dampen and enhance the sensation of pain, depending on the receptor subtypes activated. Given the common noradrenergic and serotonergic pathways implicated in chronic pain and depression, antidepressants are the most effective treatment to deal with chronic pain of diverse origins, with or without co-existing depression (Blier & Abbott, 2001; Campbell et al., 2003; Mico et al., 2006a). At the supraspinal level, these compounds increase noradrenaline and serotonin levels in the synaptic clefts while simultaneously enhancing the activity of the descending inhibitory bulbospinal pathways, thereby producing analgesia.

4.2 The opioid system

Some preclinical studies have demonstrated a functional relationship between endogenous opioid peptides and the analgesic effect of antidepressant drugs (Table 3). For example, the opioid antagonist naloxone or nor-binaltorphimine antagonize the analgesic effect of several TCAs and monoamine reuptake inhibitors in models of acute and chronic pain (Ardid & Guilbaud, 1992; Valverde et al., 1994). As opioid and monoaminergic systems appear to share common molecular mechanisms mediating nociception, opioid compounds are frequently co-administrated with antidepressants for pain relief. However, the validity of this therapeutic strategy for the treatment of mood disorders with comorbid pain remains unclear (Alba-Delgado et al., 2011; Berrocoso & Mico, 2009a; 2004; 2009; Rojas-Corrales et al., 2002; 2004). Moreover, the opioid doses required to produce antidepressant-like effects are higher than those required to produce analgesic effects, suggesting that these two processes are mediated by distinct mechanisms (Berrocoso & Mico, 2009a; Rodriguez-Munoz et al., 2011).

The influence of antidepressants on opioid signalling is region-specific. Indeed, the administration of antidepressants increases opioid receptor density in brain areas implicated in pain and depression (Ortega-Alvaro et al., 2004; Reisine & Soubrie, 1982). For example, chronic citalopram administration increases naloxone binding in cortical membranes (Antkiewicz-Michaluk et al., 1984), while imipramine and fluoxetine increase neuronal μ-opioid receptor expression in the prefrontal cortex, hippocampus and caudate putamen (de Gandarias et al., 1999; 1998). There is data revealing considerable variation in opioid receptor responses to antidepressant treatment depending on treatment duration, dose, the brain region analyzed and the antidepressant's mode of action. Importantly, opioids can also modify the action of antidepressants and a significant attenuation of the behavioural effects of two TCAs, clomipramine and desipramine, was observed in mice treated with the non-selective opioid antagonist naloxone (Devoize et al., 1984). This antagonistic effect was corroborated in subsequent studies, demonstrating a reduction in the antidepressant efficacy of tricyclic and non-tricyclic antidepressants in response to opioid pretreatment (Baamonde et al., 1992; Berrocoso et al., 2004; Besson et al., 1999; Tejedor-Real et al., 1995).

4.3 Other mechanisms involved

In addition to the monoaminergic and opioid systems, some antidepressants seem to exert their analgesic effect acting by other lesser-known mechanisms (see revision in Table 3). This is not surprising because other neurotransmission systems have been involved in the etiopathogenesis of pain and also in depression. Most evidences indicate the involvement of ionic channels (such as calcium, potassium and sodium) and neurotransmitter receptors (gamma-aminobutyric acid or GABA, N-methyl-D-aspartate, or NMDA and substance P) in the analgesic mechanism of action of antidepressants. It is interesting to note that among antidepressants, TCAs are those that act on multiple nociceptive targets both at central and

Mechanism of action	TCAs	SSRIs	NRIs	SNRIs	DNRIs	Other ADs	References
+ δ and μ-opioid receptors	Amitriptyline Mipramine Clomipramine Maprotiline Desmethylclo Imipramine Desipramine Nortriptyline Amoxapine	Paroxetine	Oxaprotiline Viloxazine	Venlafaxine	Nomifensine	Nefazodone Mirtazapine Mianserin	(Gray et al., 1998; Hamon et al., 1987; Marchand et al., 2003; Ortega-Alvaro et al., 2004; Schreiber et al., 1999; Schreiber et al., 2002; Valverde et al., 1994)
− Na^+ channel	Amitriptyline Imipramine Trimipramine Desipramine Doxepin	*Not known*	*Not known*	Venlafaxine	*Not known*	*Not known*	(Sudoh et al., 2003)
+ K^+ channel	Amitriptyline Clomipramine	Citalopram Fluoxetine	*Not known*	*Not known*	*Not known*	*Not known*	(Galeotti et al., 2001)
− Ca^{2+} channel	Amitriptyline Clomipramine Imipramine Trimipramine Desipramine Doxepin	Citalopra m	Oxaprotiline	*Not known*	*Not known*	*Not known*	(Antkiewicz-Michaluk et al., 1991; Beauchamp et al., 1995; Lavoie et al., 1994)
+ A1-adenosine receptor	Amitriptyline	*Not known*	*Not known*	*Not known*	*Not known*	*Not known*	(Esser & Sawynok, 2000; Sawynok et al., 1999; Sawynok et al., 2008; Sawynok et al., 2005)
↑ Adenosine levels	Amitriptyline	*Not known*	*Not known*	*Not known*	*Not known*	*Not known*	
$GABA_B$ receptor ↑ function	Amitriptyline Desipramine	Fluoxetine	*Not known*	*Not known*	*Not known*	*Not known*	(McCarson et al., 2006; McCarson et al., 2005; Sands et al., 2004)
− NMDA receptor	Amitriptyline Desipramine Clomipramine	*Not known*	*Not known*	Milnacipran	*Not known*	*Not known*	(Cai & McCaslin, 1992; Eisenach & Gebhart, 1995; Mjellem et al., 1993; Skolnick et al., 1996; Su & Gebhart, 1998)
↓ Substance P synthesis	Imipramine Clomipramine	*Not known*	*Not known*	*Not known*	*Not known*	*Not known*	(Bianchi et al., 1995; Iwashita & Shimizu, 1992)

Abbreviations: ADs, antidepressants; DNRIs, dopamine and noradrenaline reuptake inhibitors; GABA, gamma-aminobutyric acid; NMDA, N-methyl-D-aspartate; NRIs, noradrenaline reuptake inhibitors; SNRIs, serotonin and noradrenaline reuptake inhibitors; SSRIs, selective serotonin reuptake inhibitors; TCAs, tricyclic antidepressants; +, activation; −, blockade; ↑, increase; ↓, decrease.

Table 3. Non-monoaminergic mechanisms implicated in the analgesic effect of antidepressants

peripheral levels (Table 3) and this may be the reason why TCAs seem to be more effective than other antidepressants with a more selective monoaminergic mechanism of action. For example, many actions have been described for amitriptyline: blocking NMDA receptors and sodium channels (Sudoh et al., 2003). Also, it decreases intracellular calcium levels in the dorsal horn (Cai & McCaslin, 1992), and increases adenosine levels and the activity of A1 receptor (Esser & Sawynok, 2000; Sawynok et al., 1999; Sawynok et al., 2008; Sawynok et al., 2005). Finally, it promotes $GABA_B$ receptor function (McCarson et al., 2005), among other actions. This may help to explain why amitriptyline is one of the most widely used antidepressants in the treatment of pain. However, it is important to bear in mind that many of these targets are closely related to monoaminergic system and that these actions could lead ultimately to the increased of noradrenaline, serotonin and dopamine levels in the synaptic cleft.

4.4 Lessons from knockout mice

Recent advances in the field of genomics have led to the creation of new preclinical models where mutations are targeted to specific genes. The use of genetically manipulated rodents, mainly mice, has contributed to a better understanding of the mechanisms underlying mood and pain disorders, and of the mechanism of action of antidepressants. Knockout (KO) phenotypes are characterized using behavioural tests to evaluate the basal nociceptive threshold following pain induction and in general, the sensorial threshold is not modified in transgenic animals, although some exceptions have been reported.

Knockout mice have been used to explore the relative contributions of serotonergic and noradrenergic pathways in antidepressant-mediated analgesia (Table 4). Using homologous recombination, a KO mouse was generated lacking the noradrenaline transporter (Xu et al., 2000), resulting in reduced noradrenaline reuptake. In the tail-flick test, these mice displayed a modest elevation in the pain threshold. Moreover, unlike wild-type mice, pre-treatment with desipramine did not enhance morphine analgesia in these mutants (Bohn et al., 2000), highlighting the importance of the noradrenaline transporter in desipramine-mediated analgesia.

The role of other noradrenergic targets in analgesia has also been studied in KO mice, including that of α- and β-adrenoceptors. The α-adrenergic receptors are pre- and postsynaptic autoreceptors that regulate neuronal activity (noradrenaline release, firing rate, etc.), and their activation also promotes antinociceptive, sedative and sympatholytic effects *in vivo*. Significantly, α_2-adrenoceptor agonists are widely used clinically to mimic these effects and the α_{2A} receptor subtype has been identified as the principal mediator of antinociception (Lakhlani et al., 1997). Indeed, amitriptyline analgesia is abolished in α_{2A}-adrenoceptor KO mice in the hot plate and tail-flick tests (Ozdogan et al., 2004), suggesting that α_{2A}-adrenoceptors play a significant role in mediating the acute analgesic effects of amitriptyline, although other neurotransmitter systems may also be involved. The expression of β-adrenoceptors in the descending noradrenergic inhibitory pathway (Nicholson et al., 2005) also suggests a role for these receptors in the analgesic effects of antidepressants and the β_2 subtype has been shown to fulfil a critical role in the antiallodynic effects of nortriptyline (Yalcin et al., 2009a), venlafaxine and desipramine (Yalcin et al., 2009b).

Target	Antidepressant	Behavioural test	Effects WT mice	KO mice	References
Monoaminergic system					
α_{2A}-adrenoceptor	Amitriptyline	Tail-flick	Analgesia	No effect	(Ozdogan et al., 2004)
	Amitriptyline	Hot plate	Analgesia	No effect	(Ozdogan et al., 2004)
β_2-adrenoceptor	Desipramine	von Frey	Analgesia	No effect	(Yalcin et al., 2009b)
	Nortriptyline	von Frey	Analgesia	No effect	(Yalcin et al., 2009a)
	Venlafaxine	von Frey	Analgesia	No effect	(Yalcin et al., 2009b)
Noradrenaline transporter	Desipramine	Tail-Flick	Analgesia	No effect	(Bohn et al., 2000)
Lmx1b *(LIM homeodomain-containing transcription factor)*	Fluoxetine	Tail-Flick	Analgesia	No effect	(Zhao et al., 2007)
	Fluoxetine	Formalin (2° phase)	Analgesia	No effect	(Zhao et al., 2007)
	Fluoxetine	von Frey	Analgesia	No effect	(Zhao et al., 2007)
	Amitriptyline	Tail-Flick	Analgesia	Analgesia	(Zhao et al., 2007)
	Duloxetine	Tail-Flick	Analgesia	No effect	(Zhao et al., 2007)
	Duloxetine	Formalin (2° phase)	Analgesia	No effect	(Zhao et al., 2007)
	Duloxetine	von Frey	Analgesia	Analgesia	(Zhao et al., 2007)
RGS9-2 *(Regulator of G-protein signalling 9-2)*	Desipramine	von Frey	Analgesia	Analgesia	(Zachariou & Terzi, 2009)
	Desipramine	Hargreaves	Analgesia	Analgesia	(Zachariou & Terzi, 2009)
Opioid system					
μ-opioid receptor	Nortriptyline	von Frey	Analgesia	Analgesia	(Bohren et al., 2010)
δ-opioid receptor	Nortriptyline	von Frey	Analgesia	No effect	(Benbouzid et al., 2008b)
Other systems					
A1-adenosine receptor	Amitriptyline	Formalin (2° phase)	Analgesia	Analgesia	(Sawynok et al., 2008)
	Amitriptyline	Formalin (2° phase)	Analgesia	Analgesia	(Sawynok et al., 2008)

Abbreviations: KO, knockout; WT, wild-type.

Table 4. Analgesic response to antidepressant drugs in knockout and wild-type mice

While the majority of studies of the serotonergic action of antidepressants have focused specifically on antidepressant effects, antidepressant-induced analgesia has been studied in mice lacking Lmx1b (Zhao et al., 2007), a LIM homeodomain-containing transcription factor required for postmitotic differentiation of serotonergic neurons (Ding et al., 2003). These mice display dysfunctional central serotonergic neurotransmission and thus, they represent a novel tool to study the mode of action of antidepressants. Indeed, the analgesic effects of fluoxetine, amitriptyline and duloxetine on phasic and tonic pain (formalin and carrageenan tests) were abolished or greatly attenuated in transgenic mice (Zhao et al., 2007). This demonstrates the contribution of serotonergic neurotransmission to antidepressant-mediated analgesia, and provides important genetic evidence regarding the modulatory role of serotonin in inflammatory and acute pain.

While the contributions of noradrenaline and serotonin to pain and depression are well established, the role of other neurotransmitter systems, including the opioid system, remains unclear. Further studies are required to elucidate the neuroanatomical and molecular links between antidepressant action and opioid signalling. Indeed, several studies have suggested that this action may be centrally mediated, *e.g.,* via noradrenergic descending pathways. The generation of mice lacking μ- (Bohren et al., 2010) and δ-opioid receptors (Benbouzid et al., 2008b) has provided a novel approach to analyse the relationship between antidepressant activity and opioid signalling. Chronic treatment with the TCA nortriptyline induces antiallodynic effects in neuropathic wild-type and δ-opioid KO mice (Benbouzid et al., 2008b; Bohren et al., 2010), but not in μ-opioid deficient mice (Bohren et al., 2010), indicating that μ-opioid receptors are not required for the analgesic effects of nortriptyline in neuropathic pain. These results highlight the functional differences between μ- and δ-opioid receptors in antidepressant-mediated analgesia. It was proposed that the analgesic effect of nortriptyline may involve signalling via the endogenous opioid system through the δ subtype (Benbouzid et al., 2008b). However, further studies will be necessary to determine whether a similar mechanism may also underlie the antidepressant effects of these compounds.

5. Conclusion

Depression and chronic pain are two multifaceted illnesses with a common and complex neurobiological basis. While several neurotransmitters have been implicated in the biological origins of both conditions, the monoaminergic system appears to be the principal pathway affected. Accordingly, the primary therapeutic approach involves the use of drugs that act on this system, normalizing monoamine levels. Antidepressants that act on noradrenergic and serotonergic systems are commonly used to treat both the emotional and somatic symptoms of depression, and they are effective as analgesics for the treatment of chronic forms of pain, such as neuropathic pain. However, further studies in the analgesic mechanism of action of antidepressants beyond the monoaminergic level might help to develop new therapeutic options and to improve the treatment and prognosis of patients.

6. Acknowledgments

This work was supported by grants from: the Fondo de Investigacion Sanitaria PI10/01221; MICINN (SAF 2009-08460); CIBERSAM G18; Junta de Andalucía, Consejería de Innovación, Ciencia y Empresa (CTS-510, CTS-7748 and CTS-4303); Catedra Externa del Dolor Grünenthal-Universidad de Cadiz; and FP7-PEOPLE-2010-RG (268377), as well as an FPU fellowship (AP2007-02397).

7. References

Abdel-Salam, O.M., Baiuomy, A.R. & Arbid, M.S. (2004). Studies on the anti-inflammatory effect of fluoxetine in the rat. *Pharmacol Res*, 49, 2, pp. 119-131.

Alba-Delgado, C., Sánchez-Blázquez, P., Berrocoso, E., Garzón, J. & Mico, J.A. (2011). Opioid System and Depression, In: *Neurobiology of Depression*, Lopez-Munoz, F. & Alamo, C., pp. 223-245, Taylor & Francis Group, LLC., 9781439838495.

Antkiewicz-Michaluk, L., Rokosz-Pelc, A. & Vetulani, J. (1984). Increase in rat cortical [3H]naloxone binding site density after chronic administration of antidepressant agents. *Eur J Pharmacol*, 102, 1, pp. 179-181.

Antkiewicz-Michaluk, L., Romanska, I., Michaluk, J. & Vetulani, J. (1991). Role of calcium channels in effects of antidepressant drugs on responsiveness to pain. *Psychopharmacology (Berl)*, 105, 2, pp. 269-274.

Aoki, M., Tsuji, M., Takeda, H., Harada, Y., Nohara, J., Matsumiya, T. & Chiba, H. (2006). Antidepressants enhance the antinociceptive effects of carbamazepine in the acetic acid-induced writhing test in mice. *Eur J Pharmacol*, 550, 1-3, pp. 78-83.

Ardid, D. & Guilbaud, G. (1992). Antinociceptive effects of acute and 'chronic' injections of tricyclic antidepressant drugs in a new model of mononeuropathy in rats. *Pain*, 49, 2, pp. 279-287.

Arnold, L.M., Keck, P.E., Jr. & Welge, J.A. (2000). Antidepressant treatment of fibromyalgia. A meta-analysis and review. *Psychosomatics*, 41, 2, pp. 104-113.

Baamonde, A., Dauge, V., Ruiz-Gayo, M., Fulga, I.G., Turcaud, S., Fournie-Zaluski, M.C. & Roques, B.P. (1992). Antidepressant-type effects of endogenous enkephalins protected by systemic RB 101 are mediated by opioid delta and dopamine D1 receptor stimulation. *Eur J Pharmacol*, 216, 2, pp. 157-166.

Baidya, D.K., Agarwal, A., Khanna, P. & Arora, M.K. (2011). Pregabalin in acute and chronic pain. *J Anaesthesiol Clin Pharmacol*, 27, 3, pp. 307-314.

Bair, M.J., Robinson, R.L., Katon, W. & Kroenke, K. (2003). Depression and pain comorbidity: a literature review. *Arch Intern Med*, 163, 20, pp. 2433-2445.

Barbui, C., Butler, R., Cipriani, A., Geddes, J. & Hatcher, S. (2007). Depression in adults: drug and physical treatments. *Clin Evid (Online)*, 2007.

Beauchamp, G., Lavoie, P.A. & Elie, R. (1995). Differential effect of desipramine and 2-hydroxydesipramine on depolarization-induced calcium uptake in synaptosomes from rat limbic sites. *Can J Physiol Pharmacol*, 73, 5, pp. 619-623.

Benbouzid, M., Choucair-Jaafar, N., Yalcin, I., Waltisperger, E., Muller, A., Freund-Mercier, M.J. & Barrot, M. (2008a). Chronic, but not acute, tricyclic antidepressant treatment alleviates neuropathic allodynia after sciatic nerve cuffing in mice. *Eur J Pain*, 12, 8, pp. 1008-1017.

Benbouzid, M., Gaveriaux-Ruff, C., Yalcin, I., Waltisperger, E., Tessier, L.H., Muller, A., Kieffer, B.L., Freund-Mercier, M.J. & Barrot, M. (2008b). Delta-opioid receptors are critical for tricyclic antidepressant treatment of neuropathic allodynia. *Biol Psychiatry*, 63, 6, pp. 633-636.

Bennett, G.J. & Xie, Y.K. (1988). A peripheral mononeuropathy in rat that produces disorders of pain sensation like those seen in man. *Pain*, 33, 1, pp. 87-107.

Berna, C., Leknes, S., Holmes, E.A., Edwards, R.R., Goodwin, G.M. & Tracey, I. (2010). Induction of Depressed Mood Disrupts Emotion Regulation Neurocircuitry and Enhances Pain Unpleasantness. *Biological Psychiatry*, 67, 11, pp. 1083-1090.

Berrocoso, E. & Mico, J.A. (2009a). Cooperative opioid and serotonergic mechanisms generate superior antidepressant-like effects in a mice model of depression. *Int J Neuropsychopharmacol*, 12, 8, pp. 1033-1044.

Berrocoso, E., Rojas-Corrales, M.O. & Mico, J.A. (2004). Non-selective opioid receptor antagonism of the antidepressant-like effect of venlafaxine in the forced swimming test in mice. *Neurosci Lett*, 363, 1, pp. 25-28.

Berrocoso, E., Sanchez-Blazquez, P., Garzon, J. & Mico, J.A. (2009). Opiates as antidepressants. *Curr Pharm Des*, 15, 14, pp. 1612-1622.

Besson, A., Privat, A.M., Eschalier, A. & Fialip, J. (1999). Dopaminergic and opioidergic mediations of tricyclic antidepressants in the learned helplessness paradigm. *Pharmacol Biochem Behav*, 64, 3, pp. 541-548.

Bianchi, M., Rossoni, G., Sacerdote, P., Panerai, A.E. & Berti, F. (1995). Effects of chlomipramine and fluoxetine on subcutaneous carrageenin-induced inflammation in the rat. *Inflamm Res*, 44, 11, pp. 466-469.

Blackburn-Munro, G. (2004). Hypothalamo-pituitary-adrenal axis dysfunction as a contributory factor to chronic pain and depression. *Curr Pain Headache Rep*, 8, 2, pp. 116-124.

Blier, P. & Abbott, F.V. (2001). Putative mechanisms of action of antidepressant drugs in affective and anxiety disorders and pain. *J Psychiatry Neurosci*, 26, 1, pp. 37-43.

Bohn, L.M., Xu, F., Gainetdinov, R.R. & Caron, M.G. (2000). Potentiated opioid analgesia in norepinephrine transporter knock-out mice. *J Neurosci*, 20, 24, pp. 9040-9045.

Bohren, Y., Karavelic, D., Tessier, L.H., Yalcin, I., Gaveriaux-Ruff, C., Kieffer, B.L., Freund-Mercier, M.J. & Barrot, M. (2010). Mu-opioid receptors are not necessary for nortriptyline treatment of neuropathic allodynia. *Eur J Pain*, 14, 7, pp. 700-704.

Bonnefont, J., Chapuy, E., Clottes, E., Alloui, A. & Eschalier, A. (2005). Spinal 5-HT1A receptors differentially influence nociceptive processing according to the nature of the noxious stimulus in rats: effect of WAY-100635 on the antinociceptive activities of paracetamol, venlafaxine and 5-HT. *Pain*, 114, 3, pp. 482-490.

Brannan, S.K., Mallinckrodt, C.H., Brown, E.B., Wohlreich, M.M., Watkin, J.G. & Schatzberg, A.F. (2005). Duloxetine 60 mg once-daily in the treatment of painful physical symptoms in patients with major depressive disorder. *J Psychiatr Res*, 39, 1, pp. 43-53.

Briley, M. (2004). Clinical experience with dual action antidepressants in different chronic pain syndromes. *Hum Psychopharmacol*, 19 Suppl 1, pp. S21-25.

Cai, Z. & McCaslin, P.P. (1992). Amitriptyline, desipramine, cyproheptadine and carbamazepine, in concentrations used therapeutically, reduce kainate- and N-methyl-D-aspartate-induced intracellular Ca2+ levels in neuronal culture. *Eur J Pharmacol*, 219, 1, pp. 53-57.

Campbell, L.C., Clauw, D.J. & Keefe, F.J. (2003). Persistent pain and depression: a biopsychosocial perspective. *Biol Psychiatry*, 54, 3, pp. 399-409.

Croft, P.R., Papageorgiou, A.C., Ferry, S., Thomas, E., Jayson, M.I. & Silman, A.J. (1995). Psychologic distress and low back pain. Evidence from a prospective study in the general population. *Spine (Phila Pa 1976)*, 20, 24, pp. 2731-2737.

de Gandarias, J.M., Echevarria, E., Acebes, I., Abecia, L.C., Casis, O. & Casis, L. (1999). Effects of fluoxetine administration on mu-opoid receptor immunostaining in the rat forebrain. *Brain Res*, 817, 1-2, pp. 236-240.

de Gandarias, J.M., Echevarria, E., Acebes, I., Silio, M. & Casis, L. (1998). Effects of imipramine administration on mu-opioid receptor immunostaining in the rat forebrain. *Arzneimittelforschung*, 48, 7, pp. 717-719.

Delgado, P.L. (2004). Common pathways of depression and pain. *J Clin Psychiatry*, 65 Suppl 12, pp. 16-19.

Descombes, S., Brefel-Courbon, C., Thalamas, C., Albucher, J.F., Rascol, O., Montastruc, J.L. & Senard, J.M. (2001). Amitriptyline treatment in chronic drug-induced headache: a double-blind comparative pilot study. *Headache*, 41, 2, pp. 178-182.

Detke, M.J., Lu, Y., Goldstein, D.J., Hayes, J.R. & Demitrack, M.A. (2002a). Duloxetine, 60 mg once daily, for major depressive disorder: a randomized double-blind placebo-controlled trial. *J Clin Psychiatry*, 63, 4, pp. 308-315.

Detke, M.J., Lu, Y., Goldstein, D.J., McNamara, R.K. & Demitrack, M.A. (2002b). Duloxetine 60 mg once daily dosing versus placebo in the acute treatment of major depression. *J Psychiatr Res*, 36, 6, pp. 383-390.

Devoize, J.L., Rigal, F., Eschalier, A., Trolese, J.F. & Renoux, M. (1984). Influence of naloxone on antidepressant drug effects in the forced swimming test in mice. *Psychopharmacology (Berl)*, 84, 1, pp. 71-75.

Ding, Y.Q., Marklund, U., Yuan, W., Yin, J., Wegman, L., Ericson, J., Deneris, E., Johnson, R.L. & Chen, Z.F. (2003). Lmx1b is essential for the development of serotonergic neurons. *Nat Neurosci*, 6, 9, pp. 933-938.

Dirksen R, V.L.E., Van Rijn CM. (1998). Selective serotonin reuptake inhibitors may enhance responses to noxious stimulation. *Pharmacology Biochemistry and Behavior*, 60, 3, pp. 719-725.

American Psychiatric Association. (2000). *Diagnostic and Statistical Manual of Mental Disorders (DSM)* American Psychiatric Publishing, Washington D.C.

Duman, R.S. & Monteggia, L.M. (2006). A neurotrophic model for stress-related mood disorders. *Biol Psychiatry*, 59, 12, pp. 1116-1127.

Dwight, M.M., Arnold, L.M., O'Brien, H., Metzger, R., Morris-Park, E. & Keck, P.E., Jr. (1998). An open clinical trial of venlafaxine treatment of fibromyalgia. *Psychosomatics*, 39, 1, pp. 14-17.

Eisenach, J.C. & Gebhart, G.F. (1995). Intrathecal amitriptyline acts as an N-methyl-D-aspartate receptor antagonist in the presence of inflammatory hyperalgesia in rats. *Anesthesiology*, 83, 5, pp. 1046-1054.

Elman, I., Zubieta, J.K. & Borsook, D. (2011). The missing p in psychiatric training: why it is important to teach pain to psychiatrists. *Arch Gen Psychiatry*, 68, 1, pp. 12-20.

Emery, E.C., Young, G.T., Berrocoso, E.M., Chen, L. & McNaughton, P.A. (2011). HCN2 ion channels play a central role in inflammatory and neuropathic pain. *Science*, 333, 6048, pp. 1462-1466.

Esser, M.J. & Sawynok, J. (2000). Caffeine blockade of the thermal antihyperalgesic effect of acute amitriptyline in a rat model of neuropathic pain. *Eur J Pharmacol*, 399, 2-3, pp. 131-139.

Fishbain, D.A. (2003). Analgesic effects of antidepressants. *J Clin Psychiatry*, 64, 1, pp. 96; author reply 96-97.

Galeotti, N., Ghelardini, C. & Bartolini, A. (2001). Involvement of potassium channels in amitriptyline and clomipramine analgesia. *Neuropharmacology*, 40, 1, pp. 75-84.

Geng, S.J., Liao, F.F., Dang, W.H., Ding, X., Liu, X.D., Cai, J., Han, J.S., Wan, Y. & Xing, G.G. (2010). Contribution of the spinal cord BDNF to the development of neuropathic pain by activation of the NR2B-containing NMDA receptors in rats with spinal nerve ligation. *Exp Neurol*, 222, 2, pp. 256-266.

Ghelardini, C., Galeotti, N. & Bartolini, A. (2000). Antinociception induced by amitriptyline and imipramine is mediated by alpha2A-adrenoceptors. *Jpn J Pharmacol*, 82, 2, pp. 130-137.

Gilbert, A.K. & Franklin, K.B. (2001). Characterization of the analgesic properties of nomifensine in rats. *Pharmacol Biochem Behav*, 68, 4, pp. 783-787.

Gold, M.S., Pottash, A.C., Sweeney, D., Martin, D. & Extein, I. (1982). ANTIMANIC, ANTIDEPRESSANT, AND ANTIPANIC EFFECTS OF OPIATES: CLINICAL, NEUROANATOMICAL, AND BIOCHEMICAL EVIDENCE. *Annals of the New York Academy of Sciences*, 398, 1, pp. 140-150.

Golden, R.N. & Nicholas, L. (2000). Antidepressant efficacy of venlafaxine. *Depress Anxiety*, 12 Suppl 1, pp. 45-49.

Goldstein, D.J., Lu, Y., Detke, M.J., Lee, T.C. & Iyengar, S. (2005). Duloxetine vs. placebo in patients with painful diabetic neuropathy. *Pain*, 116, 1-2, pp. 109-118.

Gormsen, L., Jensen, T.S., Bach, F.W. & Rosenberg, R. (2006). Pain and depression. *Smerter og depression*, 168, 20, pp. 1967-1969.

Gray, A.M., Spencer, P.S. & Sewell, R.D. (1998). The involvement of the opioidergic system in the antinociceptive mechanism of action of antidepressant compounds. *Br J Pharmacol*, 124, 4, pp. 669-674.

Gutierrez, M., Ortega-Alvaro, A., Gibert-Rahola, J. & Mico, J.A. (2003). Interactions of acute morphine with chronic imipramine and fluvoxamine treatment on the antinociceptive effect in arthritic rats. *Neurosci Lett*, 352, 1, pp. 37-40.

Hamon, M., Gozlan, H., Bourgoin, S., Benoliel, J.J., Mauborgne, A., Taquet, H., Cesselin, F. & Mico, J.A. (1987). Opioid receptors and neuropeptides in the CNS in rats treated chronically with amoxapine or amitriptyline. *Neuropharmacology*, 26, 6, pp. 531-539.

Hansen, R.A., Gartlehner, G., Lohr, K.N., Gaynes, B.N. & Carey, T.S. (2005). Efficacy and safety of second-generation antidepressants in the treatment of major depressive disorder. *Ann Intern Med*, 143, 6, pp. 415-426.

Ikeda, T., Ishida, Y., Naono, R., Takeda, R., Abe, H., Nakamura, T. & Nishimori, T. (2009). Effects of intrathecal administration of newer antidepressants on mechanical allodynia in rat models of neuropathic pain. *Neurosci Res*, 63, 1, pp. 42-46.

Iwashita, T. & Shimizu, T. (1992). Imipramine inhibits intrathecal substance P-induced behavior and blocks spinal cord substance P receptors in mice. *Brain Res*, 581, 1, pp. 59-66.

Iyengar, S., Webster, A.A., Hemrick-Luecke, S.K., Xu, J.Y. & Simmons, R.M. (2004). Efficacy of duloxetine, a potent and balanced serotonin-norepinephrine reuptake inhibitor in persistent pain models in rats. *J Pharmacol Exp Ther*, 311, 2, pp. 576-584.

Jakobsen, J. & Lundbaek, K. (1976). Neuropathy in experimental diabetes: an animal model. *Br Med J*, 2, 6030, pp. 278-279.

Jones, C.K., Peters, S.C. & Shannon, H.E. (2005). Efficacy of duloxetine, a potent and balanced serotonergic and noradrenergic reuptake inhibitor, in inflammatory and acute pain models in rodents. *J Pharmacol Exp Ther*, 312, 2, pp. 726-732.

Kroenke, K., Spitzer, R.L., Williams, J.B., Linzer, M., Hahn, S.R., deGruy, F.V., 3rd & Brody, D. (1994). Physical symptoms in primary care. Predictors of psychiatric disorders and functional impairment. *Arch Fam Med*, 3, 9, pp. 774-779.

Lakhlani, P.P., MacMillan, L.B., Guo, T.Z., McCool, B.A., Lovinger, D.M., Maze, M. & Limbird, L.E. (1997). Substitution of a mutant alpha2a-adrenergic receptor via "hit and run" gene targeting reveals the role of this subtype in sedative, analgesic, and anesthetic-sparing responses in vivo. *Proc Natl Acad Sci U S A*, 94, 18, pp. 9950-9955.

Lavoie, P.A., Beauchamp, G. & Elie, R. (1994). Absence of stereoselectivity of some tricyclic antidepressants for the inhibition of depolarization-induced calcium uptake in rat cingulate cortex synaptosomes. *J Psychiatry Neurosci*, 19, 3, pp. 208-212.

Le Bars, D., Gozariu, M. & Cadden, S.W. (2001). Animal models of nociception. *Pharmacol Rev*, 53, 4, pp. 597-652.

Leino, P. & Magni, G. (1993). Depressive and distress symptoms as predictors of low back pain, neck-shoulder pain, and other musculoskeletal morbidity: a 10-year follow-up of metal industry employees. *Pain*, 53, 1, pp. 89-94.

Leo, R.J. & Barkin, R.L. (2003). Antidepressant Use in Chronic Pain Management: Is There Evidence of a Role for Duloxetine? *Prim Care Companion J Clin Psychiatry*, 5, 3, pp. 118-123.

Leo, R.J. & Brooks, V.L. (2006). Clinical potential of milnacipran, a serotonin and norepinephrine reuptake inhibitor, in pain. *Curr Opin Investig Drugs*, 7, 7, pp. 637-642.

Lynch, M.E. (2001). Antidepressants as analgesics: a review of randomized controlled trials. *J Psychiatry Neurosci*, 26, 1, pp. 30-36.

Marchand, F., Ardid, D., Chapuy, E., Alloui, A., Jourdan, D. & Eschalier, A. (2003). Evidence for an involvement of supraspinal delta- and spinal mu-opioid receptors in the antihyperalgesic effect of chronically administered clomipramine in mononeuropathic rats. *J Pharmacol Exp Ther*, 307, 1, pp. 268-274.

Mathew, R.J., Weinman, M.L. & Mirabi, M. (1981). Physical symptoms of depression. *Br J Psychiatry*, 139, pp. 293-296.

McCarson, K.E., Duric, V., Reisman, S.A., Winter, M. & Enna, S.J. (2006). GABA(B) receptor function and subunit expression in the rat spinal cord as indicators of stress and the antinociceptive response to antidepressants. *Brain Res*, 1068, 1, pp. 109-117.

McCarson, K.E., Ralya, A., Reisman, S.A. & Enna, S.J. (2005). Amitriptyline prevents thermal hyperalgesia and modifications in rat spinal cord GABA(B) receptor expression and function in an animal model of neuropathic pain. *Biochem Pharmacol*, 71, 1-2, pp. 196-202.

McDermott, A.M., Toelle, T.R., Rowbotham, D.J., Schaefer, C.P. & Dukes, E.M. (2006). The burden of neuropathic pain: results from a cross-sectional survey. *Eur J Pain*, 10, 2, pp. 127-135.

McMahon, S.B.a.K., M. (2006). Wall and Melzack's Textbook of Pain, Elsevier Chrurchill Livingstone.

McQuay, H.J., Tramer, M., Nye, B.A., Carroll, D., Wiffen, P.J. & Moore, R.A. (1996). A systematic review of antidepressants in neuropathic pain. *Pain*, 68, 2-3, pp. 217-227.

Merskey, H. (1994). Logic, truth and language in concepts of pain. *Qual Life Res*, 3 Suppl 1, pp. S69-76.

Mico, J.A., Ardid, D., Berrocoso, E. & Eschalier, A. (2006a). Antidepressants and pain. *Trends Pharmacol Sci*, 27, 7, pp. 348-354.

Mico, J.A., Berrocoso, E., Ortega-Alvaro, A., Gibert-Rahola, J. & Rojas-Corrales, M.O. (2006b). The role of 5-HT1A receptors in research strategy for extensive pain treatment. *Curr Top Med Chem*, 6, 18, pp. 1997-2003.

Mjellem, N., Lund, A. & Hole, K. (1993). Reduction of NMDA-induced behaviour after acute and chronic administration of desipramine in mice. *Neuropharmacology*, 32, 6, pp. 591-595.

Moore, R.A., Wiffen, P.J., Derry, S. & McQuay, H.J. (2011). Gabapentin for chronic neuropathic pain and fibromyalgia in adults. *Cochrane Database Syst Rev*, 3, pp. CD007938.

Nemeroff CN, E.R., Willard LB, (2003). Comprehensive pooled analysis of remission data: venlafaxine vs SSRIs. . Presented at the 156th annual meeting of the American Psychiatric Association. San Francisco, Calif.

Nicholson, R., Dixon, A.K., Spanswick, D. & Lee, K. (2005). Noradrenergic receptor mRNA expression in adult rat superficial dorsal horn and dorsal root ganglion neurons. *Neurosci Lett*, 380, 3, pp. 316-321.

Omoigui, S. (2007). The biochemical origin of pain: the origin of all pain is inflammation and the inflammatory response. Part 2 of 3 - inflammatory profile of pain syndromes. *Med Hypotheses*, 69, 6, pp. 1169-1178.

Onghena, P. & Van Houdenhove, B. (1992). Antidepressant-induced analgesia in chronic non-malignant pain: a meta-analysis of 39 placebo-controlled studies. *Pain*, 49, 2, pp. 205-219.

Ortega-Alvaro, A., Acebes, I., Saracibar, G., Echevarria, E., Casis, L. & Mico, J.A. (2004). Effect of the antidepressant nefazodone on the density of cells expressing mu-opioid receptors in discrete brain areas processing sensory and affective dimensions of pain. *Psychopharmacology (Berl)*, 176, 3-4, pp. 305-311.

Ozdogan, U.K., Lahdesmaki, J., Mansikka, H. & Scheinin, M. (2004). Loss of amitriptyline analgesia in alpha 2A-adrenoceptor deficient mice. *Eur J Pharmacol*, 485, 1-3, pp. 193-196.

Pedersen, L.H. & Blackburn-Munro, G. (2006). Pharmacological characterisation of place escape/avoidance behaviour in the rat chronic constriction injury model of neuropathic pain. *Psychopharmacology (Berl)*, 185, 2, pp. 208-217.

Pedersen, L.H., Nielsen, A.N. & Blackburn-Munro, G. (2005). Anti-nociception is selectively enhanced by parallel inhibition of multiple subtypes of monoamine transporters in rat models of persistent and neuropathic pain. *Psychopharmacology (Berl)*, 182, 4, pp. 551-561.

Raison, C.L., Capuron, L. & Miller, A.H. (2006). Cytokines sing the blues: inflammation and the pathogenesis of depression. *Trends Immunol*, 27, 1, pp. 24-31.

Reisine, T. & Soubrie, P. (1982). Loss of rat cerebral cortical opiate receptors following chronic desimipramine treatment. *Eur J Pharmacol*, 77, 1, pp. 39-44.

Reisner, L. (2003). Antidepressants for chronic neuropathic pain. *Curr Pain Headache Rep*, 7, 1, pp. 24-33.

Robinson, M.J., Edwards, S.E., Iyengar, S., Bymaster, F., Clark, M. & Katon, W. (2009). Depression and pain. *Front Biosci*, 14, pp. 5031-5051.

Rodriguez-Munoz, M., Sanchez-Blazquez, P., Vicente-Sanchez, A., Berrocoso, E. & Garzon, J. (2011). The Mu-Opioid Receptor and the NMDA Receptor Associate in PAG Neurons: Implications in Pain Control. *Neuropsychopharmacology*.

Rojas-Corrales, M.O., Berrocoso, E., Gibert-Rahola, J. & Mico, J.A. (2002). Antidepressant-like effects of tramadol and other central analgesics with activity on monoamines reuptake, in helpless rats. *Life Sci*, 72, 2, pp. 143-152.

Rojas-Corrales, M.O., Berrocoso, E., Gibert-Rahola, J. & Mico, J.A. (2004). Antidepressant-like effect of tramadol and its enantiomers in reserpinized mice: comparative study with desipramine, fluvoxamine, venlafaxine and opiates. *J Psychopharmacol*, 18, 3, pp. 404-411.

Roseboom, P.H. & Kalin, N.H. (2000). Neuropharmacology of venlafaxine. *Depress Anxiety*, 12 Suppl 1, pp. 20-29.

Rowbotham, M.C., Goli, V., Kunz, N.R. & Lei, D. (2004). Venlafaxine extended release in the treatment of painful diabetic neuropathy: a double-blind, placebo-controlled study. *Pain*, 110, 3, pp. 697-706.

Saarto, T. & Wiffen, P.J. (2005). Antidepressants for neuropathic pain. *Cochrane Database Syst Rev*, 3, pp. CD005454.

Saarto, T. & Wiffen, P.J. (2007). Antidepressants for neuropathic pain. *Cochrane Database Syst Rev*, 4, pp. CD005454.

Sands, S.A., McCarson, K.E. & Enna, S.J. (2004). Relationship between the antinociceptive response to desipramine and changes in GABAB receptor function and subunit expression in the dorsal horn of the rat spinal cord. *Biochem Pharmacol*, 67, 4, pp. 743-749.

Sansone, R.A. & Sansone, L.A. (2008). A longitudinal perspective on personality disorder symptomatology. *Psychiatry (Edgmont)*, 5, 1, pp. 53-57.

Sawynok, J., Reid, A.R. & Esser, M.J. (1999). Peripheral antinociceptive action of amitriptyline in the rat formalin test: involvement of adenosine. *Pain*, 80, 1-2, pp. 45-55.

Sawynok, J., Reid, A.R. & Fredholm, B.B. (2008). Caffeine reverses antinociception by amitriptyline in wild type mice but not in those lacking adenosine A1 receptors. *Neurosci Lett*, 440, 2, pp. 181-184.

Sawynok, J., Reid, A.R., Liu, X.J. & Parkinson, F.E. (2005). Amitriptyline enhances extracellular tissue levels of adenosine in the rat hindpaw and inhibits adenosine uptake. *Eur J Pharmacol*, 518, 2-3, pp. 116-122.

Schreiber, S., Backer, M.M. & Pick, C.G. (1999). The antinociceptive effect of venlafaxine in mice is mediated through opioid and adrenergic mechanisms. *Neurosci Lett*, 273, 2, pp. 85-88.

Schreiber, S., Bleich, A. & Pick, C.G. (2002). Venlafaxine and mirtazapine: different mechanisms of antidepressant action, common opioid-mediated antinociceptive effects--a possible opioid involvement in severe depression? *J Mol Neurosci*, 18, 1-2, pp. 143-149.

Skolnick, P., Layer, R.T., Popik, P., Nowak, G., Paul, I.A. & Trullas, R. (1996). Adaptation of N-methyl-D-aspartate (NMDA) receptors following antidepressant treatment: implications for the pharmacotherapy of depression. *Pharmacopsychiatry*, 29, 1, pp. 23-26.

Smith, G.C., Clarke, D.M., Handrinos, D. & Dunsis, A. (1998). Consultation-liaison psychiatrists management of depression. *Psychosomatics*, 39, 3, pp. 244-252.

Spetea, M., Rydelius, G., Nylander, I., Ahmed, M., Bileviciute-Ljungar, I., Lundeberg, T., Svensson, S. & Kreicbergs, A. (2002). Alteration in endogenous opioid systems due to chronic inflammatory pain conditions. *European Journal of Pharmacology*, 435, 2-3, pp. 245-252.

Su, X. & Gebhart, G.F. (1998). Effects of tricyclic antidepressants on mechanosensitive pelvic nerve afferent fibers innervating the rat colon. *Pain*, 76, 1-2, pp. 105-114.

Sudoh, Y., Cahoon, E.E., Gerner, P. & Wang, G.K. (2003). Tricyclic antidepressants as long-acting local anesthetics. *Pain*, 103, 1-2, pp. 49-55.

Sumpton, J.E. & Moulin, D.E. (2001). Treatment of neuropathic pain with venlafaxine. *Ann Pharmacother*, 35, 5, pp. 557-559.

Tasmuth, T., von Smitten, K., Blomqvist, C. & Kalso, E. (1998). [Chronic pain and other symptoms following treatment of breast cancer]. *Duodecim*, 114, 1, pp. 52-54.

Taylor, K. & Rowbotham, M.C. (1996). Venlafaxine hydrochloride and chronic pain. *West J Med*, 165, 3, pp. 147-148.

Tejedor-Real, P., Mico, J.A., Maldonado, R., Roques, B.P. & Gibert-Rahola, J. (1995). Implication of endogenous opioid system in the learned helplessness model of depression. *Pharmacol Biochem Behav*, 52, 1, pp. 145-152.

Thase, M.E., Entsuah, A.R. & Rudolph, R.L. (2001). Remission rates during treatment with venlafaxine or selective serotonin reuptake inhibitors. *Br J Psychiatry*, 178, pp. 234-241.

Valverde, O., Mico, J.A., Maldonado, R., Mellado, M. & Gibert-Rahola, J. (1994). Participation of opioid and monoaminergic mechanisms on the antinociceptive effect induced by tricyclic antidepressants in two behavioural pain tests in mice. *Prog Neuropsychopharmacol Biol Psychiatry*, 18, 6, pp. 1073-1092.

Xu, F., Gainetdinov, R.R., Wetsel, W.C., Jones, S.R., Bohn, L.M., Miller, G.W., Wang, Y.M. & Caron, M.G. (2000). Mice lacking the norepinephrine transporter are supersensitive to psychostimulants. *Nat Neurosci*, 3, 5, pp. 465-471.

Yalcin, I., Choucair-Jaafar, N., Benbouzid, M., Tessier, L.H., Muller, A., Hein, L., Freund-Mercier, M.J. & Barrot, M. (2009a). beta(2)-adrenoceptors are critical for antidepressant treatment of neuropathic pain. *Ann Neurol*, 65, 2, pp. 218-225.

Yalcin, I., Tessier, L.H., Petit-Demouliere, N., Doridot, S., Hein, L., Freund-Mercier, M.J. & Barrot, M. (2009b). Beta2-adrenoceptors are essential for desipramine, venlafaxine or reboxetine action in neuropathic pain. *Neurobiol Dis*, 33, 3, pp. 386-394.

Yokogawa, F., Kiuchi, Y., Ishikawa, Y., Otsuka, N., Masuda, Y., Oguchi, K. & Hosoyamada, A. (2002). An investigation of monoamine receptors involved in antinociceptive effects of antidepressants. *Anesth Analg*, 95, 1, pp. 163-168, table of contents.

Zachariou, V. & Terzi, D. (2009). RGS9-2 modulates the anti-allodynic and anti-hyperalgesic actions of tricyclic antidepressants and opioids in a mouse model for neuropathic pain. *Proceedings of* Neuroscience Meeting Planner, Society for Neuroscience. Chicago.

Zhao, Z.Q., Chiechio, S., Sun, Y.G., Zhang, K.H., Zhao, C.S., Scott, M., Johnson, R.L., Deneris, E.S., Renner, K.J., Gereau, R.W.t. & Chen, Z.F. (2007). Mice lacking central serotonergic neurons show enhanced inflammatory pain and an impaired analgesic response to antidepressant drugs. *J Neurosci*, 27, 22, pp. 6045-6053.

9

Antidepressant Drug Use in Patients with Diabetes Mellitus Type 1 – The Effect of Medication on Mental Problems and Glycemic Control

Jana Komorousová[1] and Zdeněk Jankovec[2]
[1]*Outpatient Department of Psychiatry, Pilsen*
[2]*Department of Internal Medicine I., University Hospital Pilsen, Czech Republic*

1. Introduction

1.1 Diabetes and mental health

Diabetes mellitus is a severe chronic life-long disease, which is diagnosed in about 6% of the population. In many aspects it is considered a psycho-somatic disease. Some mental disorders, especially depression, are more common in diabetic patients compared to the rest of the population. Diabetes mellitus affects psyche of the patients, but at the same time mental state of the patients influences the course of diabetes. The causal links are different depending on the type of diabetes and mental disorder. Nonetheless, the association is observed on a level of emotions and mental processes, but also in biochemical and hormonal aspects. In this article we will focus only on diabetes mellitus type 1.

From the moment of diagnosis, diabetes introduces substantial changes in life of a patient. His life-style should be adjusted to them in order to make the course of the disease as favorable as possible. This disease demands maintaining a regular daily regime regarding food and physical activity. The patients must watch their body-weight and measure blood glucose several times a day. Blood pressure and blood lipid level belong to strictly monitored parameters in diabetic patients. Their increase in combination with diabetes significantly influences the cardio-vascular risk of the patients.

Diabetes mellitus type 1 is caused by a selective destruction of beta cells in islets of Langerhans by an immunologic process in genetically predisposed individuals. It is specific by onset in younger age and dependence on insulin since the beginning of the treatment. [Bartoš, 2003]

1.2 Diabetes and depression

The relationship between depression and diabetes is bilateral. Recently, they have been identified as reciprocally interacting risk factors - the presence of diabetes deteriorates the prognosis of depression, while the presence of depression worsens the prognosis of diabetes. [Höschl, 2005]

Prevalence of a more or less severe depression is approximately double in patients with diabetes compared to a general population. On average, it is present in 14% (9 to 27%) of diabetics in the Czech Republic. [Češková, 2004] Depressive reactions in diabetic patients show a higher recurrence tendency in comparison with general population. Depression is more frequent in women. Depression usually follows the diagnosis of the disease in this type of diabetes. Diabetes as a primary disease is typically superimposed by depression as a reactive state. Depression is usually a result of exposure to psycho-social factors that are related to hardship caused by chronic disease. It is necessary to look for associations at the level of emotions and mental processes. For many patients it is difficult to maintain a regular life-rhythm. Their roles in social environment may change as well. Moreover, the patients often loose energy more rapidly. It often takes years until a man accepts and fixates a change in his lifestyle to which he is accustomed. It is even possible that the internal and mental manifestations of diabetes share a common origin. It can be explained through a correlation of insulin resistance and changes in central serotonin system. [Horáček, 1997] Hyperglycemia, hyperinsulinemia and impaired peripheral insulin receptor sensitivity is often found in patients with depression. Decreased insulin sensitivity is associated with lower serotoninergic activity. [Höschl, 2004]

Many chronic autoimmune diseases, including the insulin-dependent diabetes mellitus, are accompanied with symptoms of depression. However, a reversed association is also possible. Autoimmune diseases are generally more common in depressed rather than non-depressed population. One of the predisposing factors of onset of an autoimmune disorder is a serious life event that can alter the cell-mediated as well as the humoral immunity.

Furthermore, symptoms of depression often overlap with poorly controlled diabetes symptoms. It is necessary to look for the etiologic connections here as well. The cardinal symptoms include low stamina, fatigue hypomimia, change in body weight, polymorphic somatic complaints, impaired concentration, etc. Even an increase in blood glucose itself can lead to a significant change in mood, including sadness and increased fatigue [Polonsky, 1999]

Several studies concerning comorbidity of type 1 diabetes and depression identified risk factors of depression development; chronic somatic comorbidity and polypharmacy, female gender, higher age, solitary life, lower than secondary education, lower financial status, cigarette smoking, obesity, diabetes complications and a higher glycosylated hemoglobin [Engum, 2005; Bell, 2005; Hermanns, 2005; Katon, 2004]

Studies dealing with consequences of comorbidity of diabetes and depression claim that depression leads to a decrease in metabolic control of diabetes, reduction of treatment response and diet measures effect, deterioration of the quality of life and increase in healthcare costs. [Lustman, 2005] In addition, depressive symptoms have an impact on later somatic problems associated with poor glycemic control, because they affect the patients' ability to care for themselves and follow diet. [McKellar, 2004] Blood glucose regulation is also significantly impaired in depressed patients, compared to individuals without depression. Insufficient regulation of blood glucose can adversely influence patient's state of mind and his response to antidepressant drugs. The incidence of microvascular complications (especially retinopathy, but also neuropathy, nephropathy, and sexual dysfunction) and macrovascular complications is also higher in diabetic patients with depression. This is related to poor metabolic control in depressed compared to the non-depressed diabetic patients.

Furthermore, it was proven that a depression increases mortality in patients with diabetes; the probability of death within 10 years is significantly increased in these patients. [Zhang, 2005]

1.3 Antidepressant drug treatment in type 1 diabetic patients

Psychiatric treatment of diabetic patients is focused on treatment of their mental disorder with respect to diabetes, and on improvement in quality of life with disease. Furthermore, the psychiatrist may try to positively influence the glycemic control. The literature is unequivocal regarding the effect of a psychiatric treatment on glycemic control. Some studies declare its benefit in glycemic control improvement, however, most of them do not confirm it. An important randomized clinical trial demonstrated that extended treatment of patients with diabetes mellitus and severe depression or dysthymia lead an improvement in mental state. However, the improvement in depression itself from the antidepressant therapy did not lead to any improvement in blood glucose, or any significant change in glycemic hemoglobin level. [Katon, 2004 b]

Antidepressant drugs are most commonly administered psychiatric medication. They are used for therapy of mental disorders, as well as e.g. treatment of painful diabetic neuropathy.

Several research efforts regarding the effect of antidepressant drug treatment on glycemic control in depressed diabetics were conducted. According to a study by Lustman et al. the glycosylated hemoglobin decreases during the open treatment phase and remains significantly reduced during depression-free maintenance, regardless of the fact whether the patients are treated by an antidepressant, sertraline in this case, or by placebo. [Lustman, 2006] Another study with sertraline demonstrated that a specific minor population of diabetics with low financial income showed a significant reduction in glycosylated hemoglobin after the initiation of pharmacologic treatment of depression in comparison with placebo. [Echeverry, 2009] Elder diabetic patients with depression, presented in another work, who went through the antidepressant treatment were less likely to die within 5 years compared to depressed diabetics without the treatment.[Bogner, 2007]

The antidepressant drugs are also used as co-analgesics (adjuvant analgesics) in the treatment of painful peripheral diabetic polyneuropathy. They are even more effective than common analgesics. The effect on pain is direct, through the intervention in neurotransmission (serotonin and noradrenaline) and indirect (antalgic) acting through a change in attention distribution, lowering the pain threshold, reducing emotional accompaniment and reducing stress response brought about by the pain. The analgesic effect of antidepressants arises more rapidly than the antidepressant effect, already at lower doses and is independent of the presence of depression in the patient. The antidepressant drugs are the treatment of the first choice in a constant burning pain. [Doležal, 2006]

When treating a diabetic patient with antidepressants, it is important to notice how the medication influences the blood glucose, body weight, blood pressure, and renal functions. If it influences glycemia, it is necessary to advise the patient ahead that a dosage change in insulin or oral antidiabetic drugs may be necessary. The body weight increases the most after tricyclic antidepressants and mirtazapine use and the least after SSRI, MAOI a trazodone. An increase in blood glucose was described in association with TCA, a decrease after SSRI and MAOI.

1.4 Use of individual antidepressant drug groups

The longest used tricyclic antidepressants (TCA) decrease insulin secretion, increase blood glucose, appetite for sweets and body weight. Amitriptyline from this group is used even for diabetic painful peripheral neuropathy treatment.

Selective serotonin reuptake inhibitors (SSRI) decrease blood glucose (even 30% decrease in fasting glycemia has been described), temporarily reduce body weight (most often described in fluoxetine), however, they increase body weight in long-term. They reduce cholesterolemia and serum triglycerides. Citalopram and sertraline have a low potential in creating drug interactions. CYP 3A4 inhibition by fluvoxamine may disrupt metabolism of oral antidiabetic drugs. CYP 2C9 inhibition by fluoxetine, fluvoxamine or sertraline can interfere with the metabolism of sulfonylurea and tolbutamide. [Češková, 2004] In combination they can lead to hypoglycemic states, as these antidepressants cause an increase in the level of the abovementioned antidiabetic drugs.

Trazodone is a postsynaptic 5HT2 blocker and a weak serotonin reuptake inhibitor (SARI). It has considerable hypnotic effects and does not have a negative influence on metabolism. [Svačina, 2004]

Moclobemide from the Monoamine Oxydase Inhibitors (MAOI) group reduces blood glucose and can thus lead to hypoglycemic states. On the other hand, it usually does not increase body weight.

Norepinephrine dopamine reuptake inhibitor (NDRI) bupropion is neutral regarding the influence on body weight. Higher doses in combination with insulin lower seizure threshold (the risk of epilepsy is increased especially in patients with concomitant mental anorexia). This effect is eliminated in the SR form. Bupropion attenuates sexual dysfunction and facilitates smoking cessation. Both effects are of great importance in diabetic patients, as they suffer from diabetes-associated sexual dysfunction and have elevated cardiovascular risk from smoking.

Noradrenergic and specific serotonergic antagonist (NaSSA) mirtazapine induces sedation and can therefore be used in insomnia. However, it increases appetite and body weight, which is undesirable in diabetic patients. Furthermore, it can lead to an increase in glycosylated hemoglobin and thus deteriorate a long-term glycemic control. [Šabaková, 2008]

From the group of serotonin norepinephrine reuptake inhibitors (SNRI), it is necessary to mention venlafaxine and duloxetine. Venlafaxine does not increase body weight. A small, but statistically significant increase in fasting glycemia was found when using duloxetine in comparison with placebo. [Fava, 2004] Venlafaxine [Kunz, 2000; Rowbotham, 2004] as well as duloxetine [Goldstein, 2005; Raskin, 2005] have a well-established effect on chronic neuropathic pain.

St John's wort extract (hypericin) does not increase body weight, however, there is a high risk of drug interactions.

Summary of antidepressant drug use is presented in table 1.

Antidepressant group (representative)	Important effects in diabetic patients	Use in neuropathy treatment
TCA (amitriptyline)	Increase glycemia, increase body weight	+
SSRI (citalopram, sertraline)	Reduce glycemia, increase body weight	-
IMAO (moclobemide)	Reduce glycemia, do not increase body weight	-
NDRI (bupropion)	Do not increase body weight	-
NaSSA (mirtazapine)	Increase body weight and glycosylated hemoglobin	-
SNRI (venlafaxine, duloxetine)	Do not increase body weight, duloxetine increases fasting glycemia	+
St. John's wort (hypericin)	Do not increase body weight, risk of drug interactions	-

Table 1. Antidepressant drug use in diabetic patients

2. Case studies

The following case studies are pointing out patients with depression anxiety problems and diabetes mellitus type 1, where the antidepressant treatment was successful regarding mental state improvement and positive effect on glycemic control.

We chose to convey the information in form of case reports, because in spite of the fact that numerous studies concerning the influence of antidepressant drug treatment on glycemic control in diabetes mellitus have been performed, their conclusions differ or are even contradictory. This work should point out the diabetics, in whom the antidepressant treatment led to an improvement in glycemic control. They are the evidence that the use of specifically selected antidepressant drugs is suitable in diabetic patients, owing to the fact that any, even temporary improvement in glycemic control is desirable.

This article is focused on type 1 diabetic patients, as this type of diabetes is less represented in studies that deal with diabetes comorbidity, mental problems and their treatment using psychiatric medication.

Patients with e.g. a change in insulin dose or insulin delivery mode were excluded in order to clearly demonstrate the effect of the antidepressant drugs. Only the patients who did not undergo any significant change in chronic internal medication, which could have a significant effect on the change in glycemic control, are presented in the case reports.

Mental state of the patients was evaluated by a clinical psychiatric examination and on the basis of patients' complaints regarding their subjective problems. The general mental state of the patients was evaluated using Clinical Global Impression - Severity (CGI-S), which is widely used for global clinical impression assessment of psychiatric patients. The scale ranges from 1 to 7 points, where 1 means "no apparent signs of illness" and 7 denotes extremely expressed symptoms. Data is acquired from information regarding behavior of the patient and a change in his state in the course of the treatment. [Busner, 2009]

Long-term glycemic control was evaluated according to the glycosylated hemoglobin level. Its values are presented according to DCCT/NGSP calibration. Other somatic and metabolic parameters that are regularly monitored in diabetic patients were also recorded, specifically body weight, blood pressure and blood level of triglycerides and cholesterol. Monitoring of these parameters served for assessment of a potential effect of administered psychiatric drugs on metabolic functions in diabetic patients.

Patient No. 1 was born in 1963. She has been treated with type 1 diabetes since 1987, i.e. when she was 24 years old. She has been treated by intensified insulin regimen since 2008. From chronic diabetic complications, she suffers from lower-extremity polyneuropathy and cardiovascular autonomous neuropathy. Furthermore, she is treated for arterial hypertension, iron deficiency anemia, and dyslipidemia. She is obese. In 2009, she went through a transient ischemic attack and suffers from migraine ever since. Her family history is positive regarding diabetes in grandfather from mother's side, negative regarding mental disorders. The patient works as a staff at a gas station. She is married, has 5 children, her marriage is conflicting.

She was first referred to a psychiatrist in March 2010, i.e. in her 48 years, because of long-term poor glycemic control and putative influence of mental and family problems.

Already at the first contact, the patient reported long-term deteriorated glycemic control and put it herself in connection with family problems that distressed her. She felt weak for about half a year, nothing amused her, she did not care about anything, nothing could make her happy, and she resigned to important things. She described her problems in relationship with her partner and acknowledged that she was overburdened by the care of her household with five children. She did not mind working, she was engaged in charity activities. CGI-S - 4 points.

In contact she seemed depressed, in tension, with paradoxically psychomotor agitation and inadequate and excess emotionality. She answered in extensive sentences and often could not adhere to her topic. The accentuation of personal histrionic features was apparent.

A diagnosis of a moderately severe depressive phase based on histrionic features of personality was set and a treatment with antidepressant drug with active substance sertraline was initiated. The daily dose of 100 mg was reached through a gradual titration 50 mg daily for the first week.

Mental state of the patient has completely restituted within the first month of antidepressant use. Mood normalized, the patient started enjoying things she liked or liked doing, tension and irritation disappeared, the psychomotor pace stabilized. Excessive emotionality within personality prevailed, but the patient was satisfied with her state. CGI-S - 2 points. Although the situation in her family did not improve, she had more strength to face the problems. Her mental state is stabilized to date. She attends our psychiatric out-patient department every three months. The antidepressant dose was continued owing to persisting unsatisfactory situation in her family.

Her glycemic control improved significantly at the beginning of the psychiatric treatment. Glycosylated hemoglobin decreased from 9.4% at the first contact in March 2010 to 8.0% in May. It rose to 8.8% in October, 9.2% in January 2011, and returned to 9.4% in May 2011.

Psychological status (treatment)	time	HbA1c
moderately severe depressive phase (sertraline treatment initiation)	03 / 2010	9.5
without depression	04 / 2010	
full compensation	05 / 2010	8.1
continuation of medication	10 / 2010	8.8
	01 / 2011	9.3
continuation of cooperation	05 / 2011	9.5

Table 2. Timeline of mental state and glycosylated hemoglobin level development - patient No.1

Body weight of the patient was 111kg at the beginning of the treatment (March 2011), it was 115kg in the end (May 2011). There was thus a small increase in the course of the treatment observed.

Blood pressure of the patient was stable, 125/70 torr since the beginning of the treatment. It was not affected by the antidepressant drug treatment.

Her serum triglyceride level was 3.66 mmol/l at the beginning of the treatment, it was 2.33 mmol/l after 6 months, it increased to 3.10 mmol/l 10 months after the beginning of the treatment and 5.98 mmol/l in the end of the treatment. The psychiatric treatment thus led to a gradual increase in serum triglyceride level. Serum cholesterol level was 5.25 mmol/l at the beginning of the treatment and remained unchanged in the course of the treatment.

The depressive disorder completely normalized owing to the antidepressant medication. Her mental state is now long-term stabilized due to the treatment. The long-term glycemic control of the diabetes rapidly improved at the beginning of the psychiatric treatment, however, it returned to its original value within 15 months.

The case of this woman confirms that depressive disorder improvement and stress reduction lead to a decrease in glycemia. The antidepressant drug itself could have played a role in glycemic control improvement. Active substances from the SSRI group may cause a decrease in glycemia, which in turn can lead to a decrease in glycosylated hemoglobin level. The effect is probably only temporary. The initial effect of a new attitude towards her therapy, i.e. psychiatric treatment initiation, can partly participate in the glycemic control improvement.

Patient No. 2 was born in 1964. She was diagnosed with diabetes mellitus type 1 in 1991, i.e. when she was 27 years old. She has been treated by intensified insulin regimen since 2003. She gradually developed chronic complications of diabetes; diabetic peripheral polyneuropathy, non-proliferative diabetic retinopathy, moreover, she was treated with a diabetic foot syndrome of neuropathic etiology in past. Furthermore, she is treated with hyperfunction of the thyroid gland and arterial hypertension since 1996. She also suffers from cervical pain. She underwent appendectomy in 1998. Her family history regarding diabetes is positive; her grandmother had a diabetes type 2. Her family history is positive regarding mental disorders; her brother and father are alcoholics. The patient is married and has two adolescent children. She is a certified shop assistant. She had worked as a ceramic printer, but she retired to a disability pension a few months before the psychiatric treatment commencement, which relieved her from overloading. She is only partly content with the relationships in her family; she feels that her children do not need her anymore and her husband devotes too little time to her. She is thus forced to look for her own activities.

She was referred to a psychiatric care in May 2005, i.e. when she was 41 years old, by her diabetologist for symptoms of anxiety and depression. At the time of referral, she was already taking an antidepressant for about half a year. She was given 100mg of sertraline by her diabetologist with an insufficient effect leading to an impaired sexual appetite as an adverse effect.

At the first visit at the psychiatrist she complained about a long-term perceived inner tension, tearfulness, inhibitedness, easy fatigability, feelings of uselessness, general dissatisfaction and sexual problems. Moreover, she regarded her diabetes disease as a heavy burden that restricted her at all times and destined her to be monitored by others. She was aware of dependence on her husband and children, which further exhausted her. Her mood was already more positive since she was taking sertraline.

In contact she seemed subdepressed, inhibited, tired, with a psychomotor retardation, slightly blunted affect, hypobulia and apathy. She answered after increased pauses before answering. CGI-S - 4 points.

Diagnosis of a moderately severe depressive phase and accented dependant personality features was made. Her medication was changed to bupropione 15mg daily because of dominant inhibitedness and fatigability. At the following visit after a month, the patient reported an improvement in sexual appetite, but increased nervousness, tension and anxiety, she was tearful and felt that she could not deal with daily life. The antidepressant was therefore changed to trazodon titrated gradually up to a dose of 150 mg a day. CGI-S - 4 points. The patient came for the next visit after 3 months, i.e. in September 2005. She reported a relief from depression, anxiety and fatigue. She also talked about an ambivalent attitude of her husband to the treatment, who perceived his wife as unnaturally sedated. The problems with sexual appetence and tearfulness prevailed. CGI-S - 4 points. Trazodon daily dose was increased to 200mg.

The patient reported a decline of all mental problems at a visit next month (October 2005), her mental state was stabilized. CGI-S - 2 points. The following month (November 2005), she complained of enhanced anxiety, nervousness and distractedness. She had no depressive moods, sleeping disorders or problems in sexual field. She complained of diarrhea and abdominal cramps of unknown etiology for several months and thus a lower appetite and a significant body weight loss. CGI-S - 3 points. The previous daily dose of trazodon 150mg was resumed and the treatment was augmented by sulpiride at a daily dose of 50mg (since November 2005). The digestive problems gradually disappeared, however, increased fatigability prevailed. CGI-S - 2 points. Trazodon was gradually withdrawn and only sulpirid treatment continued (since April 2005). The patient consequently reported a complete amelioration of mental problems and disappearance of digestive problems and was satisfied with her medication. She insisted on its continuation in spite of the fact that it caused a mild menstrual disorder. Stability of her state lasted until a visit in October 2007 despite the fact that her 18 year-old daughter delivered her first granddaughter, which was a significant strain.

At her following visit in December 2007 she complained about depressive moods and worsening of feelings of refusal from her daughter and husband that were producing fear from future and loneliness. CGI-S - 3 points. Sertraline treatment at a dose of 50mg per day was initiated, owing to objective deterioration of the depressive disorder and a concern about further mood depression. Consequently, the mental state improved significantly again, the patient even started to look for own activities more and was generally satisfied with her life. CGI-S - 1 point. This lasted from January until September 2008. Meanwhile, the patient tried to discontinue sertraline, but she felt more even-tempered while using it and therefore decided to use it chronically.

In September 2008, the patient came for a visit complaining about subjectively deteriorated short-term memory and concentration. CGI-S - 2 points. She was educated about cognitive training and was given a preparation with an extract from Ginkgo biloba at a daily dose gradually increased to 160mg. The dose was reduced to 80mg after approximately 6 months and continued until October 2010. All this time she felt psychically stabilized, even though she developed some serious somatic problems associated with diabetes - Charcot osteopathy.

Psychological status (treatment)	**time**	**HbA1c**
moderately severe depressive phase (sertraline use)		
depression (bupropione initiation)	05 / 2005	9.2
depression (trazodon initiation)	06 / 2005	
	08 / 2005	8.5
improvement (trazodon dose increase)	09 / 2005	
further improvement	10 / 2005	
anxiety, diarrhea (sulpirid initiation)	11 / 2005	
	03 / 2006	8.1
without problems	04 / 2006	
	05 / 2006	8.7
	12 / 2006	8.2
	06 / 2007	8.7
	09 / 2007	8.2
without problems	10 / 2007	
depression (sulpiride + sertraline)	12 / 2007	
without problems	01 / 2008	8.3
	04 / 2008	7.6
	07 / 2008	8.3
memory deterioration (ginkgo initiation)	09 / 2008	7.8
	04 / 2009	8.6
	06 / 2009	8.5
	09 / 2009	8.9
	03 / 2010	8.5
without problems (sulpiride + sertraline)	05 / 2010	
	07 / 2010	8.1
cooperation continuation	10 / 2010	8.5

Table 3. Timeline of mental state and glycosylated hemoglobin level development - patient No.2

At a visit in October 2010, she agreed on a gradual withdrawal of the nootropic agent. CGI-S - 1 point. She requested chronic use of the other treatment. At present, the patient comes for psychiatric visits every six months and feels mentally stabilized despite lasting somatic problems.

Her glycemic control at the first psychiatric visit (i.e. May 2005) was 9.1% HbA1c. The value decreased to 8.4% in August same year, and 8.0% in March 2006. The value was higher again (8.7%) in May 2006. The glycosylated hemoglobin decreased to 8.1% again in December 2006. It was 8.7% in June 2007, 8.1% in September 2007, 8.2% in January 2008, 7.6% in April, 8.2% in July, and 7.8% in September. The value was 8.6% in April 2009, 8.4% in June, and 8.9% in September. The glycosylated hemoglobin was 8.4% in March 2010, and 8.0% in July. The glycosylated hemoglobin was 8.4% at the last blood examination in October 2010.

Body weight of the patient was 79 kg at the beginning of the treatment (May 2005), 80 kg after 3 months, than it decreased to 72 kg and stayed until May 2006. It increased to 77 kg in September 2006 and 80 kg in April 2009. It was 82 kg in the end of the follow-up in February 2011. The body weight of the patient thus decreased at the beginning of the treatment, it returned to its original value after 4 years and subsequently kept gradually increasing.

Blood pressure of the patient hovered around 120/60 torr during the whole treatment. It did not change due to antidepressant therapy.

Her serum triglyceride level was 0.76 mmol/l at the beginning of the treatment and 0.59 mmol/l in the end of the follow-up, it did not change owing to the psychiatric treatment. Serum cholesterol level was 5.58 mmol/l at the beginning of the treatment and 5.95 mmol/l in the end of the follow-up, there was no significant change due to the psychiatric treatment.

Mental state of the patient improved, although very slowly, since the beginning of the treatment. It was necessary to change repeatedly her psychiatric drugs for insufficient effect and intermittent decompensations of her mental state. Even her glycemic control was slightly improving at the beginning, subsequently, a tendency of glycosylated hemoglobin to fluctuate was observed at times of varying mental state compensation as well as in long periods of mental stability. Her mental state, despite periods of subcompensation, is significantly improved after several years of psychiatric treatment than it was before treatment commencement. Glycosylated hemoglobin level is also lower than prior to treatment despite its fluctuations. It did not return to the original high value.

This case demonstrates the influence of fluctuating mental compensation on fluctuation in long-term glycemic control, although it is not possible to observe a direct temporal relationship. It is acknowledged that a change in glycosylated hemoglobin always occurs with a delay after a change in condition of a patient, i.e. treatment change, attitude towards treatment change, better self-monitoring, etc. The delay duration ranges usually in weeks. No exact correlation of individual changes in time can be observed in the relationship of mental compensation and glycemic control.

Patient No. 3 was born in 1966. She was diagnosed with diabetes mellitus in 1989, i.e. in her 23 years. Regarding organ complications of diabetes she suffers from diabetic nephropathy and retinopathy. She was also diagnosed with pulmonary fibrosis, she went through a lung biopsy in 1989. Her condition is stable with no functional impairment. She has been treated for iron deficiency anemia since 1995. Her grandfather had a diabetes mellitus type II. Regarding psychiatric family history, her sister had collapse states and epilepsia in her childhood and her father suffers from dementia. The patient is married and has three children. She was just after maternity leave at time of psychiatric treatment. She did not work, she took care after her ill father. She was employed as a secretary in past. She was content in her partner life, but she was overburdened by care of her father and had conflicts with her mother-in-law.

She herself requested psychiatric care for feelings of anxiety/depression and painful diabetic polyneuropathy in May 2005, i.e. in her 39 years. She reported progressing feelings of anxiety, fear of closed-in places and tight clothing, tearfulness, sleeping disorder, hypobulia, constipation and headache for about one and a half year on the first examination. She felt overburdened, hurried and tired. She was losing her sexual appetite.

A psychomotor retardation, depressive mood, apathy, hypobulia and labile emotionality was evident in contact. The patient was significantly influenced by an apparent inner tension. CGI-S - 5 points.

A diagnosis of anxious depressive disorder was made and sertraline treatment at a daily dose of 100mg with a gradual titration from 50mg per day was started (May 2005).

At a visit the following month (June 2005) the patient reported an alleviation from anxiety. She was less agitated and more satisfied, she did not get disturbed so easily, but her anxiety prevailed in stress situations. The headache disappeared almost completely. CGI-S - 2 points. She was in an even better condition in July 2005; even sleeping and sexual appetite normalized. She was able to manage better her stress situations and was able to look for their solutions in more tranquility. In September, she complained about a slight deterioration of anxiety as a reaction to a stress at home, she was tearful and subdepressive. CGI-S - 3 points. Sertraline dose was therefore increased to 150mg per day. Consequently, her mental state stabilized again.

In January 2006, the patient complained about gastric problems that lasted for about a week and came always after sertraline ingestion. The problems comprised of a stomachache, nausea and even vomiting. From the psychiatric point of view, her mental stability prevailed, anxious states came occasionally and she was able to solve them easily. Withdrawal of the psychiatric medication was impossible owing to the short duration of mental state stabilization. Sulpirid at a daily dose of 50mg was added because of tendencies of the patient to somatize her problems.

Then in February, the patient complained about deterioration of her problems with vertigo, which she had had before, but had never spoken about. Meanwhile, her diabetologist changed the medication to 25mg of amitriptyline per day. After all examinations performed during hospitalization to find the origin of the vertigo, it was found to be psychogenic. The change in medication caused a mental decompensation of the patient, the symptoms of anxiety, tearfulness and inability to solve common problems returned, the headache came back. Moreover, she was terrified by her mental state deterioration, it was completely unexpected for her and she lost confidence in the medication. CGI-S - 4 points. Amitriptiline was continued and the dose was increased to 50mg per day. The patient was educated in detail regarding the action of the medication and encouraged to endure until onset of antipsychotic medication effects. She felt already well at a visit next month, in March 2006; she was without depression and headache, the vertigo attenuated. CGI-S - 2 points. In May, she was without depression and sleeping disorder, however the headache worsened slightly and occasionally she had an episode of anxiety, which was difficult to manage. Sometimes she was more easily distressed. CGI-S - 3 points. The dose of amitriptiline was thus increased to 75mg per day. In July 2006, the mental state of the patient was well compensated, she was without depression, sleeping disorder and headache, occasional anxiety was well tolerated. CGI-S - 2 points. The patient was satisfied and asked for termination of psychiatric consultations. She wished to continue the medication under a supervision of her diabetologist. She promised she would come for a psychiatric visit in case of mental state deterioration or for treatment withdrawal after about one year. In the end, amitriptiline was discontinued by her diabetologist in January 2008, because of fatigability and insufficient effect on pain in lower extremities from diabetic painful polyneuropathy.

Glycosylated hemoglobin was 14.6% prior to psychiatric treatment commencement in May 2005. It was 14.1% in June, 12.4% in November. It was 10.3% in February 2006, 11.4% in May, 10.8% in August and 10.9% in December 2006. Glycosylated hemoglobin was 9.7% in March 2007, 10.5% in June, and 14.3% again in October 2007.

Psychological status (treatment)	Time	HbA1c	CGI-S
anxiety depression problems (sertraline treatment initation)	05 / 2005	14.6	5
anxiety only in stress	06 / 2005	14.1	2
Improvement	07 / 2005		2
anxiety improvement, sebdepression (sertraline dose increase)	09 / 2005		3
without problems	11 / 2005	12.4	3
gastric problems (sulpiride initiation)	01 / 2006		3
vertigo (amitriptyline initiation), deterioration	02 / 2006	10.3	4
Improvement	03 / 2006		2
deterioration (amitriptyline dose increase)	05 / 2006	11.4	3
without problems, cooperation termination	07 / 2006		2
	08 / 2006	10.8	2
	12 / 2006	10.9	
	03 / 2007	9.7	
	06 / 2007	10.5	
	10 / 2007	14.3	
medication withdrawal	01 / 2008		

Table 4. Timeline of mental state and glycosylated hemoglobin level development - patient No.3

Body weight of the patient was 78 kg at the beginning of the treatment (May 2005), it was gradually increasing to 80 kg during the year, in the course of the next year it was decreasing to 74 kg in the end of the year (January 2010).

Blood pressure of the patient ranged from 120/70 to 130/70 torr during the whole course of the treatment. It did not change owing to the antidepressant drug treatment.

The serum triglycerides level was 1.66 mmol/l at the beginning of the treatment, 2.2 mmol/l in the end, there was therefore a mild increase observed. Serum cholesterol was 5.68 mmol/l at the beginning of the treatment and 5.84 mmol/l in the end, the increase due to psychiatric treatment was thus only insignificant.

Mental state of the patient slowly improved, it was necessary to change medication because of insufficient effect, but also due to the fact that the patient reported only a part of her problems, negated the rest and these emerged later as chronic problems. Later, the patient refused to attend psychiatric out-patient clinic. She explained it by good stability of her state. She wanted to be followed only by her diabetologist, where the psychopharmacological treatment continued for another year and a half and was then withdrawn. The mental state in a long-term is not stable, neither on medication, nor after its withdrawal, however, she did not come back to psychiatrist's care. Her glycemic control improved significantly at the beginning of the treatment, however, it returned to its original value after the antidepressant withdrawal.

In this case the effect of supportive counseling was quite substantial, although it was not the case of systemic psychotherapy. The patient was in a difficult life situation and apart of medication she was receiving the support she needed. It can also be seen here, that the patient did not have the insight into her mental problems, it was necessary to keep asking about them repeatedly.

Patient no. 4 was born in 1970 and suffers from diabetes mellitus type 1 since 1996, i.e. since his 26 years. He did not have any organ complications diagnosed at time of psychiatric treatment. He is also treated for arterial hypertension and hypercholesterolemia. There was no family history of diabetes nor mental disorder. The patient works a clerk, is single, childless, lives alone.

He has been in psychiatric care since December 2005, i.e. since he was 35 years old. He was referred by his diabetologist for about 2 years of incompliance in diabetes treatment, active refusal of maintaining the daily regimen and hospitalization for treatment correction. The diabetologist referred him to psychiatry for a suspicion of a mental illness.

The patient admitted a deterioration of his mental state lasting for about 2 years on examination. He is afraid of a large number of people, gets easily distressed, is emotionally labile, has depressive moods with feelings of hopelessness that come unreasonably. He has his insight into the fact that he lacks the motivation for diabetes treatment. This condition lasts for about 2 years already. He used to cope with his disease well before. At present he has conflicts with the doctors at the department of Diabetology.

In contact he was tense, anxious, with labile emotionality, depression, even resonant mood, apathetic. CGI-S - 5 points.

A diagnosis of anxiety depression disorder was made and a sertraline treatment at a dose gradually up to 100mg per day was initiated. At a visit two weeks after, the patient felt better, he was subdepressed, less anxious, but he complained that he was not motivated by any life goal; he lives from one day to another, is indifferent. CGI-S - 3 points. He felt significantly better in January 2006, he reported better cooperation with doctors at the department of Diabetology. He was getting insight into his share in the conflicts. CGI-S – 2 points. The mental state of the patient was completely restituted in February, he felt happy, he perceived occasional fluctuation of his mood as natural, he reported significant improvement in his glycemic control. He was very satisfied with the improvement and it motivated him to further improve the cooperation. Again, he found meaning in good treatment and control of his basic disease. CGI-S – 1 point. At a visit in August 2008, he reported that apart from further improvement he is successful in losing weight - he gained a few kilograms in previous two years. After mutual agreement, the patient was referred to diabetology out-patient clinic with set medication. He should come for a psychiatric check up if needed. He did not come and spontaneously discontinued the medication in the end of 2007, supposedly for financial reasons.

His long-term glycemic control at the beginning of the treatment was very unsatisfactory, the glycosylated hemoglobin level was 10.7% in January 2006, it decreased to 9.3% already in March, 9.6% in June, 9.9% in October. In January 2007 the level was 10.1%, followed by 9.9% in April, 9.6% in August, 10.1% in November, and finally 10.8% in March 2008.

Psychological status (treatment)	Time	HbA1c	CGI-S
anxiety depression problems (sertraline treatment) initation	12 / 2005		5
Improvement	01 / 2006	10.7	2
full compansation	02 / 2006		1
	03 / 2006	9.3	1
	06 / 2006	9.6	1
compliance improvement	08 / 2006		1
cooperation termination	10 / 2006	9.9	
continuation in medication	01 / 2007	10.1	
	04 / 2007	9.9	
	08 / 2007	9.6	
	11 / 2007	10.1	
medication withdrawal	12 / 2007		
	03 / 2008	10.8	

Table 5. Timeline of mental state and glycosylated hemoglobin level development - patient No.4

Body weight of the patient was 97 kg at the beginning of the treatment (December 2005), it was 93 kg in the end (March 2008). A weight loss 4 kg was thus observed in the course of the treatment.

Blood pressure of the patient ranged from 140/80 torr at the beginning of the treatment to 130/70 torr in its end. It thus mildly decreased owing to the antidepressant drug therapy in the course of the treatment.

Serum triglyceride level was 1.28 mmol/l at the beginning of the treatment, 1.23 mmol/ in the end, it did not change due to the psychiatric therapy. Serum cholesterol level was 4.56 mmol/l at the beginning of the treatment, it decreased significantly to 3.58 mmol/l after 3 months and then mildly increased again up to 5.1 mmol/l in the end of the treatment.

The mental state of the patient improved quite rapidly and a significantly better cooperation in maintaining diabetic regimen was associated with it. Glycosylated hemoglobin at the beginning of the treatment decreased significantly, however, after the antidepressant medication withdrawal it returned to its original value prior to the treatment.

This case demonstrates that a mental disorder can induce incompliance of a patient and poor glycemic control. It is also evident here that the mental state deteriorated after the termination of the cooperation with a psychiatrist, or psychotherapy withdrawal.

3. Discussion

To our knowledge, there has not been found another scientific work that would deal with mechanisms of the effect of antidepressant drugs on glycemic control. The effect of mental state improvement using antidepressants is doubtless. It leads to attenuation of chronic stress and improvement in compliance with the diabetes treatment. Biochemical context is surely also in play. More research needs to be done in this field.

The medication of choice in all patients was sertraline for its efficacy against a wide spectrum of anxiety-depression symptoms. We often choose it for its safety regarding adverse effects and drug interactions. The individual patients were subsequently treated by various antidepressant drugs as individualized care was emphasized. The medication was thus selected according to specific problems and history of patients. Patients with varied initial glycemic control and a different change in glycemic control in course of the treatment and after the treatment termination are deliberately described here in order to be able to show multiple aspects of antidepressant drug effect in diabetic patients with a mental disorder. This variability was also chosen in order to enable demonstration of several possible pitfalls in treatment of these patients.

In spite of the fact that evaluation of the effect of individual groups of antidepressants in diabetic patients was not an objective of this work, it is suitable to share some experience from our psychiatric out-patient department. Drugs of choice are antidepressant drugs from the group of SSRI, especially aforementioned sertraline, for their effectiveness in the treatment of anxiety and depression problems, low risk of drug interactions and a small influence on body weight of patients. A potential contribution of SSRI to blood glucose decrease can also be beneficial in these patients. [Češková, 2004] Another commonly used drug is trazodone (SARI) for its good hypnotic and anxiolytic effect as well as the fact that it has no influence on body weight and sexual appetence. Venlafaxine (SNRI) is also frequently used for its good therapeutic effect on anxiety and depression symptoms and minimal metabolic adverse effects. Duloxetine from the same group of antidepressants is used for its effect on neuropathic pain alleviation. Unfortunately, it is not available to psychiatrists in the Czech Republic, only to neurologists. Tricyclic antidepressants, especially amitriptiline, are used mainly in the patients with painful diabetic neuropathy and associated sleep disorders. However, a frequent appetite and body weight increase limit their use. Antidepressants from the MAOI group (moclobemide) are scarcely used for their unconvincing clinical antidepressant effectiveness although they do not have any negative metabolic adverse effects. Bupropion (NDRI) has a good effect on inhibitedness and does not influence body weight, nonetheless, quite common and considerable increase in tension and anxiety constitute limiting adverse effects for its use. Mirtazapine (NaSSA) is an unsuitable drug for diabetic patients for augmented appetite, weight gain and glycosylated hemoglobin level increase. [Šabaková, 2008]

Other somatic and metabolic parameters, which could have been influenced by the treatment, were monitored in the course of treatment of all abovementioned patients. [Svačina, 2004] The most significant change in monitored parameters was in the measurements of body weight of the patients, although the change was completely inconsistent. In the first patient, the body weight gradually increased. In the second one, it decreased at first, then returned to its original value. In the next patient, it slowly increased at first and then decreased significantly. In the last patient, the body weight significantly decreased during the whole course of the psychiatric treatment. The blood pressure values remained basically unchanged, as well as their blood cholesterol level. Only the serum triglyceride level increased in two patients in the course of the treatment, however, it was not possible to prove a direct association with antidepressant drug treatment here.

The focus of this work on antidepressant drugs does not allow broader addressing of issues concerning the origin of the mental problems, e.g. the influence of diabetes as a chronic disease, life crisis, etc. [Rossová, 1992] Even these factors undoubtedly significantly influence the treatment using antidepressant drugs and their effect on glycemic control.

Another important factor in this context is premorbid personality structure. It is acknowledged that antidepressant drug treatment of mental state decompensation is controversial in personal psychopatology. It could thus also have a smaller effect on glycemic control.

The psychiatric care cannot be perceived merely as the effect of psychotropic drugs. The counseling with a doctor have a certain psychotherapeutic potential, although it is not a form of systemic psychotherapy. A certain part of the session is psychoeducation and motivational and supportive interview. [Beran, 2000] Even this aspect needs to be taken in account when we evaluate the effect of antidepressants on a glycemic control in patients in psychiatric care.

Some patients with the described problems can profit from antidepressant medication, some from the systemic psychotherapy, some from the combination of the two. The indication of both should be wise. The antidepressant drugs are especially important in patients with a somatic disease as is diabetes mellitus, as these patients require quite lengthy psychotherapeutic work because of their significant orientation on somatic problems and laboratory findings. The need for mental state improvement, cooperation and glycemic control is often urgent. The treatment is thus often started with antidepressants and the psychotherapy is added after at least a partial improvement of the mental state.

Another issue is the eventual withdrawal of the medication. This is commonly dictated by the same rules as in other patients with mental illness. For some patients a long-term medication is beneficial, in spite of the fact that their mental problems long have disappeared. However, it was demonstrated that the patients should be left in the care of a psychiatrist during the whole time of medication administration.

Also, when initiating psychotherapeutic medication, all patients should be examined and educated by a psychiatrist. It is beneficial when the treatment can be indicated by a diabetologist to enable a fast treatment initiation, however, it has been proven that even psychoeducation and education regarding treatment is a very important part of a successful therapy and should therefore be performed by a professional. The advantage of a psychiatrist is also the ability to choose from a broader spectrum of psychiatric drugs.

4. Conclusion

The case studies demonstrate that the effect of an antidepressant drug on glycemic control improvement in patients with comorbid psychiatric disorder is possible.

Mental state of diabetic patients when treated by antidepressant drugs changes similarly as in the rest of the population, i.e. rapidly in some, slowly in others, and in some a change in medication is needed. The glycemic control improvement is associated especially with the mental state improvement. In most patients the improvement in glycemic control was evident at the beginning of the treatment. The fact that the diabetic patient is introduced with a completely new treatment modality of his disease, i.e. psychiatric treatment, plays a positive role. The patients with a lasting improvement in their mental state have a high probability of persisting improved glycemic control. The deterioration of the basic disease can be expected in the diabetic patients, who mentally deteriorate some time after the antidepressant treatment withdrawal.

It is necessary to treat mental disorders in diabetic patients, as the antidepressant drug treatment has a positive effect not only on their mental state, which is associated with their compliance, but also it can positively influence the glycemic control, which is desirable even if the improvement were only temporary. Correctly selected antidepressants should not have an adverse effect on other somatic and metabolic parameters. Mental problems of diabetic patients should be treated by a psychiatrist educated in the problems of diabetes, because psychoeducation and a support of the patient are appropriate parts of the treatment.

5. References

Bartoš V, Pelikánová T. a kol.: Praktická diabetologie. Maxdorf 2003.

Bell RA, Smith SL, Arcury TA, et al: Prevalence and correlates of depression symptoms among rural order afrikan americans, native americans, and whites with diabetes. Diabetes Care. 2005 Apr;28(4): ss. 823-829.

Beran J. Základy psychoterapie pro lékaře. Grada 2000.

Bogner HR, Morales KH, Post EP, Bruce ML: Diabetes, depression , and death: a randomized controlled trial of a depression treatment program for older adults based in primary care. Diabetes Care. 2007 Aug;ahead of print.

Busner J, Targum SD: The Clinical Global Impressions Scale: Applying a Research Tool in ClinicalPractice. Psychiatry 2009, ISSN 1550-5952.

Češková E: Deprese a somatická onemocnění. In: Lékařské listy 4/2004, s. 16.

Doležal T, Hakl M, et al: Metodické pokyny pro farmakoterapii akutní a chronické nenádorové bolesti. Čas. Farmakoterapie. 2006(3), ss. 287-299.

Echeverry D, Duran P, Bonds C, et al: Effect of pharmacological treatment of depression on A1c and quality of life in low-income Hispanics and African Americans with diabetes: a randomized, double-blind, placebo-controlled trial. Diabetes Care. 2009 Dec; 32(12): ss. 2156-60. Epub 2009 Sept 3.

Engum A, Mykletun A, Midthjell K, et al: Depression and Diabetes: A large population-based study of sociodemographic, lifestyle, and clinical factors associated with depression in tipe 1 and 2 diabetes. Diabetes Care. 2005 Aug;28(8): ss. 1904-1909.

Fava M, Mallinckrodt CH, et al: The Effect of Duloxetine on Painful Physical Symptoms in Depressed Patients: Do Improvements in These Symtoms Result in Higher Remission Rate? J Clin Psychiatry 65: 4 April 2004.

Goldstein DJ, et al: Duloxetine vs. placebo in patients with painful diabetic neuropathy. Pain 116 (2005), ss. 109-118.

Hermanns N, Kulzer B, Krichbaum M, et al: Affective and anxiety disorders in a German sample of diabetic patients, comorbidity and risc factors. Diab. Med. 2005 Mar;22(3): ss. 293-300.

Horáček J, Kuzmiaková M: Je deprese poruchou inzulinových receptorů? Psychiatrie. 1997, č. 3-4; ss. 121-126.

Höschl C: Psychiatrie. Tigris Praha, 2004: ss. 133-138.

Höschl C: Konceptuální model deprese a její léčba. Depresivní stavy. Depresivní nemocný v nepsychiatrických ordinacích. Výběr z přednášek odborného sympózia konaného v květnu 2005 v Praze. Medical Tribune, 2005; ss. 34-37.

Katon WJ, von Korff M, Ciechanowski P, et al: Behavioral and clinical factors associated with depression among individuals with diabetes. Diabet Care. 2004 Apr;27(4): ss. 914-920.

Katon WJ, von Korff M, Lin EH B, et al: The Pathways Study. A randomized trial of collaborative care in patients with diabetes and depression. Arch Gen Psychiatry. 2004; 61: ss. 1042-1049.

Kunz NR, et al: Efect of Venlafaxine XR on Diabetic Neuropthic Pain. Eur Neuropsychofarmacol. 2000;10(3): s. 389.

Kvapil M: Základní principy edukace diabetiků 2. typu. Postgraduální medicína, 7/2001, roč. 3; ss: 760-763.

Lustman PJ, Clouse RE: Depression in diabetic patients, the relationship between mood and glykemic control. Diabetes complications. 2005 Mar-Apr; 19(2): ss. 113-22.

Lustman PJ, Clouse RE, Nix BD, et al: Sertraline for prevention of depression recurrence in diabetes mellitus: a randomized, double-blind, placebo controlled trial. Arch Gen Psychiatry. 2006 May; 63(5): ss. 521-9.

McKellar JD, Humphreys K, Piette JD: Depression increases diabetes symptoms by complicating patients' self-care adherence. Diabetes Educ. 2004 May-Jun;30(3): ss. 485-492.

Polonsky WH: Diabetes Burnout. American Diabetes Association, 1999.

Raskin J, et al: A double-blind, randomized multicenter trial comparing duloxetine with placebo in the management of diabetic peripheral neuropatic pain. Pain Med. 2005 Sept-Oct; 6(5): ss. 346-56.

Rossová EK: Hovory s umírajícími. Signum Unitatis, 1992.

Rowbotham MC, Goli V, Kunz NR, Lei D: Venlafaxine extended release in the treatment of painful diabetic neuropathy: a double-blind, Placebo-controlled study. Pain. 2004 Aug;110(3):697-706.

Svačina Š: Metabolické účinky psychofarmak, Triton 2004: 72-77.

Šabaková J., Rušavý Z., Jankovec Z., Diabetici léčení v psychiatrické ambulance - prospektivní sledování. XLIV. Diabetologické dny, Luhačovice, 17.-19.4.2008. Diabetologie, Metabolismjus, Endokrinologie, Váživa 11.2008; Suppl 1: s.53-54.

Zhang X, Norris SL, Gregg EW, et al: Depressive symptoms and mortality among persons with and without diabetes. American Journal of Epidemilogy. 2005 Apr; 161(7): ss. 652-660.

10

Effects of Fluoxetine and Venlafaxine on the Salivary Gland – Experimental Study

Silvana da Silva, Luciana Reis de Azevedo,
Antônio Adilson Soares de Lima, Beatriz Helena Sottile França,
Maria Ângela Naval Machado, Aline Cristina Batista Rodrigues Johann and
Ana Maria Trindade Grégio
The Pontifical Catholic University of Paraná,
Brazil

1. Introduction

Depression is the most common form of affective disorders and may range from discrete to severe. Various studies have worked with the hypothesis that depression arises from the deficiency of monoamines (noradrenaline, serotonin and dopamine), the most adequate treatment being to raise the supply of these neurotransmitters in the central nervous system (CNS). Statistical data have shown that depression has increased as a result of the longer life expectancy and is common among the elderly population (Glassman et al., 1984).

The treatment of psychiatric disorders and affective disturbances mainly involves antidepressant, antipsychotic and anxiolytic drugs. Studies relate that patients with psychiatric alterations that make use of these drugs complain of a dry mouth (Thomsom et al., 2000). Depressive alterations accompanied by the symptom of a dry mouth are 20% more frequent in women than in men (Bogetto et al., 1998) and the most affected age group ranges from 30 to 59 years (Scully, 2003).

Antidepressants have an affinity for the adrenergic and cholinergic receptors present in the salivary glands and present an anticholinergic effect. The action of antidepressant drugs may be related to this affinity and the reduction of the cholinergic and sympathetic influx to the CNS. The main side effect of these drugs is inhibition of the secretagogue effect caused by cholinergic stimulation, thus causing hyposalivation (Grégio et al., 2006). Other side effects include: nausea, dizziness, somnolence, sweating and tremors (Horst & Preskorn, 1998).

Fluoxetine is a selective serotonin reuptake inhibitor (SRI) and, among others of the same class, is the result of research to find medications as effective as the tricyclic medications, but with fewer tolerability and safety problems. This drug does not inhibit the reuptake of other neurotransmitters, having no affinity for the adrenergic, muscarinic, cholinergic, H1-histaminic or dopaminic receptors (Goldstein & Goodnick, 1998). Although they are considered safe drugs and present easily attainable therapeutic doses, the SRIs present significant side effects, such as: nausea, diarrhoea, headaches, insomnia and xerostomia (Papakostas, 2008).

Venlafaxine is an antidepressant drug with a completely different chemical structure from that of other antidepressant agents. Its action mechanism resembles that of other known antidepressant, such as: fluoxetine, sertraline and paroxetine, since it is directly associated with potentiating neurotransmitter activity in the CNS (Makhija & Vavia, 2002; Owens et al., 2008).

This drug is presented as a selective serotonin and noradrenalin reuptake inhibitor, and presents weak activity as a dopamine reuptake inhibitor, being clinically significant only at high doses (Goldstein & Goodnick, 1998). It does not present affinity for adrenergic receptors α1 and muscarinic or histaminic receptors (Diaz-Martinez et al., 1998; Goldstein & Goodnick, 1998). Consequently, it is less likely to produce side effects related to these pharmacologic properties (Denys et al., 2003).

In a Cochrane systematic review (1966-2004), the adverse effects of fluoxetine (dry mouth sensation, dizziness and sudoresis) were compared with the adverse effects of the most recent antidepressants (venlafaxine, reboxetine, phenelzine, nefazodone) and they have shown to be less pronounced than in the latter (Cipriani et al., 2005).

Normal salivation is essential for oral health due to its important contributions to the oral defence mechanisms. Diminished salivary secretion could lead to caries disease and deterioration of the mucosa (Mandel & Wotman, 1976; Mandel, 1980; Narhi, 1994).

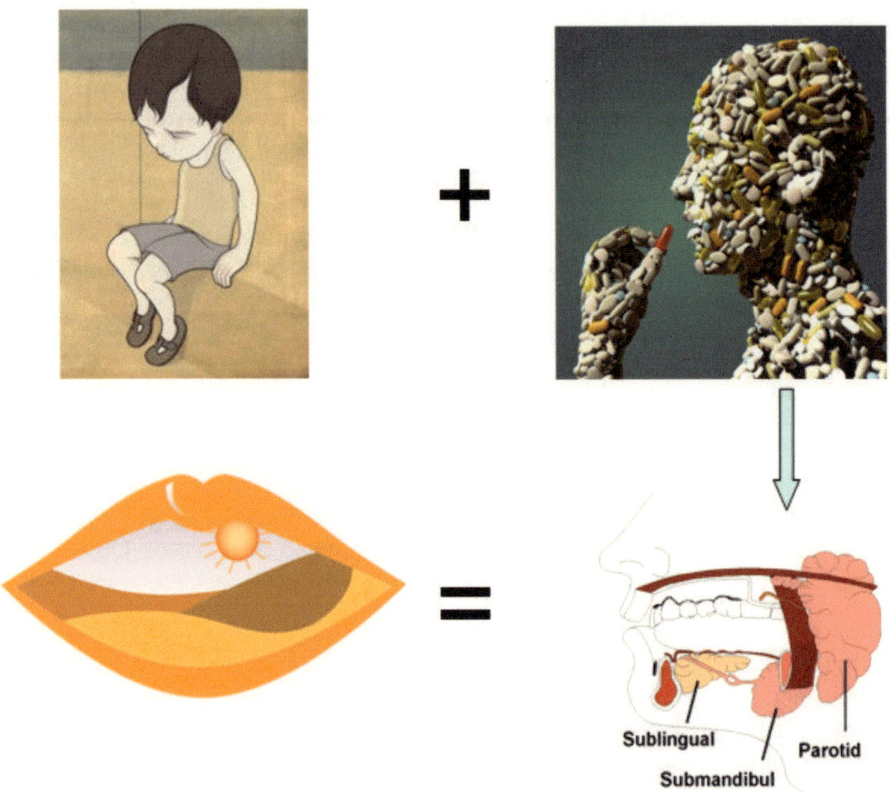

Fig. 1. Depression = affective disorders = depressive patient takes antidepressants drugs that cause dry mouth: alteration on salivary glands (parotid, sublingual and submandibul).

Salivary secretion is neurologically controlled by stimulation of reflex action. The salivary glands are enervated by the sympathetic and parasympathetic autonomic nervous system (ANS). Sympathetic enervation is linked by means of the type α2 and β2 adrenergic receptors (Baum, 1987), while parasympathetic enervation is linked to the muscarinic receptor M3. The primary acinar content is modified as it passes through the system of salivary gland ducts. This process occurs because the cells of the duct receive stimuli from the sympathetic and parasympathetic pathways (Scully, 2003).

Grégio et al. (2006), when studying the effects of the chronic use of the association of a benzodiazepine (Diazepam®) and an antidepressant (Tryptanol®) on the parotid glands of rats, observed hyposalivation and hypertrophy of serous cells. These findings suggested a possible inhibition of the activity of the myoepithelial cells, originating from nervous stimulation, a decrease in the number of such cells with the chronic use of psychotropic drugs or an alteration in the number of acinar and ductal cells.

The aim of the present study was to verify the action of two drugs in the antidepressant class, fluoxetine and venlafaxine, on the salivary flow rate, as well as to make a histomorphometric analysis of the rat parotid glands submitted to chronic treatment with such drugs.

2. Material and methods

This study was approved by the Research Ethics Committee of Tuiuti University of Paraná, under the registration number CEP-UTP 55/2003.

The animal model enrolled in this investigation consisted of male rats (Rattus norvegicus albinus, Wistar strain) obtained from the Central Animal Facility of the Pontifical Catholic University of Paraná. The animals weighed approximately 250g and were maintained in cages with water and food ad libidum on a light/dark cycle of 12 hours.

Sixty animals, divided into six groups were used, each group consisting of 10 animals (Table 1). The experimental groups received two antidepressants drugs, injectable solution of fluoxetine (lot 20040625, Galena Química e Farmacêutica Ltda., Campinas, Brazil) and venlafaxine (lot D/VN/002/02, Galena Química e Farmacêutica Ltda., Campinas, Brazil). Controlled groups S30 and S60 received solution injectable from physiological serum and the P60 group received a gel base prepared with 1% from pilocarpine hydrochloride (Gerbras Química e Farmacêutica Ltda., São Paulo, Brazil).

Groups	Drug	Treatment time	Dose	Administration via
1. Experimental (FS)	Fluoxetine	1-30 days	20mg/kg	Intraperitoneal
	Physiological Serum	31-60 days	0.1 mL	Intraperitoneal
2. Experimental (VS)	Venlafaxine	1-30 days	40mg/kg	Intraperitoneal
	Physiological Serum	31-60 days	0.1 mL	Intraperitoneal
3. Experimental (F30)	Fluoxetine	1-30 days	20mg/kg	Intraperitoneal
4. Experimental (V30)	Venlafaxine	1-30 days	40mg/kg	Intraperitoneal
5. Control (S30)	Physiological Serum	1-30 days	0.1 mL	Intraperitoneal
6. Control (S60)	Physiological Serum	1-60 days	0.1 mL	Intraperitoneal

Table 1. Controls and experimental groups in accordance with the drug, treatment, time, dose and administration.

2.1 Sialometry

According to described methodology of Onofre et al. (1997), saliva samples were collected 30 hours after the end of treatment. The animals had received two drops of 4% pilocarpine hydrochloride eye drops (Allergan pilocarpina® 4%, Allergan Produtos Farmacêuticos Ltda., Guarulhos, Brazil), to stimulate salivation. After one minute, saliva was collected in a collecting pot that was weighed on a high precision scale - Belmark® U210A (Bel Engenharia, Piracicaba, Brazil), obtaining thus a salivary flow rate (SFR).

The values of amount of saliva were obtained in accordance with the described formula below (Banderas-Tarabay et al., 1997; Olsson et al., 1991).

$$\text{weight of pot after collection (g) - weight of pot before collection (g)} = \\ = \frac{\text{weight saliva}}{\text{time (1 min)}} = \text{salivary flow rate (ml/min)} \qquad (1)$$

2.2 Parotidean gland exsiccation and size measurement

Glands were obtained from each group right after the saliva collection. Rats were weighted and anaesthetised by intraperitoneal administration of 100 mg/kg sodium thiopental (Thionembutal®, Abbott Laboratórios do Brazil Ltda.) and killed.

The right and left parotid glands were dissected and carefully removed. Fresh gland masses were determined with a BelMark® U210A precision scale. After this, the millimetric longitudinal dimensions were achieved using a high precision digital calliper - Mitutoyo 500 Mical® (Mitutoyo Co., Tokyo, Japan). The average of the glands size and the glands mass was carried through, for attainment of variable so size (GS) and mass (M) for each rat. After the measurement of the part, gland tissue was fixed in 10% neutral formalin solution and embedded in paraffin. Four μm sections were obtained and submitted for routine haematoxylin-eosin (in accordance with the routine of the Laboratory of Experimental Pathology of the PUCPR).

The microscopy Olympus® BX50 (Olympus Corporation, Ishikawa, Japan) was used with the objective of 40X and 100X (oil immersion). The images were captured with a digital camera - Sony® CCD-IRIS DXC-107A (Sony Eletronics Incorporation, Tokyo, Japan) connected to the microscope and a microcomputer. With a programme for analysis of images (Image-Pro® Plus, Cybernetics, Silverspring, U.S.A.), the histological analysis front to the use of antidepressants was evaluated.

2.3 Histomorphometry of parotid glands

To establish the comparisons among the groups with regard to the cellular volume (CV), the variable presented had been used in the study of Onofre et al. (1997).

Processed gland volume (vp) was calculated for each animal using the following equation:

$$Vp=m/\ d\times rf \qquad (2)$$

M is fresh mass, d is density and rf is the shrinkage caused by histological processing. For these calculations we used d=1.089 g/cm^3 and rf=0.7 using the method of Onofre et al. (1997).

For the stereological evaluation of acinar volume density (Vvi) and total volume (Vti) an objective of 40X it was used connected to the programme Image-Pro® Plus, where if it obtained a vertical grating with ten horizontal lines and ten vertical lines, determining one hundred points of which forty had been chosen randomly. In these, 40 chosen points had counted how many points coincided with acini (Pi). The Vvi by means of the formula was calculated then:

$$Vvi=Pi/Pt \tag{3}$$

Pt mentions the number to it of selected points 40.

Having obtained the Vvi and processed gland volume (Vp) values, we calculated the total acinar volume (Vti) by the formula:

$$Vti = Vvi \times Vp \tag{4}$$

Nuclear volume was determined from the measurement of the orthogonal diameters of 50 nuclei per gland using a microscopy technique as stated before. We calculated the mean radius of the geometric mean diameter by:

$$r2 = d1 \times d2 \tag{5}$$

The nuclear volume was calculated by the formula for the volume of a sphere:

$$V=4/3 \times \pi \times r3 \tag{6}$$

The cytoplasmic volume was calculated as of the nucleus densities and the cytoplasm of acinar cells (Weibel, 1969). In this respect, the points over nuclei (Pn) were counted and over the cytoplasm (Pcyti) in 40 histological fields of the cells under study. The corrected nuclear volume density (pncorr) was calculated by the equation:

$$pncorr = (Pn/Pn+Pcyti)/Ko \tag{7}$$

Ko is the correction factor and is calculated by the formula:

$$Ko = 1+3t/2d \tag{8}$$

d is the mean nuclear diameter and t is section thickness.

The corrected cytoplasm volume density is:

$$pcyticorr = 1 - pncorr \tag{9}$$

By dividing pcyticorr by pncorr the cytoplasm/nucleus ratio (RC/N) of the acinar cells was obtained. On the basis of nuclear volume (Vni) and the C/N ratio, the cytoplasmic volume (Vcyti) was calculated by the equation:

$$Vcyti = Vni \times RC/N \tag{10}$$

This then permitted calculating the cell volume by:

$$Vc= Vni + Vcyti \tag{11}$$

2.4 Statistical analysis

To rest the presupposition of normality of the variables for each group, the Komolgorov-Smirnov test was used. The Levene test verified the homogeneity of the variances among the groups. When the analysis of variance Anova found differences among the means of the groups and treatments, the Tukey HSD multiple comparisons test was used for the variables that presented homogeneity of variances among the groups. For the variables that did not present homogeneity of variances among the groups, the Games-Howell test was used.

For all the tests the level of significance of 5% ($p<0.05$) was applied.

3. Results

All the groups presented normality of distribution of the data for the variables GS, M, SFR and CV of the studied glands ($p>0.05$), with the exception of the variable SFR in the group S60, the variable GS in groups FS and S30 and the variable M in the group F30.

The variables GS and M showed homogeneity of variance ($p>0.05$) and the variables SFR and CV did not present homogeneity of variance ($p<0.05$).

3.1 Groups treated for 30 days

There was a statistically significant difference between the means of the variable GS among the following groups: F30 (p=0.0002), V30 (p=0.0112), when compared with group S30 (control).

For the variable M, there was a statistically significant difference for the following groups: F30 and V30 (p=0.0011), F30 and S30 (p=0.0190), the highest mean being found for the group F30 and the lowest mean for the group V30.

There was a statistically significant difference for the variable CV between the following groups: F30 (Figure 3) and S30 (p=0.0005), V30 and S30(p=0.0004).

The variable SFR presented a statistically significant difference between groups: F30 and S30 (p=0.0031).

Table 2 shows the means and standard deviations of the studied variables in accordance with the groups treated for 30 days.

Groups	C30		F30		V30	
Variables	Mean	SD	Mean	SD	Mean	SD
SFR (mL/min)$^{\delta}$	0.051	0.026	0.014	0.006	0.026	0.022
CV (mm^3)$^{\delta}$	6965.683	3792.951	10384.311	4869.539	11945.927	7891.179
Gland size (mm)	7.036	0.506	9.501	1.404	8.696	1.409
Mass (mg)	0.075	0.010	0.103	0.032	0.064	0.018

serum - 30 days), F (fluoxetine - 30 days) and V (venlafaxine -30 days). SD = standard deviations.
δ: Values obtained from the study by Da Silva et al. (2009).
SFR - Stimulated salivary flow rate.
CV – Cellular volume.
* Statistically significant difference among groups ($p<0.05$).

Table 2.Values of studied variables in accordance with groups treated with C (physiological

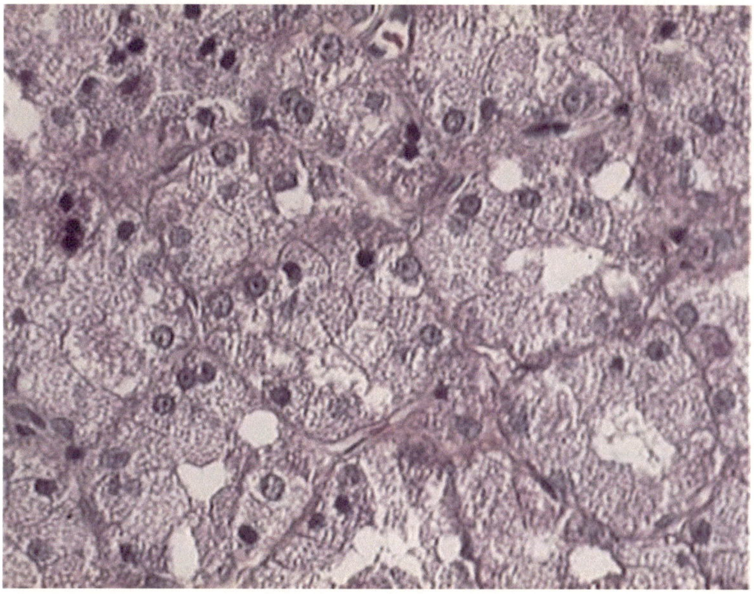

Fig. 2. Histological aspect of the salivary gland of the fluoxetine 30 group showing disorganised glandular parenchyma. There was a loss of borders to the serous cells, which were also increased in size, with a consequent reduction or disappearance of the central lumen (H.E.; original magnification: 400X).

Figures 3 and 4 show rat parotid glands from groups venlafaxine 30 and saline 30, respectively.

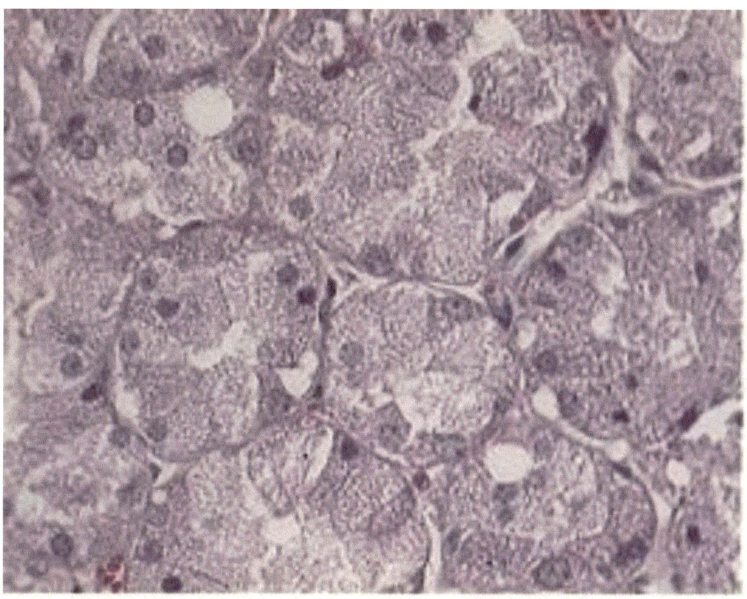

Fig. 3. Histological aspect of the salivary gland of the venlafaxine 30 group. There was a loss of borders to the serous cells, which were also increased in size, with a consequent reduction or disappearance of the central lumen (H.E.; original magnification: 400X).

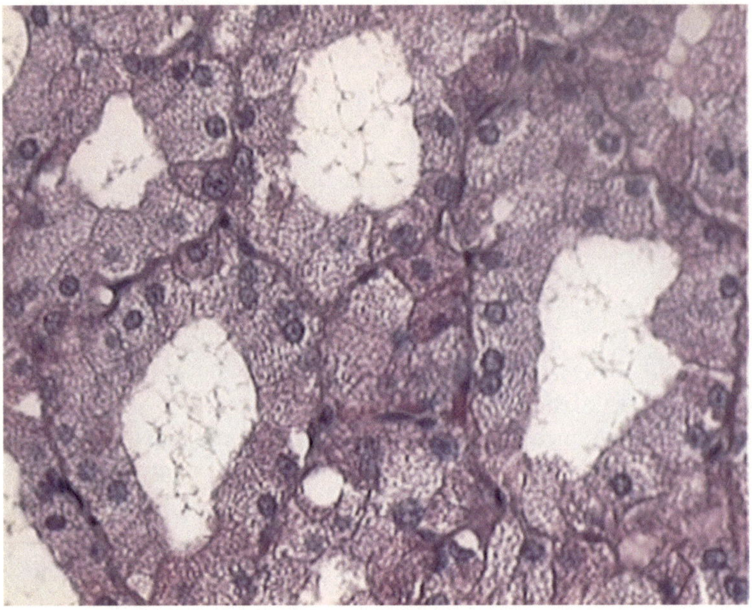

Fig. 4. Group saline 30. Well-structured glandular parenchyma divided into lobules. Inside the lobules, intercalary ducts were covered by cuboidal cells while striated ducts were found covered by columnar cells. (H.E.; original magnification: 400X).

3.2 Groups treated for 60 days

Table 3 shows the means and standard deviations of the studied variables in accordance with the groups treated for 60 days.

For SFR, there were statistically significant differences between the following groups: V60 and C 60 (p=0.000).

The variable GS did not show statistically significant differences among the groups. There were statistically significant differences for the variable M between groups VS and S60 (p=0.0132).

The variable CV did not showed statistically significant differences between groups C60, F60 and V60.

Groups /Variables	C60		F60		V60	
	Mean	SD	Mean	SD	Mean	SD
SFR (mL/min) δ	0.052	0.029 [a]	0.036	0.017	0.020	0.004 [a]
CV (mm^3) δ	6505.564	3343.475 [b]	6809.347	3189.246 [c]	7525.112	3196.085
Gland size (mm)	7.885	0.628	8.350	0.077	8.040	0.949
Mass (mg)	0.074	0.021	0.095	0.014	0.101	0.016

δ: Values obtained from the study by Da Silva et al (2009).
SFR - Stimulated salivary flow rate.
CV - Cellular volume.
a,b,c, groups followed by the same letter differed statistically from each other.
* Statistically significant difference among groups ($p<0.05$).

Table 3.Values of studied variables in accordance with groups treated with C (physiological serum -60 days), F (fluoxetine - 60 days) and V (venlafaxine -60 days). SD = standard deviations.

4. Discussion

The anticholinergic effects of drugs that act on the CNS have not yet been completely explained. The majority of authors opt for defining the autonomic capacity of these drugs in linking to the adrenergic and cholinergic receptors, altering the quality and quantity of salivary flow. But several other factors must be considered, because in addition to interaction with and affinity to the sympathetic and parasympathetic CNS and ANS, other neurotransmitters, proteins and amino acids are capable of resulting in alteration of activity in the salivary glands (Scully, 2003).

This study observed that fluoxetine (F30) produced an increase in GS and M of the rat parotid salivary glands, in addition to increasing CV in comparison with the control group S30. This effect probably occurred because the drugs with central action promote an action of salivary gland hypertrophy (Grégio et al., 2006). This result corroborates those of Martinez-Madrigal & Micheau (1989), who characterised hypertrophy of the glands by widening of the acini and accumulation of secretion granules, caused by drugs with central action.

The anticholinergic action of psychotropic drugs (Martinez-Madrigal & Micheau, 1989; Scully, 2003) was proved once again, because in the group treated with fluoxetine for 30 days (F30), the animals' SFR was lower in comparison with the control group (S30), thus justifying the increase in GS and M, as there was retention of saliva in the acini lume and little of it being released.

The antidepressants SRIs when compared to the tricyclic drugs have not presented significant effect on the flow rate, probably due to lack of anticholinergic activity. The flow reduction could occur through the serotonin receptor action presented at the peripheric microcirculation (Hunter & Wilson, 1995; Siepmann et al., 2003). According to Schubert & Izutsu (1987), the salivary flow can be affected by drugs through alteration of the blood flow to the salivary glands. For Grubb & Karas (1998) the seratonin has important physiology participation in the autonomic regulation since the CNS controls the sympathetic, the parasympathetic and the serotonin mechanisms, and therefore probably a decrease or activation of the release of serotonin at the CNS would result in the alteration of both sympathetic and parasympathetic systems. This hypothesis contributes to our finding regarding the reduction of the SFR caused by fluoxetine.

The uncertainty with regard to the exact biochemical mode of action of antidepressants frequently causes the development of new drugs to be empirical. This leads to the introduction of a heterogeneous group of compounds (to which venlafaxine belongs), the atypical antidepressants. In practice, the most recent drugs may definitively be superior to the tricyclic drugs in terms of side effects and acute toxicity, but they have not been shown to have a faster action or be more effective (Goldstein & Goodnick, 1998; Siepmann et al., 2003).

With regard to the results obtained for venlafaxine (V30), both GS and CV had higher values in comparison with the control group, and in addition there was diminished SFR when compared with the control (S30), once again demonstrating the anticholinergic action of psychotropic drugs and the effect of acinar cell hypertrophy (Grégio et al., 2006; Martinez-Madrigal & Micheau 1989).

Venlafaxine has fewer anticholinergic and adrenergic α-blocker effects than the other antidepressive (Denys et al., 2003). This would cause a reduction in the adverse effects, because at low doses this drug predominantly blocks serotonin and noradrenalin reuptake, and at high doses it also inhibits dopamine reuptake. This hypothesis reinforces the great expectation in the use of venlafaxine in comparison with fluoxetine, and is in agreement with the present study findings, since the value of SFR for venlafaxine (V30) was higher when compared with the SFR value for fluoxetine (F30). Furthermore, fluoxetine has metabolite of prolonged action and is pharmacologically active (Goldstein & Goodnick, 1998).

The acinar cells present adrenergic α and β receptors, vasoactive intestinal peptide receptors (VIP), acetylcholine and P substance. The receptors for β adrenergic and for VIP, activate the cyclic AMP cascade, activating the G protein, which activates the adenylate cyclase enzyme. Whereas the α adrenergic receptors and the receptors for acetylcholine and P substance activate the inositol 1, 4, 5 triphosphate cascade (IP3) and of diacylglycerol. These biochemical reactions and interaction sequences influence both salivary secretion and composition (Berne et al., 2000).

Because venlafaxine is a weak serotonin and noradrenalin reuptake inhibitor, it has fewer side effects than fluoxetine (De Nayer et al., 2002). Another hypothesis which could contribute to explaning the result,besides the others mentioned before, is that the majority of types of serotoninergic receptors are coupled to the G proteins, affecting adenylate cyclase activity. This enzyme, in turn, converts ATP into the second messenger, cyclic AMP (Gould & Manji, 2002) which, as a central effect, presents activation of the protein kinase A (PKA), an enzyme that regulates ionic channels, which are responsible for the entry and exit of water and electrolytes from cells (Walton & Dragunow, 2000).

On the other hand, the CV of rat parotid glands in the group treated with venlafaxine (V30) was greater than in the group treated with fluoxetine (F30). This is probably owing to the fact that venlafaxine (because it also inhibits noradrenalin reuptake and this being the mediator of the sympathetic ANS, which in turn tends to modulate the composition of saliva) induces the protein secretion mechanism (Berne et al., 2000) which may be accumulating inside the salivary gland, resulting in cellular hypertrophy.

The groups FS and VS presented lower SFR values than the group S60, proving that after suspension of the drug, withdrawal symptoms may occur, which appear within one to 10 days and persists for up to three or four weeks. The most frequent symptoms are dizziness, vertigo, ataxia, gastrointestinal disorders, flu symptoms, sensorial disturbances, sleep alterations, psychic alterations and anticholinergic effects. As happens with other psychoactive substances, these symptoms may be the result of adaptive alterations, which most frequently involve the adjustment of the receptors to compensate for the pharmacological activity of the drug, described as a rebound effect (Goldstein & Goodnick, 1998).

The advances in research on the psychopharmacology of antidepressants have offered patients with very different pharmacokinetic profiles. In spite of this, the action mechanisms proposed for each of them remain linked to monoaminergic theories of increased amounts of neurotransmitters in the synaptic gap and the subsensitisation of presynaptic receptors (Paykel, 1992).

In terms of the number of drugs available, there has been a considerable enlargement of the therapeutic arsenal, both with expansion in the number of compounds of the same pharmacological group, and in the appearance of drugs with different action profiles from those of the original ones. The more recent compounds are more selective, leading to greater tolerability and adherence to treatment (Goldstein & Goodnick, 1998).

It is verified an effort in the sense of increasingly improving the action in receptor sites determinant of clinical efficacy, avoiding those responsible for side effects (Hunter & Wilson, 1995). However, new inquiries have become necessary due the complexity of the involved events in the saliva secretion mechanism.

5. Conclusion

It could be concluded that both fluoxetine and venlafaxine reduced the SFR and caused hypertrophy of the rat parotid gland, with fluoxetine having a more pronounced anticholinergic action.

6. Acknowledgment

The authors thank the biologist Ana Paula Camargo Martins - technician responsible for the Experimental Pathology Laboratory at PUCPR and the scientific initiation students of PUCPR (PIBIC) Miriam Vanessa Zaclikevis and Anna Clara Duszczak D'Agulham for their valuable contribution towards concluding this work.

7. References

Banderas-Tarabay, J.; Gonzalez-Begne, M.; Sanchez-Garduno, M.; Millan-Cortez, E.; Lopez-Rodriguez, A. & Vilchis-Velazquez, A. (1997). The flow and concentration of proteins in human whole saliva. *Salud Pública de México*, Vol.39, No.5, (September - October 1997), pp.433-441, ISSN 0036-363

Baum, B. (1987). Neurotransmitter control of secretion. *Journal of Dental Research*, Vol.66, No.Spec., (February 1987), pp.628-632, ISSN 0022-0345

Berne, R.; Matthew, N.; Koeppen, B. & Staton, B. (2000). *Fisiologia*. Guanabara Koogan, ISBN 85-277-0559-1, Rio de Janeiro

Bogetto, F.; Maina, G.; Ferro, G.; Carbone, M. & Gandolfo, S. (1998). Psychiatric comorbidity in patients with burning mouth syndrome. *Psychosomatic Medicine*, Vol.60, No.3, (June 1998), pp.378-385, ISSN 0033-3174

Cipriani A, Brambilla P, Furukawa TA, Geddes J, Gregis M, Hotopf M, et al. (2005). Fluoxetine versus other types of pharmacotherapy for depression, *Cochrane Database of Systematic Reviews*. In: The Cochrane Library. Vol. 4, (Oct 2005), pp.19 – 4 , ISSN: 1465-1858

De Nayer, A.; Geerts, S.; Ruelens, L.; Schittecatte, M.; De Bleeker, E.; Van Eeckhoutte, I.; Evrard, J.; Linkowski, P.; Fossion, P.; Leyman, S. & Mignon, A. (2002). Venlafaxine compared with fluoxetine in outpatients with depression and concomitant anxiety. *The International Journal of Neuropsychopharmacology*, Vol.5, N.2, (June 2002), pp.115-20, ISSN 1461-1457

Denys, D.; van der Wee, N.; van Megen, H. & Westenberg, H. (2003). A double blind comparison of venlafaxine and paroxetine in obsessive-compulsive disorder. *Journal of Clinical Psychopharmacology*, Vol.23, No.6, (December 2003), pp.568-575, ISSN 0271-0749

Diaz-Martinez, A.; Benassinni, O.; Ontiveros, A.; Gonzalez, S.; Salin, R.; Basquedano, G. & Martinez, R. (1998). A randomized, open-label comparison of venlafaxine and fluoxetine in depressed outpatients. *Clinical Therapeutics*, Vol.20, No.3, (June 1998), pp.467-476, ISSN 0149-2918

Glassman, A.; Carino, J. & Roose, S. (1984). Adverse effects of tricyclic antidepressants: focus on the elderly. *Advances in Biochemical Psychopharmacology*, Vol.39, (1984), pp.391-398, ISSN 0065-2229

Goldstein, B. & Goodnick, P. (1998). Selective serotonin reuptake inhibitors in the treatment of affective disorders--III. Tolerability, safety and pharmacoeconomics. *Journal of Clinical Psychopharmacology*, Vol.12, No. 3 Suppl B, (1998), pp.S55-87, ISSN 0271-0749

Gould, T. & Manji, H. (2002). Signaling networks in the pathophysiology and treatment of mood disorders. *Journal of Psychosomatic Research*, Vol. 53, No.2, (August 2002), pp.687-697, ISSN 0022-3999

Grégio, A.; Durscki, J.; Lima, A.; Machado, M.; Ignácio, S. & Azevedo, L. (2006). Association of amitryptiline and Diazepam on histomorphometry of rat parotid glands. *Pharmacologyonline*, Vol.2, (2006), pp.96-108, ISSN 1827-8620

Grubb, B. & Karas, B. (1998). The potential role of serotonin in the pathogenesis of neurocardiogenic syncope and related autonomic disturbances. *Journal of Interventional Cardiac Electrophysiology*, Vol.2, No.4, (December 1998), pp.325-332, ISSN 383-875X

Horst, W. & Preskorn, S. (1998). Mechanisms of action and clinical characteristics of three atypical antidepressants: venlafaxine, nefazodone, bupropion. *Journal of Affective Disorders*, Vol.51, No.3, (December 1998), pp.237-254, ISSN 0165-0327

Hunter, K. & Wilson, W. (1995). The effects of antidepressant drugs on salivary flow and content of sodium and potassium ions in human parotid saliva. *Archives of Oral Biology*, Vol.40, No.11, (November 1995), pp.983-989, ISSN 0003-9969

Makhija, S. & Vavia, P. (2002). Once daily sustained release tablets of venlafaxine, a novel antidepressant. *European Journal of Pharmaceutics and Biopharmaceutics*, Vol.54, No.1, (July 2002), pp.9-15, ISSN 0939-6411

Mandel, I. & Wotman, S. (1976). The salivary secretions in health and disease. *Oral Sciences Reviews*, No.8, (1976), pp. 25-47, ISSN 0300-4759

Mandel, I. (1980). Sialochemistry in diseases and clinical situations affecting salivary glands. Critical reviews in clinical laboratory sciences, Vol.12, No.4, (1980), pp.321-366, ISSN 1040-8363

Martinez-Madrigal, F. & Micheau, C. (1989). Histology of the major salivary glands. *The American Journal of Surgical Pathology*, Vol.13, No.10, (October 1989), pp.879-899, ISSN 0147-5185

Narhi, T. (1994). Prevalence of subjective feelings of dry mouth in the elderly. *Journal of Dental Research*, Vol.73, No.1, (January 1994), pp.20 25, ISSN 0022 0345

Olsson, H.; Spak, C. & Axell, T. (1991). The effect of a chewing gum on salivary secretion, oral mucosal friction, and the feeling of dry mouth in xerostomic patients. *Acta Odontologica Scandinavica*, Vol.49, No.5, (October 1991), pp.273-279, ISSN 0001-6357

Onofre, M.; de Souza, L.; Campos, A. & Taga, R. (1997). Stereological study of acinar growth in the rat parotid gland induced by isoproterenol. *Archives of Oral Biology*, Vol.42, No.5, (May 1997), pp.333-338, ISSN 0003-9969

Owens, M.; Krulewicz, S.; Simon, J.; Sheehan, D.; Thase, M.; Carpenter, D.; Plott, S. & Nemeroff, C. (2008). Estimates of serotonin and norepinephrine transporter inhibition in depressed patients treated with paroxetine or venlafaxine. *Neuropsychopharmacology*, Vol.33, No.13, (December 2008), pp.3201-3212, ISSN 0893-133X

Papakostas, G.; Homberger, C. & Fava, M. (2008). A meta-analysis of clinical trials comparing mirtazapine with selective serotonin reuptake inhibitors for the treatment of major depressive disorder. *Journal of Psychopharmacology*. Vol.22, N.8, (November 2008), pp.843-848, ISSN 0269-8811

Paykel, E. (1992). *Handbook of affective disorders* (2nd edition). The Guilford Press, ISBN 0898626749, New York

Schubert, M. & Izutsu, K. (1987). Iatrogenic causes of salivary gland dysfunction. *Journal of Dental Research*, Vol.66, No.Spec., (February 1987), pp.680-688, ISSN 0022-0345

Scully, C. (2003). Drug effects on salivary glands: dry mouth. *Oral Diseases*, Vol.9, No.4, (July 2003), pp.165-176, ISSN 1354-523X

Siepmann, M.; Grossmann, J.; Muck-Weymann, M. & Kirch W. (2003). Effects of sertraline on autonomic and cognitive functions in healthy volunteers. *Psychopharmacology*, Vol.168, No.3, (July 2003), pp.293-298, ISSN 0033-3158

Thomsom, W.; Chalmers, J.; Spencer, A. & Slade, G. (2000). Medication and dry mouth: findings from a cohort study of older people. *Journal of Public Health Dentistry*, Vol.60, No.1, (Winter 2000), pp. 60:12-20, ISSN 0022-4006

Walton, M. & Dragunow, I. (2000). Is CREB a key to neuronal survival? *Trends in Neurosciences*, Vol.23, No.2, (February 2000), pp.48-53, ISSN 0166-2236

Weibel, E. (1969). Stereological principles for morphometry in electron microscopic cytology. *International Review of Cytology*, Vol.26, (1969), pp.235-302, ISSN 0074-7696